THE HEINEMANN

ILLUSTRATED DICTIONARY

HEALTH & SOCIAL CARE

Yvonne Nolan

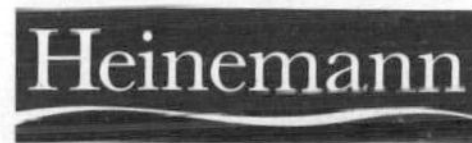

Heinemann is an imprint of Pearson Education Limited, a company incorporated in England and Wales, having its registered office at Edinburgh Gate, Harlow, Essex, CM20 2JE. Registered company number: 872828

www.heinemann.co.uk

Heinemann is a registered trademark of Pearson Education Limited.

First published 2009
13 12 11 10 09
10 9 8 7 6 5 4 3 2 1

British Library Cataloguing in Publication Data is available from the British Library on request.

ISBN: 978 0 435 401 054

Designed and typeset by Tek-Art, Crawley Down, West Sussex
Original illustrations © Pearson Education Limited, 2009
Picture research by Elena Wright
Cover design by Pearson Education
Cover Illustration Pearson Education
Printed in Italy by Rotolito Lombarda S.p.A

Websites
There are links to relevant websites in this book, given at the end on an entry. In order to ensure that the links are up to date, that the links work, and that the sites are not inadvertently linked to sites that could be considered offensive, we have made the links available on our website at www.heinemann.co.uk/hotlinks http://www.heinemann.co.uk/hotlinks. When you access the site the express code is 1054T.

Acknowledgements
The author would like to acknowledge the following who have provided invaluable assistance in the publishing of this book in particular: Beryl Stretch for all of her hard work, diligence and invaluable assistance in checking entries and comments on content. The author would also like to thank Jane Kellas, Venus Training and Consultancy; Frances Sussex, Quality Manager in the Teaching and Learning Unit at City and Islington College; and Jan Doorly, Juliet Mozley and Bruce Nicholson for editorial support.

Photo acknowledgements
The authors and publisher would like to thank the following for permission to reproduce photographs:

Alamy/Adrian Sherratt; Alamy/Picture Partners; Alamy/67photo; Alamy/Charles Mistral; Alamy/David R. Frazier Photolibrary, Inc.; Alamy/David Tipling; Alamy/Medical-on-Line; Alamy/Phototake Inc.; Arclight/Alamy; Art Directors and Trip; Babor UK and Ireland; Bill Anderson/Science Photo Library; Brand X Pictures; Brand X Pictures/Joe Atlas; Charles Bowman/Alamy; Corbis; Corbis/epa/Waltraud Grubitzsch; Corbis/Jules Perrier; Corbis/Mediscan; Corbis/Tom Stewart; Cordelia Molloy/Science Photo Library; David H. Lewis/iStockphoto; Digital Stock; Digital Vision; Digital Vision/Rob van Petten; Dmitriy Shironosov/Shutterstock; Eyewire; f1 online/Alamy; Getty Images/Visuals Unlimited; Getty Images/Chris Baker; Getty Images/Thinkstock; Image Source Limited; iofoto/iStockphoto; iStockphoto; iStockPhoto/Maartje van Caspel; Justin Horrocks/iStockphoto; Karin Lau/iStockphoto; Kristy Batie/Shutterstock; LWA-Dann Tardif/Corbis matka_Wariatka/Shutterstock; Pearson Education/Jules Selmes; Pearson Education Ltd/Lord & Leverett; Pearson Education Ltd/Mind Studio; Pearson Education Ltd/Gareth Boden; Pearson Education Ltd/Jules Selmes; Pearson Education Ltd/Lord & Leverett; Pearson Education Ltd/MindStudio; Pearson Education Ltd/Studio 8; Pearson Education Ltd/Tudor Photography; Pearson Education/Debbie Rowe; Pearson Education/Peter Evans; Pearson Education/Richard Smith; PhotoDisc; PhotoDisc/Jim Wehtje; Photodisc/Kevin Peterson; Photos.com; Richard Smith/Pearson Education Ltd; Science Photo Library/ Gusto; Science Photo Library/Ian Boddy; Science Photo Library/Ian Hooton; Science Photo Library/National Cancer Institute; Sean Warren/iStockphoto; The Illustrated London News Picture Library; webphotographer/iStockphoto; Westholme.

How to use this book

Cross references

As you work your way through the dictionary you will find that any words that have their own entry in the dictionary are highlighted in purple so that you can easily identify the links to entries. An example is shown below for the entry blood groups which shows links to **red blood cells**, **proteins**, **antigens**, **immune response** and **blood transfusions**.

blood groups

Different types of **blood**. **Red blood cells** contain **proteins** that can act as **antigens** and bring about an **immune response**. The ability to define blood into groups that contain specific proteins means that it is possible for individuals to receive **blood transfusions** of a compatible type.

Websites

There are links to relevant websites in this book, given at the end of an entry. In order to ensure that the links are up to date, that the links work, and that the sites are not inadvertently linked to sites that could be considered offensive, we have made the links available on our website at www.heinemann.co.uk/hotlinks. When you access the website use the express code given on the imprint of this book.

Legislation grid

The legislation grid on page 309 gives details of relevant legislation covered in this book. It covers all four countries of the United Kingdom.

Introduction

This dictionary is designed to be a practical, handy reference for you as you work or study. There is so much to remember in Health and Social Care, that we all need a quick refresher from time to time. You may also find the dictionary helpful if you want to just find out some general information quickly, rather than having lots of details, or it could help you to start out learning about something you will go on to follow up in more detail.

The dictionary is intended to be useful for people working in many different roles in health and social care. Regardless of whether you work in the community, in a residential setting, in daycare or in a hospital, I hope that you will find the entries helpful.

There are over 1,500 entries in the dictionary covering everything from Asthma to zygote. There are links to relevant websites in this book. To ensure that links are kept up to date details of all the websites referred to in the book are provided on the Heinemann website. Details of how to access the Heinemann website are provided on the imprint page of this book.

You will find that any words that have their own entry in the dictionary are highlighted so that you can easily identify the links to entries.

You will find a grid giving you the major pieces of legislation, for different parts of the UK, that you are likely to come across in your work. There is also a brief note of the main features of each Act.

As health and social care undergoes major changes in the move to personalisation, the demands on staff are constantly increased and keeping up to date becomes more and more important whatever level you are working at.

I hope that you will find that the dictionary is useful in many different ways and that you will find that you are referring to it regularly to check up, recall, or to find out something new. Above all, I hope that it contributes to helping you to offer the best possible service to the people you work for.

Yvonne Nolan

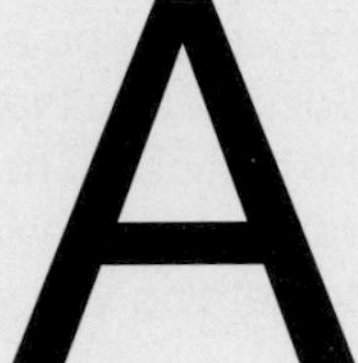

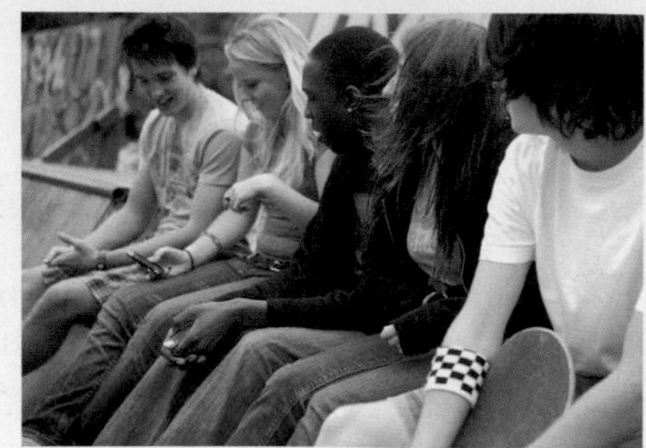

ABC of resuscitation

The three steps for attempting to **resuscitate** a person in an emergency.

- Airway: Tip the head back and raise the chin – this opens the airway and prevents the **tongue** from falling to the back of the throat.
- Breathing: Using the correct technique it is possible to breathe directly into the person's mouth and so into the **lungs**, thus keeping the **blood oxygenated** through artificial ventilation.
- Circulation: Using the correct technique, in conjunction with artificial ventilation, a person's **circulation** can be maintained by using **chest** compressions to push blood through the **heart** and round the body.

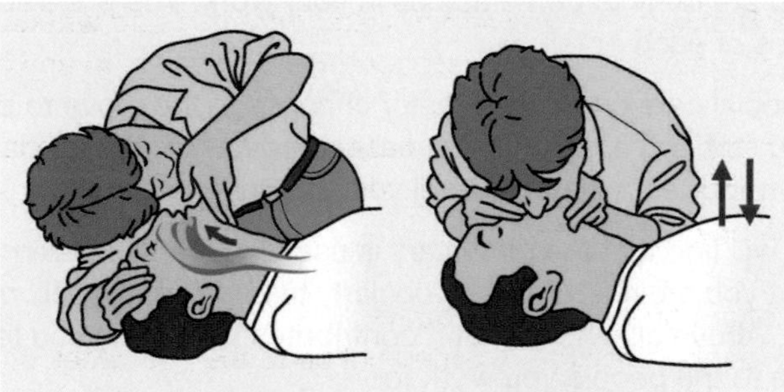

A – Airway **B – Breathing**

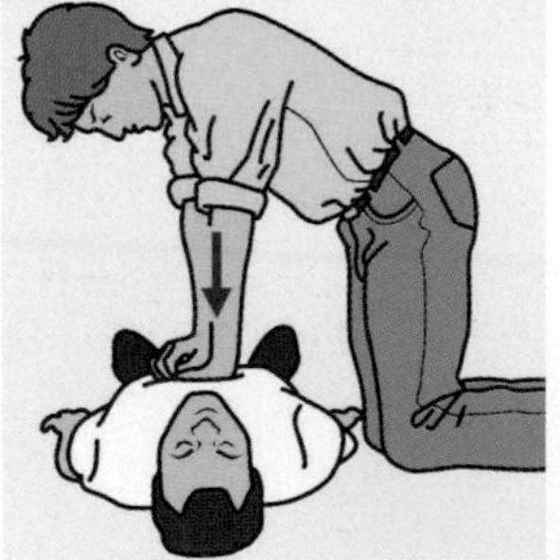

C – Circulation

The ABC of resuscitation.

B C D E F G H I J K L M N O P Q R S T U V W XYZ

abdomen
The area of the body that lies between the **chest** and the **pelvis**. It contains most of the major **organs**: **stomach**, **intestines**, **liver**, **pancreas** and **spleen**. It is commonly referred to as the 'belly' or 'tummy'.

abortion
The termination of a **pregnancy** usually (90% of cases) in the first 13 weeks of pregnancy. A spontaneous abortion that occurs naturally is known as a **miscarriage**. Abortions can be performed surgically or with the use of drugs to induce **labour**. There are legal restrictions surrounding both the reasons for performing an abortion and the stage of **foetal development** at which it is allowed. Many people hold strong views about abortion, and there are two main attitudes:

- 'pro-choice' people believe that every pregnant woman has a right to choose whether to continue with the pregnancy
- 'pro-life' people believe that the foetus is a separate individual and has the right to be born.

More information can be found at www.fpa.org.uk

Abortion Act 1967
An Act of **Parliament** which identified for the first time the circumstances in which abortion would be legal in most of the UK (not Northern Ireland). Before this Act was passed, abortions had been **illegal** and were carried out by so-called 'back-street' abortionists, many of whom were untrained and worked in unhygienic conditions. Under the Abortion Act, two **doctors** must agree to any abortion on the basis that either:

- continuing with the **pregnancy** would cause greater risk to the physical, emotional or **mental health** of the pregnant woman or her existing children than terminating the pregnancy

or

- there is a risk of abnormality in the **foetus**.

This Act allowed for abortions to be carried out up to the 28th week of pregnancy. The limit was lowered to 24 weeks by the Human Fertilisation and Embryology Act 1990.

abscess
An **infection** in one place, usually resulting in an **inflamed** swelling filled with pus.

absolute poverty
Lack of the basic essentials for day-to-day living and Insufficient **resources** to live a safe and healthy life. Poverty can also be defined within the context of the **society** in which people live. *See* **relative poverty**.

B C D E F G H I J K L M N O P Q R S T U V W XYZ

abuse
Deliberate **harm** of, or failure to care for, a child or **vulnerable adult**. Abuse can be one of five types. *See* **signs and symptoms of abuse**.

Type of abuse	Examples
Physical	Punching, hitting, kicking, slapping, burning, scalding, restricting
Emotional	**Intimidating**, **bullying**, swearing, threatening, humiliating, undermining (all abuse also has an emotional element)
Sexual	Any of the following with a child, or an adult who does not consent: intercourse, intimate **touching**, showing pornographic material, involving in pornography, sexual contact of any kind, sexual comments
Financial	Taking money, accessing **pensions**, accessing bank accounts, inappropriate selling, persuading people to hand over money or financial control
Neglect	Deliberate failure to provide care, protection from harm, adequate **food**, warmth, and adequate clothing, or failure to maintain the person's cleanliness

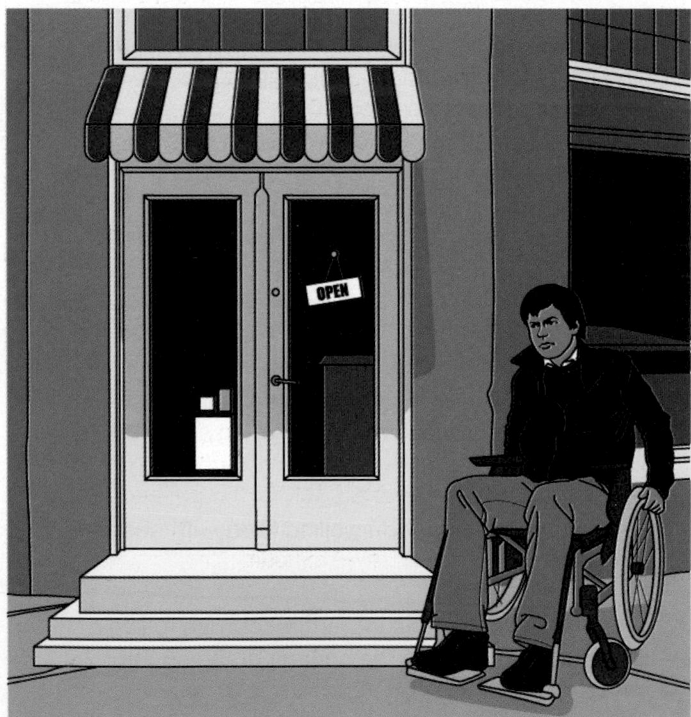

An individual has the right to set boundaries as to what is acceptable in terms of dignity.

access
The ability to reach the **services**, **facilities** and **information** people need in order to lead the life they wish. Access requires the use of the right language, the right format (e.g. audio, **Braille** or large print), suitable wheelchair access, suitable transport, clarity, the right level of **communication**, and trust in **confidentiality**. *See* **barriers**.

accident
An incident that is not planned and does not happen deliberately, and has the potential to cause **harm**. All accidents that occur in a care setting must be **recorded** in an **accident book**.

accident book

A book or form used to **record** any accident occurring in any **workplace** or place to which the public has **access**. Entries must record details of the person or people involved, the date, time and location of the accident, a description of the circumstances and details of the action taken.

accountable

Prepared to accept **responsibility** for actions and to justify and explain why, and how, things have or have not been done. In a **work** situation, people can be accountable directly to a line manager. However, in **health** and **social care** there is also accountability to the people who use **services** and to the general public who pay for them.

Acheson Report

A **report** written by Sir Donald Acheson in 1998 about **inequalities** in **health** across the UK. The report identified significant differences in health between rich and poor people and concluded that **poverty** was a major cause of poor health, as were lack of **understanding** about **nutrition** and about the importance of eating a balanced **diet**. The report recommended a ban on **smoking** in public places, increases in state **benefits**, and **education** to improve health. Acheson identified many **housing** estates as '**food** deserts' with no **access** to good quality, affordable, fresh food locally and a lack of public transport making travel difficult.

Beeches Residential Home

Report of an Accident, Dangerous Occurrence or Near Miss

Date of incident 06/07/05 **Time of incident** 10:00

Location of accident, etc. Dayroom

In the event of the casualty being absent from normal duties, please fill in the date of the first absence and date of return to work

Date off work 07/07/05 **Date return to work** 08/08/05

Details of the person injured or involved in the accident, dangerous occurence or near miss

Full name, address and post code: Daisy May, 39 Draft Street, Portsmouth PO1 1XX

Age: 26

Sex (M or F): F

Occupation of injured person or status if not an employee (e.g. Resident, Visitor) Staff Nurse

Nature of injury Burn to hand

Management of injury (Please tick appropriate box)

First aid only ✓ Advised to see doctor ☐

Casualty sent to hospital ✓ Admitted to hospital for more than 24 hours ☐

Account of accident, dangerous occurrence or near miss

Describe what happened and how. In the case of an accident, state what the injured person was doing at the time.

Daisy was handing out cups of tea to the residents when Mr Jones, who is blind, knocked in to her, causing her to spill tea on her left hand.

Witnesses (Please give names, address and occupation)

Health Care Support Worker
Kate Hill, 17 Beenthere Street
Portsmouth PO2 37Y

Remedial action taken

(**Note:** All accidents, other than minor incidents, will require an accident investigation form to be completed.)

Kate Hill immersed Daisy's hand in cold water for ten minutes, wrapped it up in a towel and took her to A&E.

Signature of person making report K Hill K. Hill **Date** 06/07/05

Signature of Safety Co-ordinator **Date**

On completion the residential home should retain a copy and send a copy to:
1. the Director of Environmental, Health and Safety Services (EHSS)
2. the Person(s) involved in the incidents

Accident report form.

acne

Acne vulgaris is the most common type of acne. It usually starts in puberty and causes red pustules. Its underlying cause is the skin's reaction to the hormone testosterone. It is a very distressing condition for young people when the face, upper back and neck are the worst affected areas. It can damage the self-esteem and confidence of many young people. Severe cases can now be treated by

B C D E F G H I J K L M N O P Q R S T U V W XYZ

medication, but there are side effects and it must be carefully monitored. Acne can leave behind facial scarring.

Acquired Immune Deficiency Syndrome (AIDS)
A terminal syndrome that affects the **immune system** and is caused by the **human immune deficiency virus (HIV)**. Usually called immunodeficiency virus. Some people can be infected with HIV without developing full-blown AIDS. Various types of cancers, infections and blood disorders may be characteristic of AIDS.

acquired immunity
Immunity achieved after birth may be active or passive. Active immunity results from the body making its own specific antibodies in response to a specific infection or immunisation (injection of dead or weakened pathogens). Passive immunity comes from receiving antibodies made elsewhere such as babies via mother's breast milk or prepared antisera.

Act of Parliament
Legislation that has gone through the process of debate and being voted on by Members of Parliament to become law.

active listening
Two-way **communication** involving a positive response to what a person is saying. Showing attentive interest, demonstrating **understanding** and encouraging the speaker to continue are all key parts of active listening. People find it easier to communicate if they receive an encouraging and interested **reaction**.

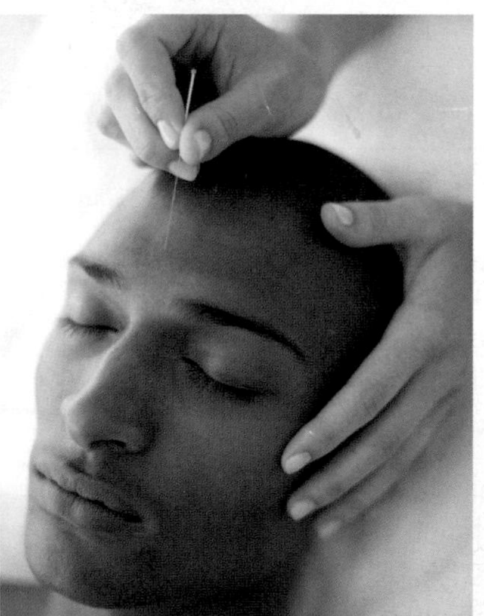

Acupuncture needles being inserted.

active support
Providing encouragement for people to live as **independently** as they can, and providing only the help that is absolutely essential in order that people can do as much as possible for themselves.

acupuncture
A treatment based on the Chinese **alternative** approach to medicine. Very fine needles are inserted at specific points in the body to treat many different conditions. There are claims that acupuncture can be effective in both physical conditions and in psychological ones such as **addictions**. Acupuncturists undertake lengthy training. The procedure is frequently used alongside mainstream medicine and many **referrals** are made by traditional **medical practitioners**.

B C D E F G H I J K L M N O P Q R S T U V W XYZ

acute
Sharp or severe in effect; intense, for example, pain.

acute illness
Illness, or disease, that begins suddenly and is usually short-term. As opposed to chronic conditions that are long-term.

addiction
Dependency on a substance, or behaviour, to the extent that it interferes with normal living. People can be physically and/or psychologically addicted to substances such as alcohol, **prescription** or **illegal drugs**, and **nicotine**. They can also be addicted to a particular behaviour, such as gambling.

additive
A substance added to another to change or improve it, most commonly found in foods. Some additives can cause allergic reactions and others can cause behaviour changes.

adipose tissue
Connective tissue where fat **cells** form an insulating layer and **energy** store under the **skin**, and protective layer around the major **organs**.

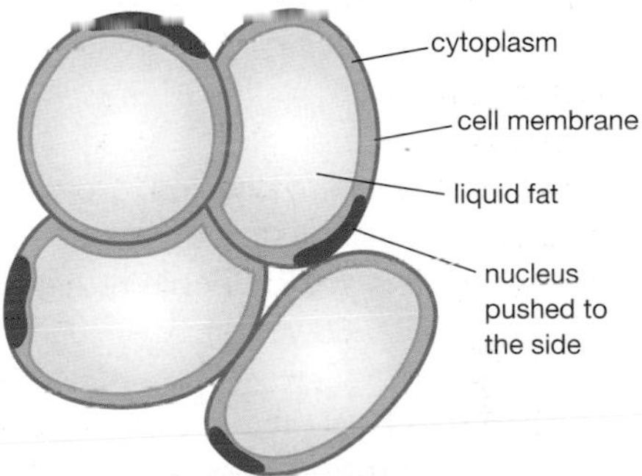

Adipose tissue.

administration
Systems and procedures that are necessary for the delivery of **services**, and the work that is done carrying out these procedures.

adolescence
One of the life stages of **human development**. Adolescence follows childhood and ends when adulthood is reached. It includes the physical changes of **puberty** and the accompanying emotional and social changes of this period.

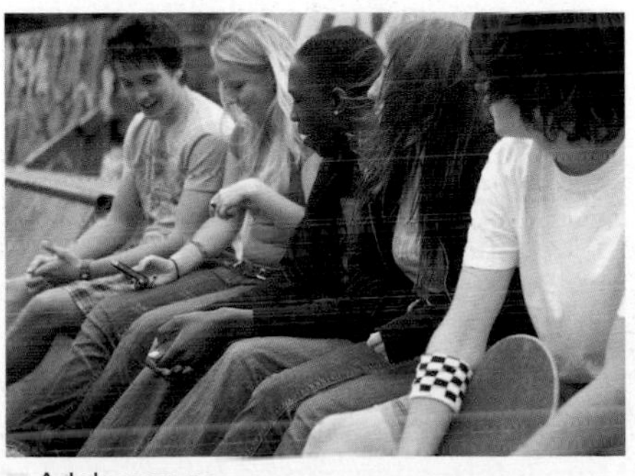

Adolescence.

adoption
A legal **process** to **change** the **parent**(s) of a child from the **birth** parent(s) to a different parent or parents, referred to as adoptive parents. Once an adoption is complete, the legal **relationship** and **responsibilities** between adoptive parents

B C D E F G H I J K L M N O P Q R S T U V W XYZ

and children is the same as between birth parents and children. Adoptions can be arranged through **local authority** children's services or through adoption agencies that are validated by the Department of Health to provide adoption **services**.

adrenal gland
An endocrine gland. There are two adrenal glands, one on top of each kidney. Each gland consists of the medulla (centre of the gland) surrounded by the cortex (outer region). The adrenal gland is responsible for regulating the body's stress response. The medulla produces adrenaline and noradrenaline (a stress hormone) and the cortex produces cortisol, aldosterone and some sex hormones. Regulation of metabolism, water balance and sexual function are carried out by these hormones.

adrenaline
The 'flight or fight' **hormone**, produced by the adrenal **gland** and released into the bloodstream as a response to a **threat**. In times of **fear** or **stress** it raises both the **heart rate** and respiratory rates, increases **blood** flow to the **muscles**, increases blood **sugar**, dilates pupils and prepares the body to fight or run.

adulthood
The **life stage** where physical growth and development is mainly completed. Adulthood does not start at a specific age in terms of growth and development, but legally it begins at 18. People move through middle adulthood (45–65) and older adulthood (over 65 years).

adverse reaction
A negative **reaction** to a substance introduced into the body. This can be a **medication** taken by mouth or **intravenously**, a cream or ointment applied to the skin, or exposure to an **environmental** substance such as pet hairs, dust mites, latex or particular metals. Reactions can take various forms; the most serious is **anaphylactic shock** that can result in **death**. Minor reactions include an irritating **rash**. Adverse reactions should always be **reported** and treated.

Advisory Conciliation and Arbitration Service (ACAS)
An **organisation** providing **support** for industrial relations between employers and employees in both private and public sectors. ACAS offers **mediation** in many **employment** disputes. The **service** will talk to both sides and offer a solution. Usually both sides will have agreed to accept any reasonable solution offered by arbitration before starting the **process**.
More information can be found at www.acas.org.uk

advocacy
Putting forward a person's views and opinions on his, or her, behalf and working for the **outcome** that the individual wishes to achieve. Advocacy can be necessary for people who are unable to act for themselves because of illness or **disability**, or because individuals lack the **confidence** to express themselves in particular situations. The essential **skill** of advocacy is ensuring that the person's views, and not the advocate's, are put forward.

aerobic exercise
Physical activity that raises the **heart** and **respiration** rate. This type of **exercise** will improve the health of the **cardiovascular system** through increased intake of **oxygen**. Running, fast walking and swimming are examples of aerobic exercise.

Age Concern
A national charity that represents the interests of older people. The organisation lobbies on behalf of older people, provides information, advice, services and support.
More information can be found at www.ageconcern.org.uk

ageing
The **process** of growing older. Ageing begins from the moment of **birth**, but the term is generally used to refer to the **changes** of later **adulthood**. This can bring physical changes such as loss of elasticity of the **skin**, stiffness of the **joints**, loss of **muscle** flexibility and tone, and loss of hair colour. It can result in sensory deterioration so that sight and/or hearing are less acute.

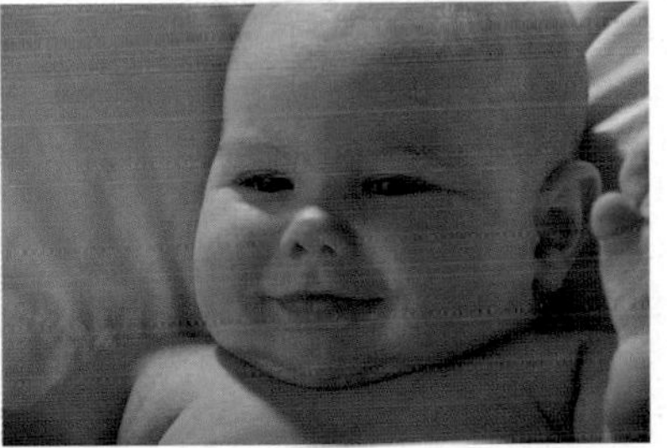

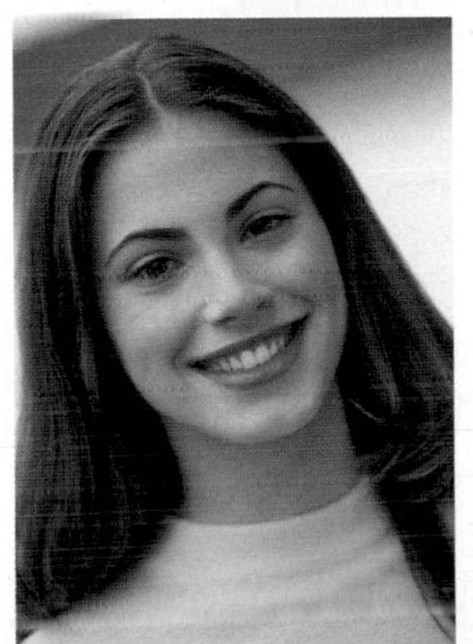

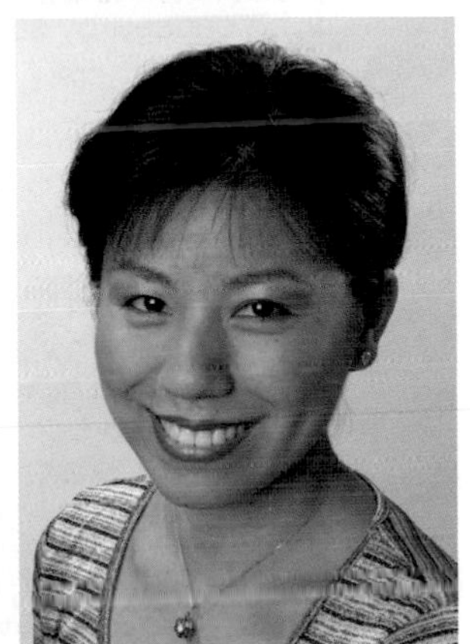

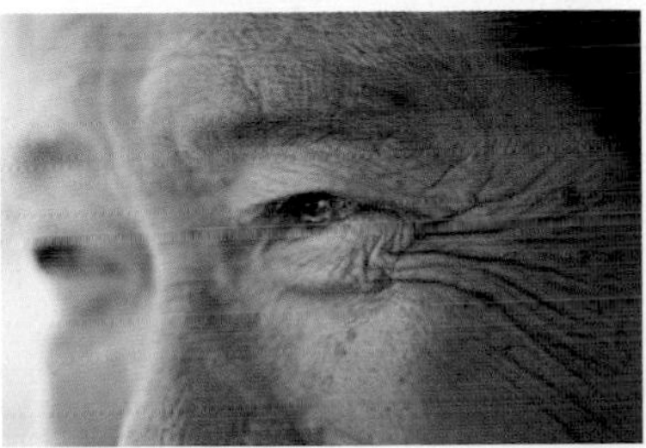

As a person ages, the skin begins to show signs of wear and tear.

There are also psychological and intellectual changes; often the life experience of ageing people brings a mature and thoughtful response to life events – commonly called wisdom – but there can also be less positive effects for some people, such as the deterioration of **memory** and **understanding**.

ageism
Discrimination on the grounds of age. Age discrimination in **employment** on the grounds of age is unlawful under the Employment Equality (Age) Regulations (2006).

agency
A general term used in **health** and **social care** to describe an **organisation** that either commissions or delivers **services**. The term can be used to describe **statutory** or **voluntary sector** organisations.

aggressive behaviour
Behaviour that is unpleasant, frightening or **intimidating**. It can cause emotional **harm** to people at whom it is directed. Such behaviour can result from a **personality** or **mental health** issue, be a side effect of some **medications**, or be caused by **substance misuse** or **fear**. It can also be an attempt to dominate others.

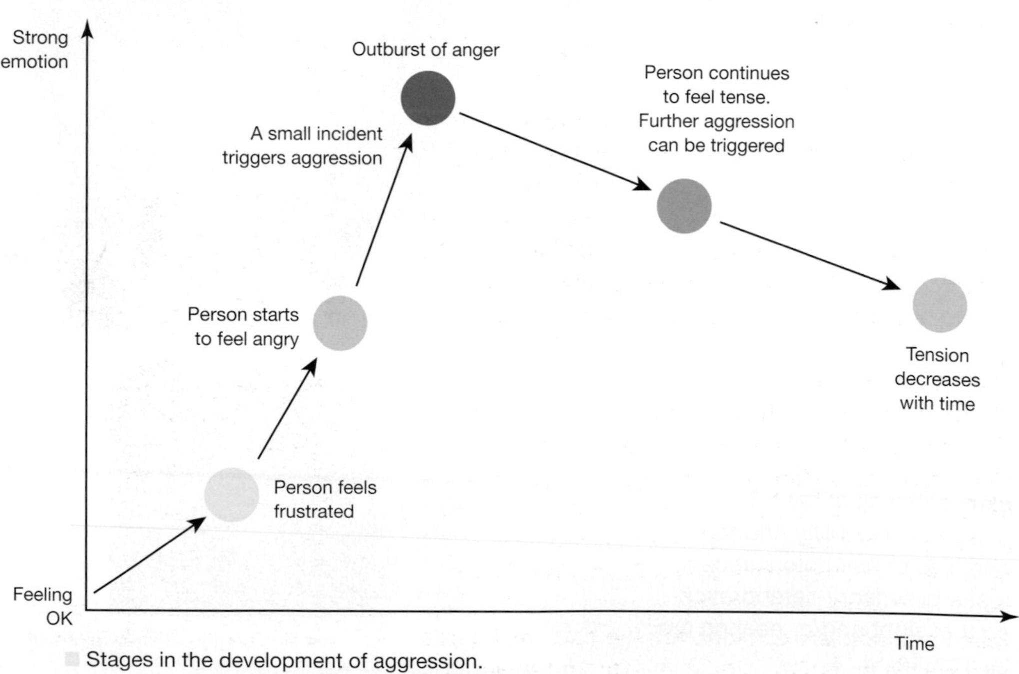

Stages in the development of aggression.

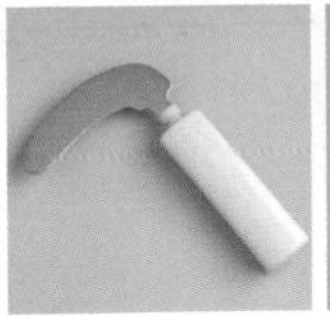
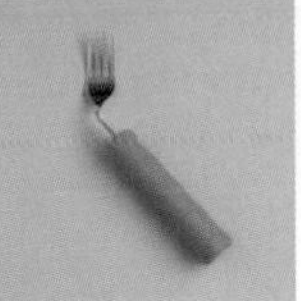
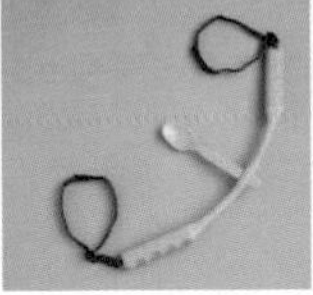
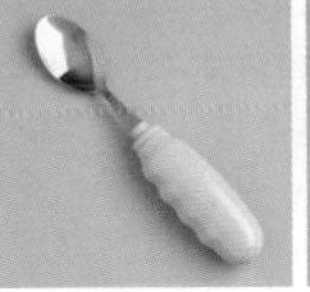
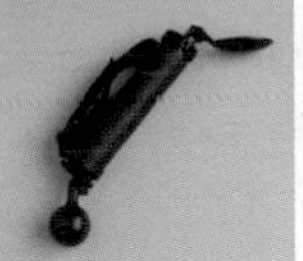
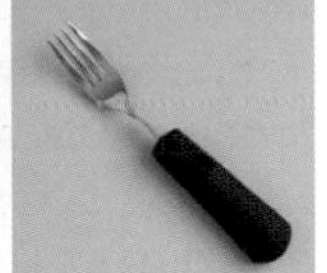

Aids for eating and drinking.

aids and adaptations
Equipment and alterations that are needed to enable people to carry out daily living and working tasks. These can include aids for walking, sitting, reaching, **bathing**, etc., and adaptations to stairs, baths, showers, workstations, etc.

alcohol
Alcohol helps people lose their inhibitions and talk openly. In moderation, it is enjoyed by many cultures around the world as a means of gathering people together for celebrations and to renew and build friendships.
Government guidelines state that men should not drink more than three to four units a day, a maximum of 28 units a week, and women should not drink more than two to three units a day, up to a maximum of 21 units a week.

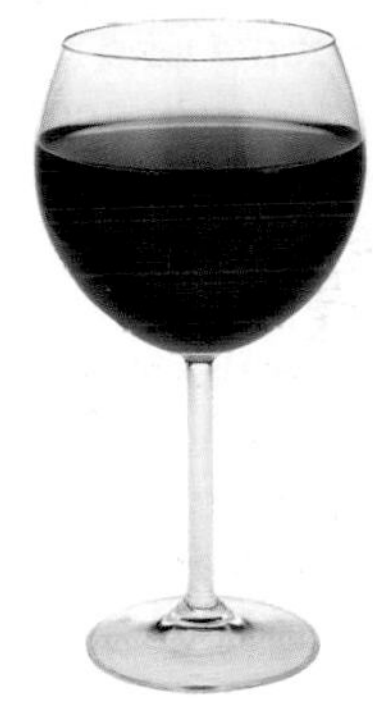

A glass of wine is equal to 1.5 units.

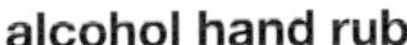

alcohol hand rub
A gel that can be used on thoroughly washed, clean hands to remove most **bacteria** if there is no immediate availability of soap and running water for **hand washing.** It is an important part of maintaining **hygiene** and minimising the spread of **infection** on hands. However, alcohol gel is not effective against some bacterial infections such as ***Clostridium difficile***.

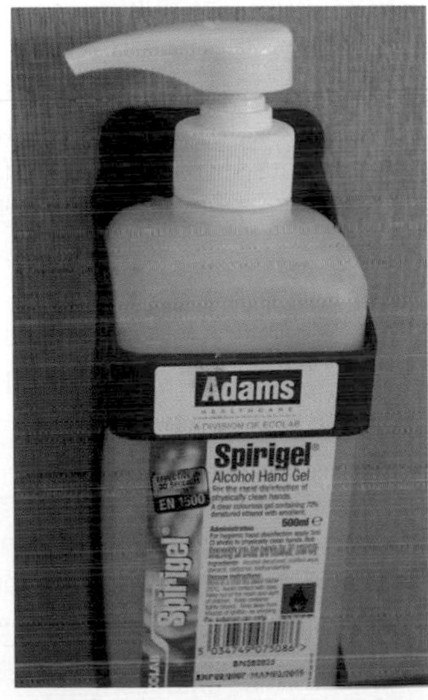

Alcohol hand rub.

alimentary canal
The various parts of the body that together process **food** and expel the resulting waste products. The alimentary canal starts with the mouth, passes through the **oesophagus**, **stomach** and **intestines**, and ends at the **anus**. Food moves along the canal by **peristalsis**, and is digested and absorbed into the body through the walls of the canal. Finally, the waste products are ejected from the body as **faeces** through the anus. See **digestive system** for diagram.

B C D E F G H I J K L M N O P Q R S T U V W XYZ

alkali
A substance with a pH greater than 7, used to neutralise acids resulting in the formation of salts.

allergen
The substance, or **organism**, that causes an allergic reaction.

allergy
An intolerance of particular substances (known as allergens) to the extent that they **trigger** a physical **reaction**. Allergic reactions can include **rashes**, **skin** blotches, **inflammation** and swelling, **vomiting**, **wheezing** and, most seriously, **anaphylactic shock**. Any known allergies must always be **recorded** in medical notes and/or **care plans**. People who have serious allergies may carry **information** identifying the allergy in case of **accidents**.
More information can be found at www.allergyuk.org

alopecia
Hair loss or baldness, ranging from a small bald patch on the head to loss of all hair over the entire body.

altered mental state
A condition usually caused by mental illness, but can also be caused by physical illness, disease, drugs or an adverse reaction to medication. As a result of any of these circumstances a person is not in touch with reality and will act accordingly.

alternative medicine
Therapies and **treatments** that are different from current medical approaches. Some of the therapies and treatments are ancient or from non-western **cultures**; for example, **acupuncture** originates in China, and **homeopathy** is based on natural ingredients that have been used for centuries. **Osteopaths** and **chiropractors** use massage and movement techniques to deal with musculo-skeletal problems.

alveoli
The single-celled berry-like structures which fill the **lungs** and across which the important **gaseous exchange** takes place by diffusion.

Alzheimer's disease
A degenerative, terminal illness that is the most common form of **dementia**. The **disease** causes physical **changes** in the **brain** that result in increasing **memory** loss, confusion, disorientation and often **delusions** or **hallucinations**. The causes are not clearly understood and there is no cure, although medication or psychosocial **treatments** can slow the progress of the disease.
More information can be found at www.alzheimers.org.uk

Alzheimers Society
A national charity that represents the interests of people with Alzheimer's disease. The organisation lobbies on behalf of people with Alzheimer's and provides advice and information. It also commissions research into the causes and treatments of the disease. More information can be found at www.alzheimers.org.uk

anaemia
A condition where **haemoglobin** levels in the blood are reduced because of a deficiency in the quality, or quantity, of red blood cells. This can cause tiredness, breathlessness and dizzy spells. There are several different types of anaemia and the most common is iron-deficiency anaemia. People can be anaemic because of a **diet** that does not contain sufficient iron, because of excessive bleeding, or because of **diseases** such as **sickle cell** or multiple myeloma.

anaesthetic
A drug that causes a loss of sensation in the body, either in a specific area (local anaesthetic) or over the whole body (general anaesthetic). Usually, a general anaesthetic is given to people undergoing major **surgery**, and a local anaesthetic is used for minor procedures. A common form of anaesthetic is an **epidural**, which is a spinal anaesthetic given during childbirth, or for chronic pain conditions, to cause a loss of sensation in the lower part of the body. Anaesthetists are usually responsible for administering anaesthetic drugs.

analysis
The **process** of considering and making judgements about a situation or a set of **information** by carefully examining all the evidence and considering issues in different ways and with different approaches contributes to analysis.

anaphylactic shock
A sudden, life-threatening, whole-body **reaction** to a foreign substance (also known as anaphylaxis). **Blood pressure** drops and airways are narrowed. Immediate medical assistance is essential. The commonest causes are **allergic** reactions to peanuts, sesame seeds, dairy **foods**, eggs, strawberries, latex or penicillin.

anatomy
The study of the structure of the human body and how the different parts relate to each other. Often studied along with physiology, which concerns the body systems and their functions.

aneurysm
A swelling in a weak area of an **artery** wall. The weak wall causes the artery to swell like a balloon. Some people have aneurysms throughout their lives and are never aware of them; however, if an aneurysm bursts, the consequences are severe as it causes major bleeding. Aneurysms usually occur in arteries, but can occasionally be found in **veins**.

anorexia nervosa
An **eating disorder** usually, but not exclusively, found in **young people**. The **symptoms** are an obsessive concern with **food** and/or **exercise**, **fear** of becoming fat, continuing weight loss even when obviously thin, **chronic** fatigue, not eating or eating very small amounts, disturbances in **menstruation** in women, and the growth of fine, downy hair covering the body. About half of people with anorexia need **hospital treatment**, and around 10 per cent die from **starvation**.
More information can be found at www.anorexiabulimiacare.co.uk

Arm bent (flexed)

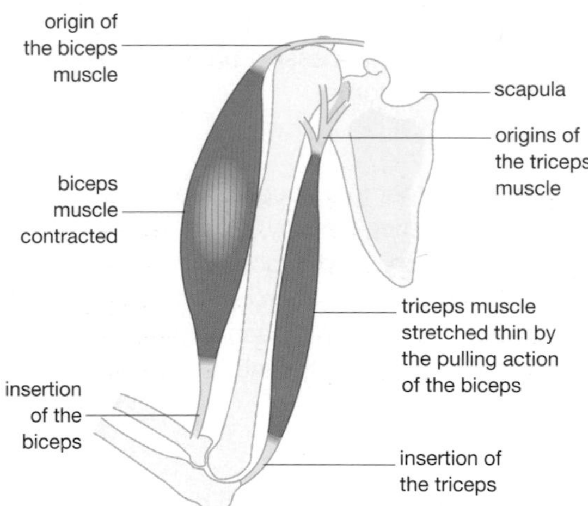

Arm straight (extended)

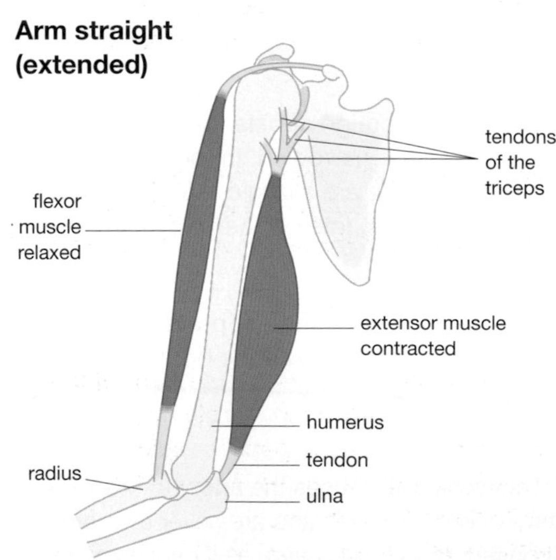

The antagonistic movement of the arm muscles.

A condition where the sense of smell is lost. It can be permanent, as the result of conditions such as nasal polyps, or temporary following a cold or sinus **infection**. The condition can be a problem for people who live alone as they are unable to detect potentially dangerous smells such as leaking gas or **food** that has begun to deteriorate.

antagonistic muscles
Muscles that work against each other in order to move a **joint**, for example biceps and triceps work in opposite ways: one contracts (shortens), the other relaxes (lengthens) in order to move the arm.

antenatal
Before birth; refers to the period of **pregnancy**, when a **foetus** is developing in the **womb**. Care is provided throughout this period by **midwives**, and **doctors** if necessary. The antenatal period ends when a woman goes into **labour**.

antibiotic
A prescribed drug that kills or prevents the growth of bacteria. Some feel the over-use of antibiotics has led to the rise of antibiotic resistant bacteria. *See* **MRSA** and **Clostridium Difficile**.

antibody
A **protein** in **blood** produced by white blood cells when the body is attacked by **bacteria, viruses** or a foreign body. Antibodies neutralise the risk posed by the invading substance, by attacking and attempting to overwhelm it.

anti-discriminatory practice
A way of **working** that actively **promotes equality**. This is about more than just not being **discriminatory**, it means being positive about equality and consciously working against any sort of discrimination.

antigen
A substance or foreign body (object coming from outside the body) that can stimulate the production of antibodies.

Anti-Social Behaviour Act (2003)
Legislation covering England and Wales that aims to tackle anti-social behaviour. It provides for **parenting orders** that set out what **parents** must do to control their children, and anti-social behaviour orders (ASBOs) that prohibit certain types of behaviour by restricting a person's **access** to places or people. The act allows for the dispersal of **groups** and of 'raves'. It also covers graffiti, **truancy** and problems caused for neighbours, for example by high hedges or intrusive noise.

Anti-Social Behaviour Orders (ASBOs)
An order given out by the Court for anti-social behaviour as all, or part of, a sentence. It states exactly what the person can and cannot do, depending on the reasons why it was given, for example an offender who has been harassing someone may be forbidden to visit the street the person lives in.

anus
The opening in the body through which **faeces** are expelled by the **process** of **defecation**. The anal sphincter **muscle** controls the opening and closing of the anus. Damage to the muscle or its controlling **nerves** can cause **incontinence**. Part of the alimentary canal.

anxiety
A normal response to a concerning or worrying situation; a more severe form of this normal emotional experience may develop into a neuroses when people become overly anxious about small, everyday events. This can result in panic attacks, breathlessness, dizziness, **vomiting** and **fear** of leaving the house. Anxiety that interferes with normal living requires investigation and **treatment**.
More information can be found at www.mentalhealth.org.uk

aorta
The main **artery** of the circulatory system, with the largest diameter and the thickest walls. It carries oxygenated blood (blood with a high concentration of oxygen) from the left ventricle of the **heart** to smaller arteries and capillaries which carry the blood to the tissues of the body.

Apgar score
A method of checking the general condition of a **baby** immediately after **birth**. Scores are given (maximum 2) for the baby's:
- **heart rate**
- breathing
- colour
- **muscle** tone
- response to stimuli.

These are measured at one minute and five minutes after delivery. A score of 6 or below, one minute after delivery, would give cause for concern; all babies should have a score of 9 or 10 within five minutes of birth.

PART A: Appraisee's Self-Evaluation

The Job
Please attach your up-to-date job description.

What you have done
What do you see as the main purpose of your job?

Does your job description need to be revised? If so what changes would you like to see?

How well did you achieve last year's objectives?

Overall, what do you feel have been your main achievements in the last year?

What new skills, knowledge, and experience have you acquired?

How you did it
What do you do well? What aspects of the job do you find most rewarding?

What aspects of your job do you find the most difficult? What have been the frustrations?

What would/could help (including any help/support from your line-manager or any training and development)?

How effective was any development or training you received?

What next?
How do you see yourself or your role developing in the next year?

Are there any development and training implications for the coming year?

Example of an appraisal form.

aphasia
Loss of the ability to speak due to damage or **disease** affecting the speech centre in the **brain**. This can happen following a **stroke** or a brain **injury**.

aphonia
Inability to speak because of an **injury** or **disease** affecting the **muscles** or **nerves** of the mouth, throat or vocal cords, such as **motor neurone disease**.

appraisal
An evaluation of **performance** at **work**. This is usually conducted by a line manager on an annual basis. **Goals** and **targets** will be set for the coming year and continuing professional development which involves **self-assessment** and the manager's **assessment** of performance progress discussed.

B C D E F G H I J K L M N O P Q R S T U V W XYZ

appropriate adult
Required by **legislation** when the police interview a **young person** under the age of 17 years or someone who has a **learning disability** or is regarded as vulnerable. Appropriate adults can be workers from the youth offending teams (YOT), social workers, parents or specially trained people on an Appropriate Adult Panel. Their role is to protect the well-being of the young or vulnerable person during an interview. The appropriate adult is not there to fulfil the same role as a legal representative whose job is to protect the interests of the persons concerned.

approved mental health professional
Under the Mental Health Act 2007, the approved mental health professional has replaced the previously used approved **social worker** as one of the specially trained people (along with a **doctor** with **mental health** training) who can take the decision to compulsorily detain someone in **hospital**.

aromatherapy
Use of essential oils to **promote** a feeling of **health** and **well-being.** Oils can be mixed with a carrier, such as almond oil, and massaged into the **skin** so that they are absorbed, or they can be given by inhalation (breathed in). *See* **massage**.

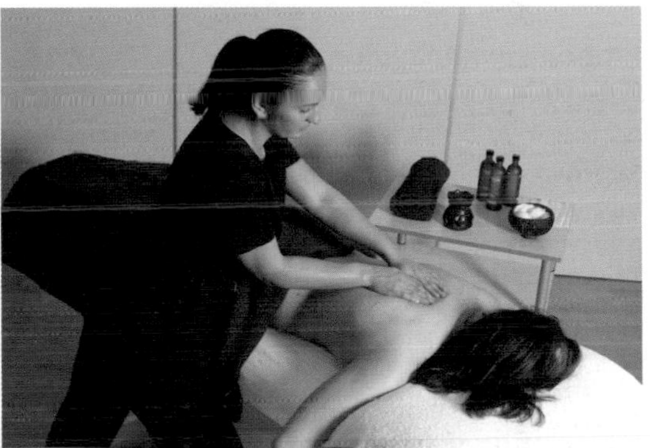
Aromatherapy massage.

arrhythmia
Irregular heartbeat. Heartbeats can vary from the normal rhythm for a range of reasons, and not all are causes for concern.
Any unusual changes to **heart** rhythm should be investigated by a **doctor**.

artery
A **blood** vessel that carries **oxygenated** blood away from the **heart** to **muscles** and **organs**. The heart **ventricles** contract to pump blood into the arteries; artery walls are elastic, so they expand and contract to maintain the blood flow around the body.

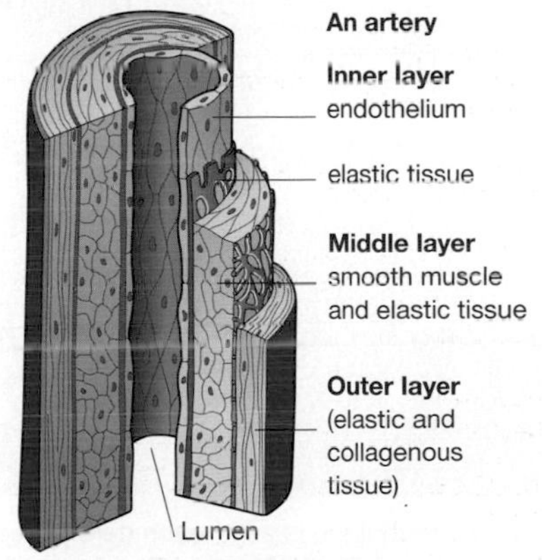

The structure of an artery.

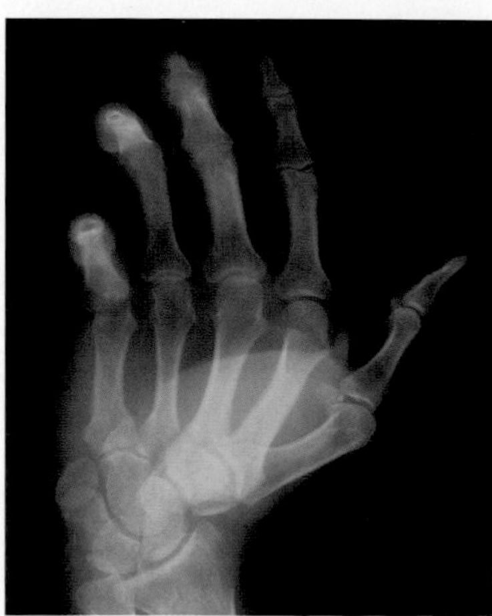

Osteo-arthritis is caused by wear and tear.

arthritis

A painful and degenerative condition affecting **joints**. There are two main types of arthritis: rheumatoid arthritis and osteo-arthritis. Rheumatoid arthritis (RA) is an auto-immune **disease** where the body's **immune system** mistakenly attacks healthy **tissue**, causing pain and **inflammation** of joints. RA is most commonly seen in hands and feet. Osteo-arthritis is not an auto-immune disease and is caused by wear and tear or **injury**, and results in **inflamed** and stiff joints. It is most commonly seen in weight-bearing joints such as hips and knees.
More information can be found at www.arthritiscare.org.uk

artificial insemination

A technique for introducing **semen** into the **vagina**. A means of assisting conception if there is a difficulty in conceiving through **sexual intercourse**. The technique is used to assist **conception**.

aseptic technique

Also called sterile technique, this is any **health care** procedure in which added precautions such as sterile **gloves**, **equipment** and instruments are used to prevent

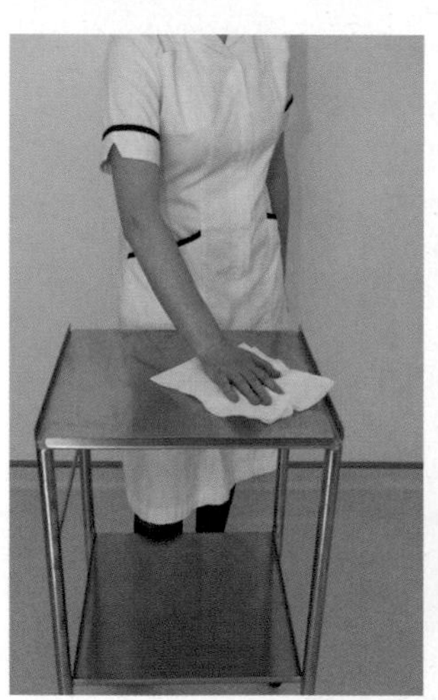

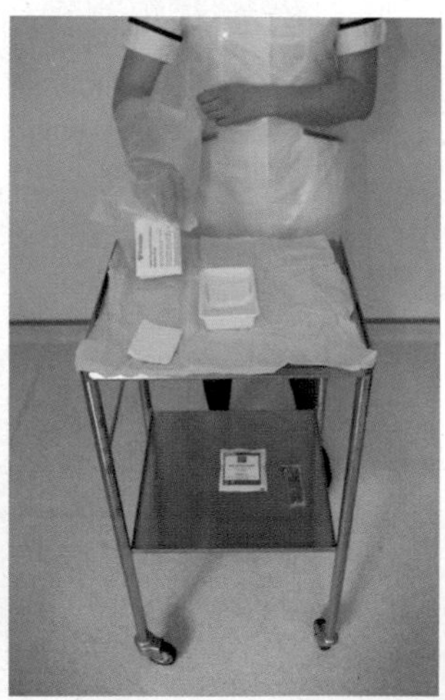

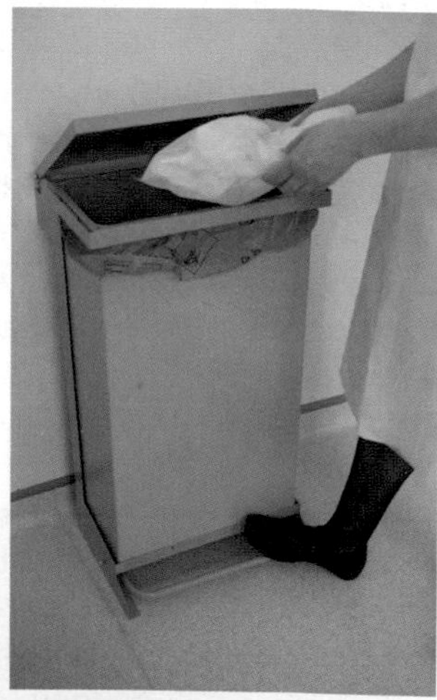

Aseptic technique is any health care procedure in which added precautions such as sterile gloves, equipment and instruments are used to prevent contamination of a person, object, or area by the micro-organisms that cause infection.

contamination of a person, object, or area by the **micro-organisms** that cause **infection.** It is used in **surgery**, or in any invasive or other procedures that carry the risk of infection.

Asperger syndrome
A condition that is on the **autistic spectrum**. People with Asperger syndrome have difficulty in social **relationships** and in **communicating** with others. They lack the ability to read the signals of **non-verbal communication**, may make inappropriate comments and find it difficult to join in discussions and conversations. Most people with the syndrome have average or above-average levels of **intelligence**.
More information can be found at www.aspergerfoundation.org.uk

assertiveness
The **skill** of being clear and firm but not aggressive in the way you **communicate** with others. You can learn the **skills** and techniques of controlling your emotions (such as anger, **fear** or tearfulness) and be calm and authoritative in your **interactions** with others.

assessment
In **social care**, the **process** of working with people to identify their **needs**, the **outcomes** they want to achieve and ways in which they want to achieve them. Assessment can also describe the process of judging progress towards achieving outcomes. Assessments can involve a **team** of **professionals** with a range of **skills**, and the process should be co-ordinated so that it does not need to be repeated several times. For adults this is done through the **single assessment process** (SAP) and for children and **young people** through the Common Assessment Framework (CAF).

asthma
A condition affecting a person's airways. An irritant (known as a **trigger**) causes the airways to narrow as the **muscles** around them tighten; the linings of the airways swell and create mucus, thus further reducing the space for air to move. People with asthma **wheeze**, have a tight **chest** and are short of breath. Asthma attacks can be triggered in many ways, but the commonest are exposure to dust, pollen, pet hair, cigarette **smoke**, sudden changes in **temperature**, colds, spores or emotional **stress**. Over 5.2 million people in the UK receive **treatment** for asthma.

Asthma UK
A national charity that represents the interests of people with asthma. The organisation lobbies on behalf of people with Asthma and provides advice and information. It also commissions research into the causes and treatments of the disease.
More information can be found at www.asthma.org.uk

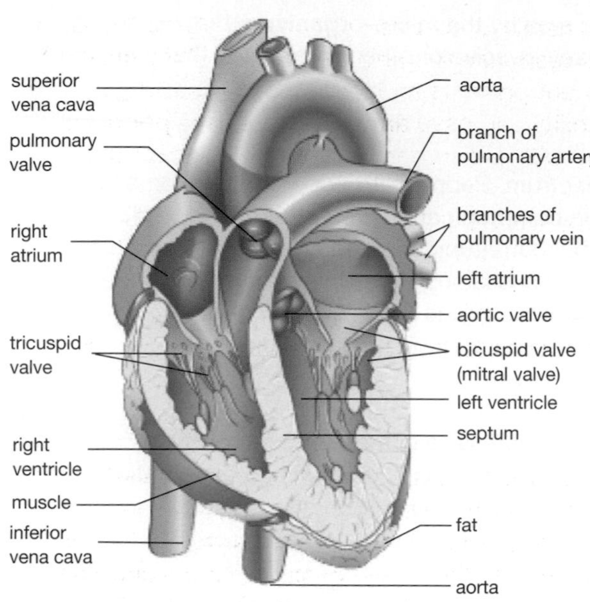

The heart

atrium
One of the upper chambers of the **heart**. **Oxygenated blood** from the **lungs** goes into the left atrium, and de-oxygenated blood that has circulated around the body goes into the right atrium.

attachment theory
Theory first proposed by John Bowlby, which highlights the importance of a child having a **significant adult** with whom to **bond**. The significant figure is usually the **mother**, but it can be any other adult. Children who are not able to bond in this way do not develop successfully as **infants**, and can have difficulties with **relationships** in later life.

attention deficit hyperactivity disorder (ADHD)
A disorder seen in children. Affected children show very limited concentration, the tendency to be easily distracted, over-activity, restlessness, disorganisation and poor **memory**. They need the **support** of a **team** of **professionals**.

Audit Commission
An **independent** body responsible for overseeing public spending in **local government**, **health**, **community safety** and **housing**. It is the role of the Audit Commission to **report** on whether public money has been spent efficiently and effectively in delivering **services**.
More information can be found at www.audit-commission.gov.uk

autistic spectrum disorder
The term autistic spectrum disorder (ASD) describes all the disorders that are on the spectrum, such as autism and **Asperger syndrome**. There are differences between the disorders on the spectrum, but all people with an ASD share a 'triad of **impairments**' in their ability to:

- **understand** and use non-verbal and verbal **communication**
- understand social behaviour, to an extent that affects their ability to **interact** with other people
- think and behave flexibly, which may be shown in restricted, obsessive or repetitive activities.

Some people with an ASD have a different perception of sounds, sights, smell, **touch** and taste, which affects their response to these sensations. They may also have unusual **sleep** and behaviour patterns and can present **challenging behaviour**. People of all levels of ability can have an ASD, and it is important that you do not assume that anyone with a disorder on the autistic spectrum also has a **learning disability**.
More information can be found at www.nas.org.uk (National Autistic Society)

autonomic nervous system
The part of the peripheral nervous system that maintains the balance of the body systems – homeostasis, controlling functions such as temperature, blood pressure and blood oxygen levels.

autonomy
The freedom to take **independent** decisions without having to ask anyone else or receive permission. People who use care **services** should be allowed to be autonomous in taking decisions about their lives. Some people who work in **health** and care are autonomous in their work, while others have to act under the direction and with the permission of other people. An example are **nurses** who work to the directions of **doctors**, whereas midwives are autonomous practitioners who can take all decisions and **responsibility** for women and **babies** during normal **pregnancy** and **birth**.

axilla
The armpit.

B

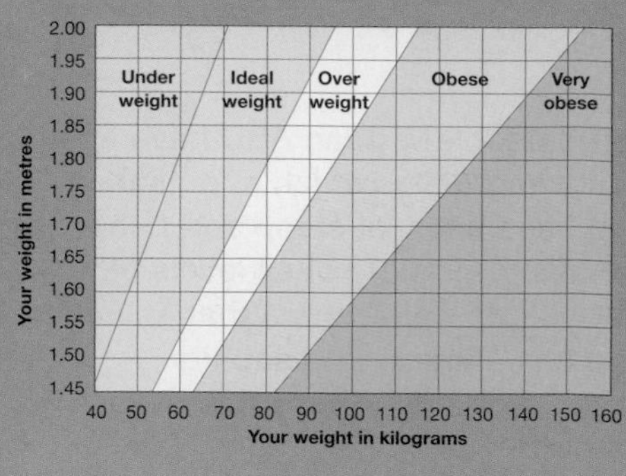

baby

Child in the first stage of **human development**, also know as an **infant**. During this stage, human babies are helpless and totally **dependent** on the care of others, usually the **mother**. This stage lasts from **birth** until the end of the second year of life, and is a period of rapid development that involves absorbing a massive amount of **information** and **learning**.

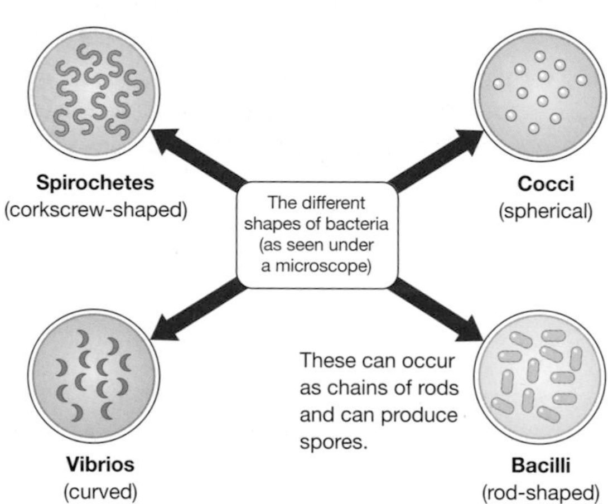

■ The different shapes of bacteria.

bacteria

Single-celled **micro-organisms** that can be **harmful** or beneficial, depending on type. Some are essential to break down dead plant and animal material to enable **recycling** to take place, and others carry illnesses such as food poisoning, typhoid and **pneumonia**. Bacteria are about one thousandth of a millimetre in length and can only be seen with a **microscope**. They take different shapes: rods (bacilli), spirals (spirochetes), spheres (cocci) and curves (vibrios).

balanced diet

See **diet**

Bandura, Albert

A Canadian **psychologist** (born 1925) who developed **social learning theory**: the theory that we **model** our behaviour on that of people around us, particularly if they are people we admire or the behaviour results in **outcomes** we consider valuable or desirable. Modelling is not just **imitating**; it involves **observing** what others do and then using that as a basis to develop new behaviours of our own.

bar chart
A widely used type of **graph** providing a clear way of viewing comparative **information.** The use of wide lines or blocks representing the different variables often makes it easier to read and interpret than a line graph.

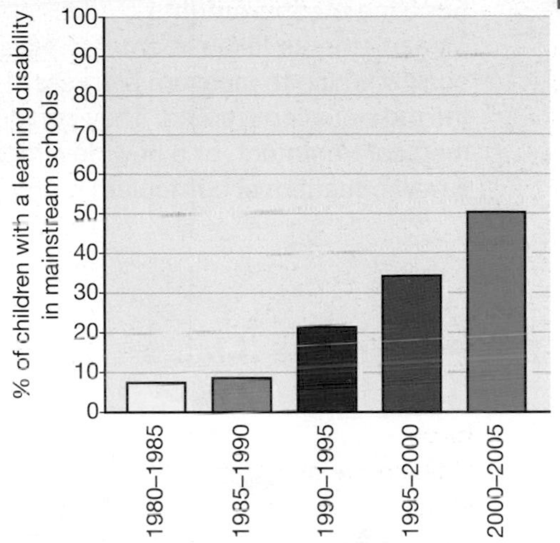

■ A bar chart showing the number of children with a learning disability in mainstream schools in Everytown over past 25 years.

Barnardos
A national children's **charity** providing a range of **services** for children and **families.** It was founded by Thomas Barnardo in 1867 and provided **residential care** for children until changes in **practice** in recent years led to a broader range of **work** with children, including **fostering** and **adoption**, counselling, **vocational training**, **participation work** and work with **disabled** children.
More information can be found at www.barnardos.org.uk

barrier
A physical or emotional difficulty that causes problems for people using **services** or **communicating** with **health** and care **professionals**. Examples of physical barriers include those related to:

- **access**
- lack of money
- geography/location.

Examples of emotional barriers include:

- lack of **confidence**
- feelings of shame, or **fear** of the **reaction** of others
- **cultural** issues in relation to communication or service **provision.**

barrier nursing
Part of **infection control** which is taken to prevent infection spreading from one patient to another or to staff. Usually involves caring for a patient in a separate room with restricted access. Staff wear disposable protective clothing and following strict infection control procedures.

barrister
A legal consultant who provides legal opinions and is instructed to represent individuals in the Crown Court and **High Court.** Barristers are not directly instructed by the individuals they represent, but by a **solicitor** on behalf of the individual. Advocates perform a similar role in Scotland, where they represent individuals in the Session Court.

baseline measurements
Measurements taken in order to establish an initial position and provide a point against which to measure progress. These measurements provide the '**norm**' for the individual concerned. They could be recorded at the start of a new course of **medical treatment**, or a new **development programme** of activities, or at the start of a new **educational curriculum** for children.

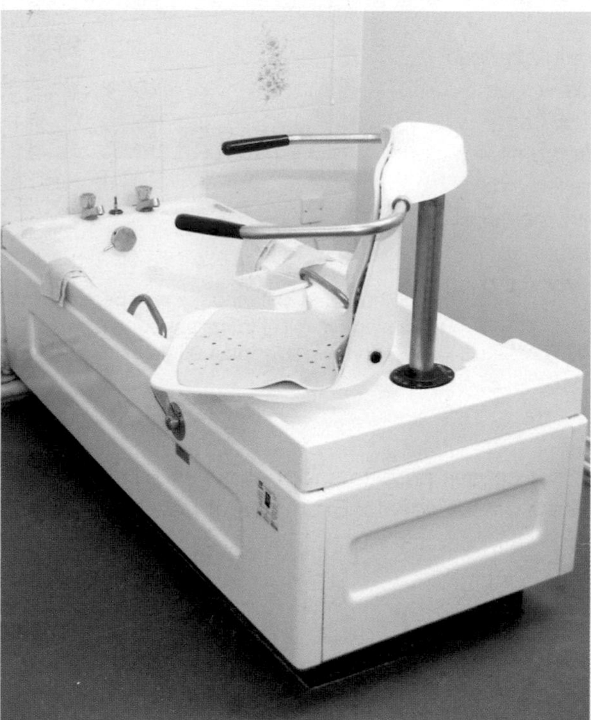
■ A bath with bath aids.

bathing
Immersion of the body in water in order to keep clean – part of **personal hygiene**. Some people may require assistance with bathing. Wherever possible people should be **supported** to have a bath or shower through the use of **hoists** and bath lifts or **shower chairs**, but sometimes it is necessary to bath people without moving them out of bed. Bed-bathing can be carried out with a bowl of warm water and soap, or with specially designed wipes or aerosol foam. Baths can be relaxing and pleasurable. Most **babies** enjoy bath-time and many adults use a bath as a way to relax.

behaviour
Actions and communications by a person that are usually an indication of how they are feeling.

behaviour management
The management of a person's behaviour based on **learning** theories. These theories suggest that **human behaviour** is changed and controlled by the consequences of an experience. We behave in particular ways because we are either 'rewarded' or 'punished' as a consequence of what we do, for example in very simple terms, if a child touches a hot iron, he or she learns that it hurts and will not do so again. Similarly, we learn that if we behave in an acceptable way we are rewarded by praise or the acceptance of others.

A common form of behaviour management is the '**positive discipline**' programmes run in many **schools**, where children and **young people** are rewarded for acceptable behaviour.

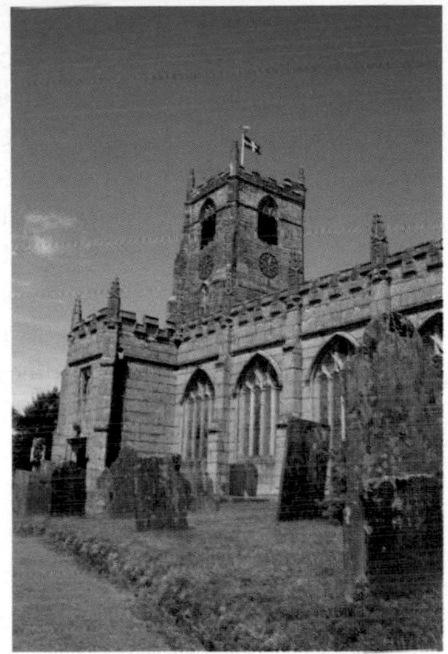

Christians worship in a church.

beliefs

Concepts that people hold to be true. Beliefs can be based in **religion** or **culture**, or can be about the types of behaviour considered to be acceptable and right. Beliefs have a significant influence on how people behave, and care **professionals** need to examine their own and **understand** how their **work** can be affected by them.

benchmarking

Measuring an action, activity or performance against a standard, for example the patient waiting times for a local health service can be compared with a national benchmark.

benefits

Financial **support** for people who are unable to work through illness or **disability**, or through a lack of **job opportunities**; or support for those who have **retired** and are receiving a **pension**. There are also benefits for **carers** who are looking after a relative or friend in need of support. These are administered and managed by the Department for Work and Pensions. 'Universal benefits' are available to everyone, for example **Child Benefit**. Other benefits are only available after an **assessment** of how much **income** and savings an individual has, for example **Housing Benefit**. These are called 'means-tested benefits'.

benign

A condition that is not aggressive or life-threatening. The term is most commonly used to describe a non-**malignant tumour**.

bereavement

The **process** of losing someone close through **death**. Everyone **grieves** and reacts to bereavement in a different way and on different timescales, but generally there are stages to the bereavement process. These may not be clear cut and may overlap.

- Initially people are stunned and numb; even where a death has been expected, there is still numbness and disbelief.
- This is often followed by a great sense of loss and searching for the person who has died. Often people will report seeing the person everywhere or dreaming about him or her.

- Some people go through a stage of being very angry about the death; sometimes it is with people who were around at the time, or with medical staff, or the person may feel guilty about not having done more to try to prevent the death.
- This stage can be followed by periods of **depression** and intense grieving before people gradually begin to accept the loss and to move on with their lives.

Not everyone goes through all these stages, and not always in this order, but most people go through something similar. It is difficult to put a timescale on the process, but it usually takes at least a year or two. A good piece of advice to anyone who has been bereaved is to 'do nothing irrevocable for two years'. Very many people will make emotionally based decisions during this time that they later regret.

Best Value

A **statutory** framework for **local government** to ensure that **public services** are delivered in the most effective way. 'Best Value' requires **local authorities** to **consult** local people and to **review** all their **services** on a regular basis. Reviews examine:

- the reasons for delivering the particular service and whether the **outcomes** to which it is **contributing** can be achieved in other ways
- **feedback** from local people about improvements needed for the service
- the current **contract** and whether it is offering the best possible value and approach to the service
- the cost of the service and whether this can be delivered in a different way at lower cost without reducing quality.
- the last Best Value Performance Indicators are in 2008 when reporting of performance will be through the new National Indicator Set (NIS).

Beveridge, William

An economist (1879–1963) who, in 1942, produced a **report** for **Parliament** that was the basis for the creation, in 1948, of the **Welfare State** and the **National Health Service**. The Beveridge Report identified the 'five great evils' of **poverty**, ignorance, squalor, **disease** and idleness and outlined how a '**national insurance**' system would fund the creation of a **health service** 'free at the point of use' and provide **pensions** and **benefits** for people in need.

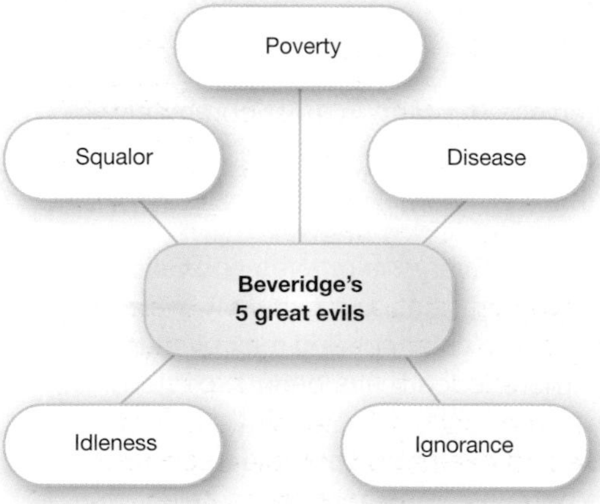

■ Beveridge's five great evils.

bias

A preference for one **group** or individual over another. In a **research** project, if there is bias in the **sample** selected, the results can be invalid.

bibliography
A list that acknowledges the books, articles, papers and other **references** used when **researching** and preparing a **report**, article, assignment, essay or book. It is usually included at the end of the work and shows the title, author, publisher and date of the work that has been used as a **reference**.

bile
A juice secreted by the **liver** and stored in the **gall bladder**. It contains salts which break down fats into small globules (emulsification) so that **digestion** can be carried out by **enzymes** secreted from other glands. Bile does not contain any enzymes.

bilirubin
A reddish-brown pigment produced as a waste product of **haemoglobin** from old red blood cells. It is part of **bile** and is responsible for the colour of faeces.

biopsy
The **process** of removing a **sample** of **human tissue** for **microscopic examination** to provide, or assist in, a **diagnosis** of **disease**.

birth
The **process** of a **foetus** leaving the **uterus** (**womb**) and beginning an independent existence as a **baby**. For humans the length of time from **conception** to birth is about 40 weeks. A normal birth begins when the uterus starts to contract. This starts the process of **labour**. Over several hours, the uterus passes through three distinct stages and gradually pushes the foetus out. During the first stage of labour, the **cervix** will gradually dilate until it is sufficiently wide for the baby's head to pass through. The baby is delivered out of the uterus during the second stage by a combination of strong contractions and pushing by the **mother**. At the end of this stage, the baby will be born, still attached to the mother by the **umbilical cord**. Following the cutting of the umbilical cord, the third stage of labour begins when the **placenta** is pushed out and the birth is complete. Some births require medical **intervention** and can require a **caesarean section** or an **instrumental delivery**.

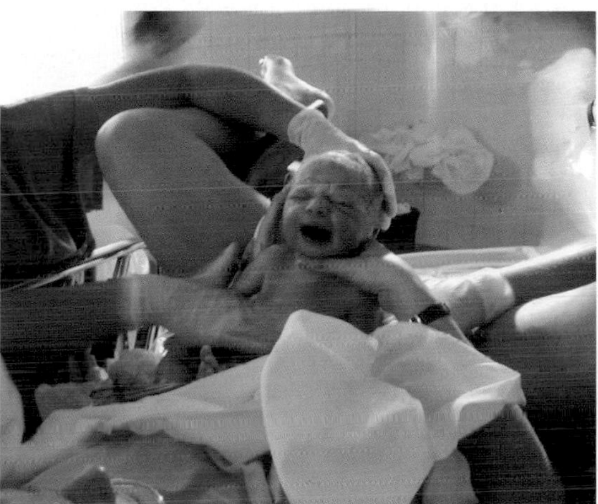

■ The three stages of labour and delivery are: dilation of cervix, birth and placenta delivery.

birth canal
The name given to the combined passageway of the uterus and vagina after the cervix has dilated. The foetus will pass through this canal to be born.

birth rate
The number of live births per 1000 of the population. Data is maintained by the Office for National Statistics.
More information can be found at www.statistics.gov.uk

Black Report (1980)
A milestone report which clearly described the health inequalities in the UK; viewed as too politically sensitive by the government of the day, the report was suppressed and its distribution strictly limited. The **Acheson Report**, published in 1998, came up with very similar conclusions.

bladder
The muscular sac within the pelvis, connected to the **kidneys** by the ureters, which stores **urine**. When the bladder is full, a message is sent to the **brain** that it needs to be emptied. As children, most of us learn to control our bladders and wait to empty them in a **toilet**. However, age, **disease** or **injury** can cause control to be lost and people become **incontinent**.

blind
Totally or almost totally unable to see. People are usually classified as blind if they have less than one tenth vision in their better eye after using any lenses or spectacles. Blindness can be **congenital** or it can develop later in life through **disease** or **injury**.

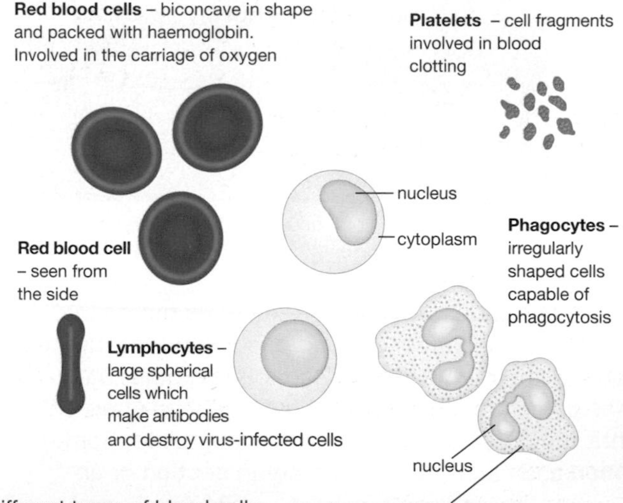
Red blood cells – biconcave in shape and packed with haemoglobin. Involved in the carriage of oxygen
Platelets – cell fragments involved in blood clotting
nucleus
cytoplasm
Red blood cell – seen from the side
Phagocytes – irregularly shaped cells capable of phagocytosis
Lymphocytes – large spherical cells which make antibodies and destroy virus-infected cells
nucleus
cytoplasm containing granules
Different types of blood cells

blood
The vital fluid in the human body. An adult has about 5.5 litres of circulating volume. Blood carries **oxygen** and **carbon dioxide** around the body, along with other substances such as **urea** and **hormones**. It also defends the body against **infections** through the **white blood cells**. The **platelets** are associated with the clotting process. Blood is made up of 45% blood cells and 55% **plasma** which is the liquid part of the blood.

blood-borne virus/infection (BBV)

Blood-borne **viruses** are diseases caused by viruses that are spread by contact with infected blood. These include hepatitis and human immune deficiency virus (**HIV**). Universal precautions such as safe disposal of sharps, wearing gloves and eye protection are important barriers to reduce risks.

blood clotting (or coagulation)

An enzyme process which converts liquid blood into a thickened mass called a clot or thrombus. Under normal circumstances, this occurs when blood is shed to prevent further blood loss and form a protection against bacterial invasion. Sometimes, this can occur inside blood vessels which have narrowed and roughened interiors often with serious consequences particularly in the heart and brain, known as cardiac or cerebral thrombosis.

blood glucose levels

The level of glucose or **sugar** in the blood should be 4–6 mmol per dm^3. **Insulin**, which is produced by the **pancreas**, controls the level of glucose in the blood. When the pancreas fails to make sufficient insulin to control blood glucose, **diabetes mellitus** develops. Blood glucose levels can be measured and **monitored** by testing a drop of blood.

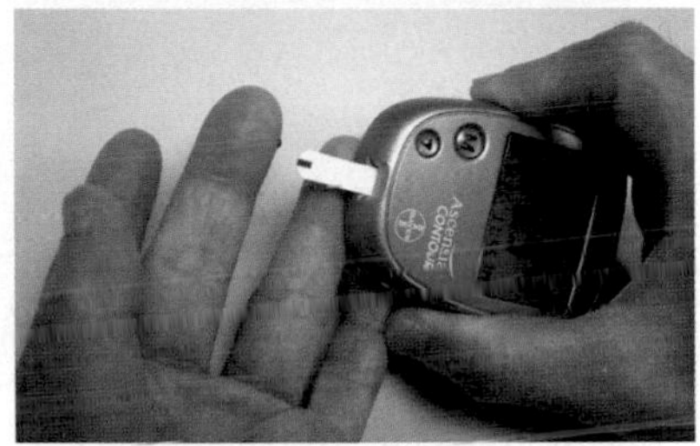

■ A blood glucose monitor.

blood groups

Different types of **blood**. **Red blood cells** contain **proteins** that can act as **antigens** and bring about an **immune response**. The ability to define blood into groups that contain specific proteins means that it is possible for individuals to receive **blood transfusions** of a compatible type. Commonly, four blood groups are identified: A, B, AB and O. This links to the proteins antigen A and antigen B. People in blood group A have antigen A in their red blood cells; those in blood group B have antigen B; those in blood group AB have both A and B antigens; those in blood group O have neither. In general, only blood of the matching group is given in transfusions.

blood pressure

The pressure of blood against the **artery** walls as it is pumped from the **heart**. Blood pressure that is too high or too low is an indicator of health concerns. Blood pressure is usually measured using a digital device that notes and **records** all **measurements**. It can also be taken manually using a **sphygmomanometer** by:

- attaching the cuff to the person's arm
- feeling the **pulse** at the inner elbow (brachial artery)

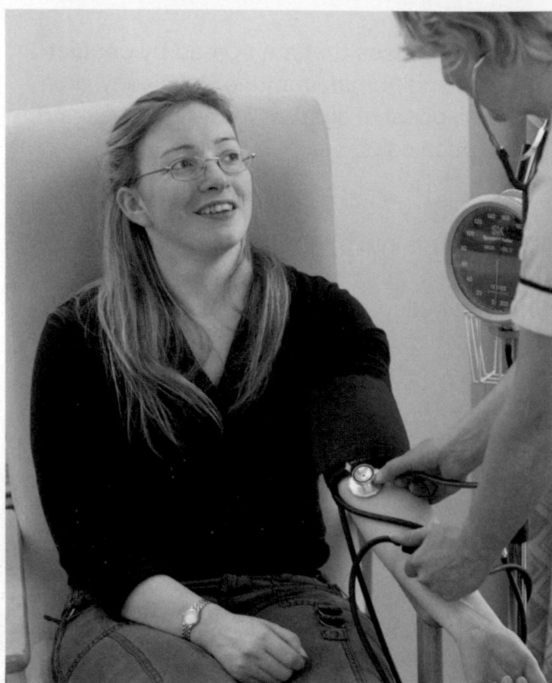
Taking a blood pressure reading using a sphygmomanometer.

- putting a **stethoscope** at the same point on the inner elbow
- pumping up the cuff until the measurement on the sphygmomanometer reaches approximately 180–200
- decreasing the air in the cuff slowly, letting it out using the valve on the sphygmomanometer until the pulse is heard through the stethoscope
- noting the reading on the sphygmomanometer at this point – the **systolic** (upper) reading (normally around 120)
- letting the air out of the cuff and listening until the pulse disappears; the reading at this point is the **diastolic** (lower) reading and should be around 80.

bloodstream
A collective term for the blood in the blood vessels and heart.

blood transfusion
The **process** of transferring blood from a donor to another individual. Knowing the **blood group** of both donor and recipient is essential for blood to be **transfused** safely. Blood can only be given to a recipient of the same blood group as the donor in order to avoid an **immune response** to the new blood. Blood is collected and stored in a blood bank under specialised conditions.

blood vessels
Channels (**arteries**, **veins** and **capillaries**) that carry blood to and from the **heart** and **body** tissues.

bodily fluids
Any liquid that is produced by the body. Apart from the **blood** this includes **urine**, **vomit** and **sputum**.

body
Refers to the main trunk of a person rather than their head and limbs.

body composition
The ratio of lean body mass to fat mass in an individual.

body language
See **non-verbal communication**.

body mass index (BMI)
A way of measuring a healthy weight. A BMI of 20–25 is ideal. It is calculated by dividing a person's body weight in kilograms by the height in metres squared MI = weight (kg)/height (m^2). Some sports people who have a large muscle mass can have a BMI in the unhealthy range so the index must be treated with caution in such cases.

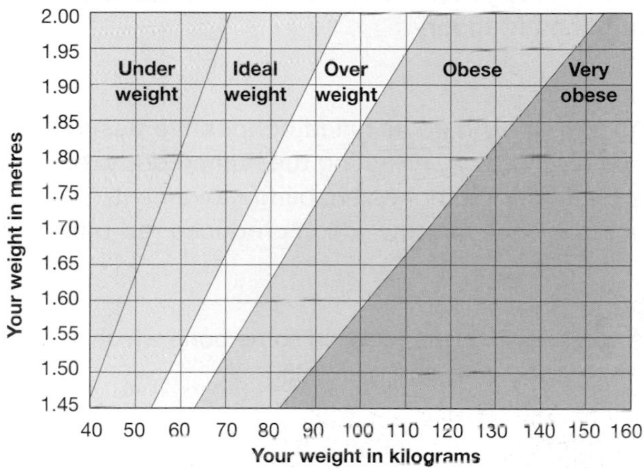

■ Ideal weight for height chart.

body temperature
The human body maintains its **temperature** through the **hypothalamus**, a part of the **brain**. Maintaining temperature is part of **homeostasis**, the **process** by which the body maintains stability. The body loses or maintains the heat it needs for a stable temperature of 37 degrees **Celsius** (98.4 Fahrenheit). A digital thermometer is used to check and **record** a person's body temperature.

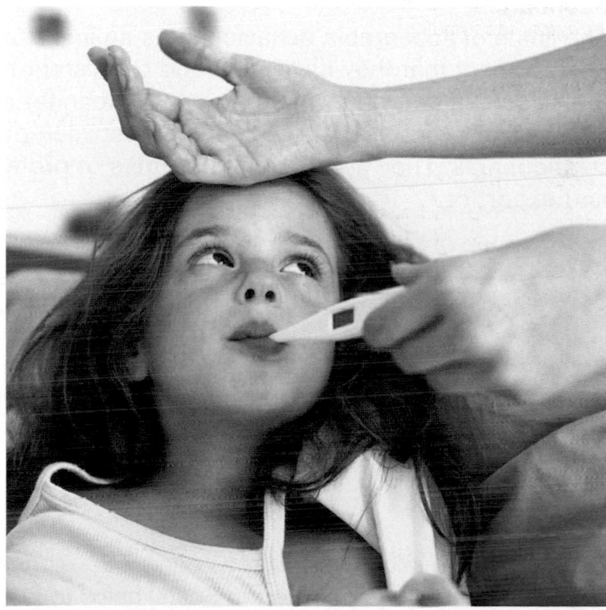

■ Checking body temperature.

A B C D E F G H I J K L M N O P Q R S T U V W XYZ

bonding
The **process** of a **newborn baby** developing a close bond with its **carer** (usually the **mother**). This is an essential part of **human development**, and **research** has shown that babies who are unable to bond with a carer will be less able to form **relationships** with others later in life. The bonding process comes about through **touch**, **eye contact** and making contact through sounds. *See* **attachment theory**.

bone
An extremely hard calcified **connective tissue** that forms the **skeleton**, supporting and protecting the human body. **Muscles**, **tendons** and **ligaments** are attached to bones enabling movement. Some of the bones in the body contain bone marrow which produces **red blood cells**.

bone marrow
A semi-liquid tissue found in some bone which manufactures red blood cells, some white blood cells and **platelets**.

borough
A town or district represented in Parliament by locally elected officials.

boundaries
The limits of acceptable behaviour. It is an important part of children's development that they have clear and consistent boundaries, so that they feel secure in knowing what they can and cannot do. **Professional boundaries** are the limits that define the difference between personal and **professional relationships**. They also identify the limits of professional **competence** and **expertise**.

bowel
A familiar term used to mean the intestines.

Bowlby, John
A psychologist who developed theories around the importance of bonding and attachment between mother and baby immediately in the period after birth. See **attachment theory**.

Braden scale
A tool used to **evaluate** the risk of a person developing **pressure ulcers/sores**. Using a scale like this (*see* **Norton Scale**) helps to identify whether an individual is at particular risk so that **preventive measures** can be put in place.

bradycardia
A heart rate that is slower than normal.

Braille
A reading and writing **system** used by people who are **blind** or **visually impaired**. The system is based on six raised dots that are used in different combinations to represent letters and numbers. The system was invented in France in the 1850s by Louis Braille, who was himself blind.

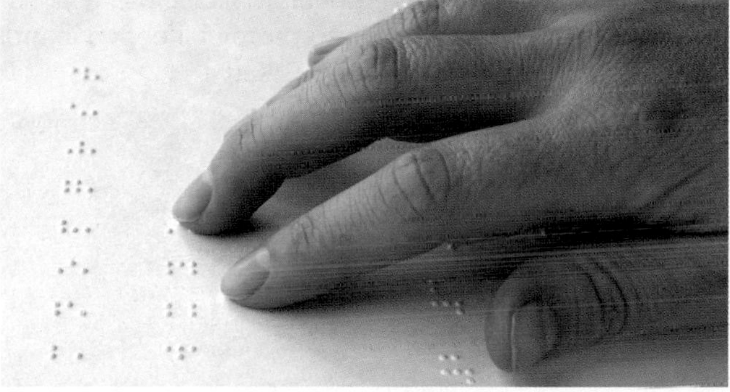

■ Braille.

brain
The most complex and highly developed part of the human body. The brain controls the functioning of the body. It is protected by the **skull** and surrounded by three membranes called the **meninges**. Specific areas of the brain control different functions such as speech, **motor control**, vision and other senses.

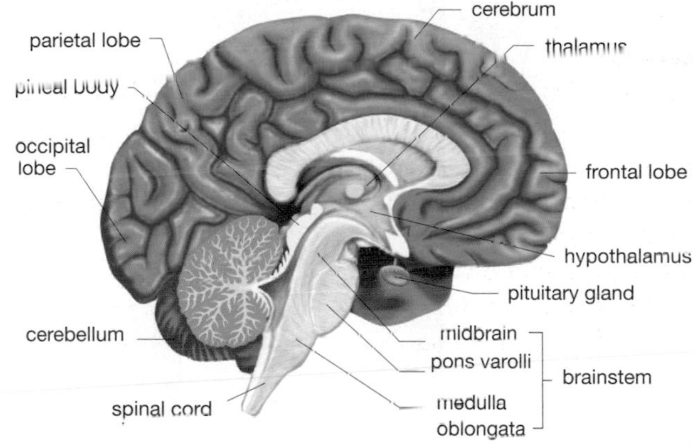

■ The brain

breathing
The alternate processes of taking air into the lungs (inhalation or inspiration) and out (exhalation or expiration).

British Medical Association (BMA)
A **professional** body for **doctors** that provides representation and **promotes** the interests of medicine and the medical profession. It is similar to a trades union and negotiates with the **government** about terms and conditions and **contracts** for doctors. The BMA is not the registration body or **regulator** of doctors; that is the role of the General Medical Council (GMC).
More information can be found at www.bma.org.uk

British Sign Language (BSL)
A fully recognised official language, and the language of **choice** for many people who are **deaf** or who have severe **hearing impairment**. The language has its own grammar and structure and is entirely visual, using signs made by the hands. A suitably **skilled** and qualified **interpreter** is needed in order to **communicate** with someone whose first language is BSL.

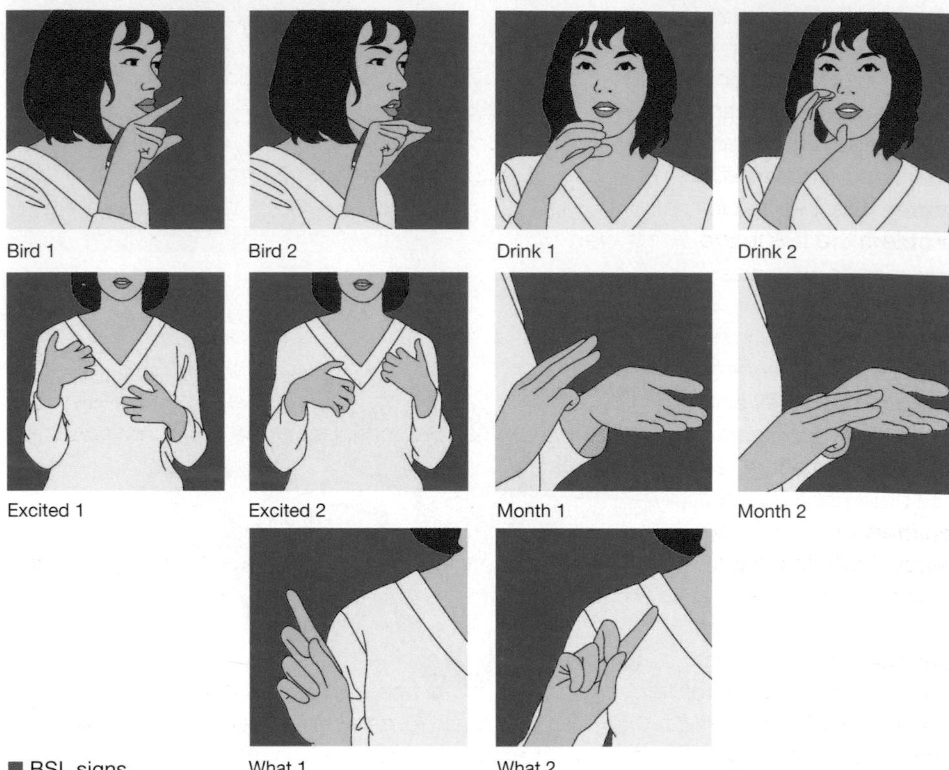

■ BSL signs.

bronchioles
Small tubes in the lungs that are formed by the branching of the bronchi. They terminate in the alveoli.

bronchitis
Inflammation of the bronchi (airways) within the **lungs**. This results in coughing and breathlessness.

bruise
Discolouration of the **skin** caused by an impact. The discolouration results from small **blood** vessels bleeding under the skin. Initially, a bruise is dark bluish black and gradually fades through green and yellow.

Bruner, Jerome
An American **psychologist** (born 1915) who developed theories about how children learn. His theories are based on **Piaget**'s work, but extended it to suggest that children learn by doing and by thinking, talking and writing about what they have been doing. He believes that **interactions** with adults are vital parts of a child **learning** to make sense of the world.

buddy
Someone who provides one-to-one **support** and friendship. Buddy schemes have been introduced in many situations where some individuals may need support, such as in **schools** where an older child can act as a 'buddy' to a younger child, or a **birthing** buddy to support a woman through **labour** (also known as a **doula**). Buddies can support people with **AIDS** or help people with **mental health problems** to live in the **community**.

budgeting
The **skills** of managing **personal finances** in order to pay bills, buy **food** and clothes and save money. Different approaches can be used to **support** people to budget effectively, but all involve planning through identifying **income** and essential items of **expenditure**. Also refers to the financial management of an organisation or department's income and expenditure.

bulimia
A psychological eating disorder characterised by uncontrollable overeating or binge eating, followed by forced **vomiting** or overuse of laxatives.

bulimia nervosa
An **eating disorder** usually characterised by low **self-esteem** and a **fear** of becoming fat. People with the disorder will eat large amounts of **food** and then make themselves **vomit** before the food can be **digested**.

bullying
The act of **intimidating**, threatening, humiliating or frightening others. Bullying can happen in any setting where people are together, such as **school**, **work** or communal living, and it is important to act against it when it is discovered. Most **workplaces** have anti-bullying policies covering staff behaviour and working **practices**, and will take action where necessary.

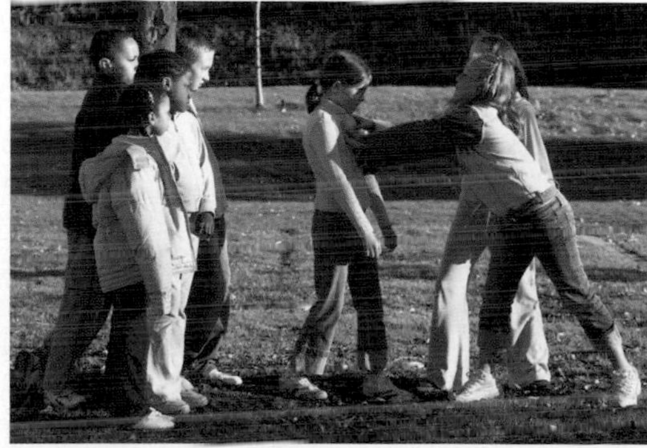
■ Bullying.

C

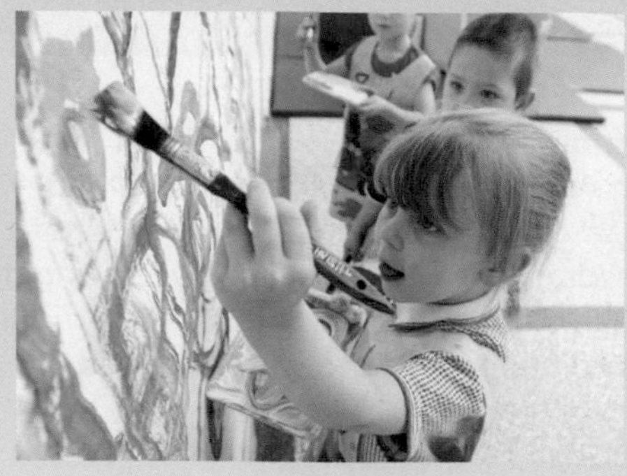

caesarean section

A surgical procedure for delivering a **baby**. Instead of being born through the **cervix** and **vagina**, the baby is removed from the **uterus** through an abdominal incision. Depending on the circumstances, the procedure can be carried out under a general **anaesthetic** where the **mother** is **unconscious**, or with an **epidural anaesthetic** where the mother is awake but feels no pain. The procedure may be necessary because of foetal distress or risk to the mother. Caesarean sections may be planned in advance in some cases because of previous history, known problems or more controversially maternal preference.

Cafcass

An organisation that provides advice to the Family Courts in England. Staffed by **social workers** called Family Courts Advisors, they champion the rights of **children** in **family court** proceedings such as **divorce** and custody or when a **local authority** applies for a child to be looked after.

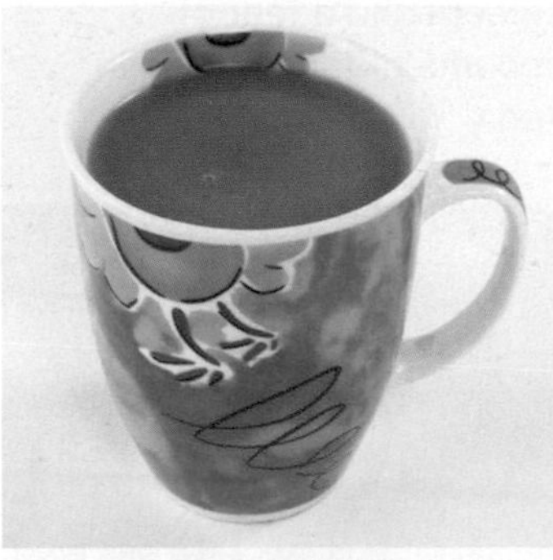

Caffeine.

caffeine

An alkaloid stimulant that can cause **irregular heart rhythm**, headache, agitation, **insomnia** and **muscle** tremors. It is commonly found in tea, coffee, cola and chocolate.

Caldicott principles

Rules that apply to the handling of **confidential** and sensitive **information**. The principles were drawn up by the 1997 committee chaired by Dame Fiona Caldicott that examined **patient**-identifiable information in the **NHS**. The principles have been adopted throughout **health** and **social care**. They are:

1. Justify the purpose.
2. Don't use patient-identifiable information unless it is absolutely necessary.
3. Use the minimum amount of identifiable information.

4. **Access** to identifiable information should be strictly on a 'need to know' basis.
5. Everyone should be aware of their **responsibilities**.
6. **Understand** and comply with the **law**.

calories
Unit of **energy**. One calorie contains the amount of energy required to raise the temperature of one gram of water by one degree **Celsius**. Often used as a description of energy values in food.

campaigns
An organised range of activities designed to achieve a particular aim.

cancer
A general description for over 100 different diseases. Cancer results from an abnormal division of **cells** that continues to grow into a **tumour** and invades neighbouring **tissues**. Cancer that develops attached to **organs** or in **soft tissue** is called a carcinoma, and one that develops in hard tissues such as **bones** is called a sarcoma. Cancers can also develop in **blood** cells and spread throughout the bloodstream. Cancers have different **treatments** and the chances of success vary depending on the type of cancer.

cannabis
An **illegal** recreational drug. It is currently classified as a 'Class C' drug which means that people possessing small amounts of the drug for personal use are unlikely to be **prosecuted**, although supplying or dealing is still a serious **offence** likely to result in a prison **sentence**. Cannabis has been found to be helpful in some medical conditions, such as **multiple sclerosis** and glaucoma.

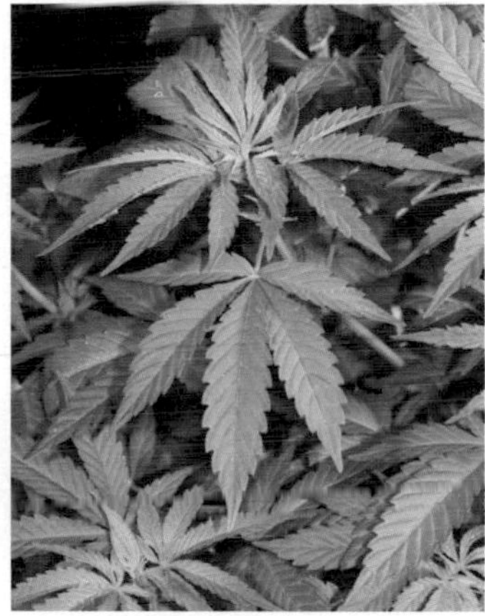
Cannabis plant.

cannula
A hollow tube inserted into the body for the purpose of introducing or removing a fluid.

capability
The ability to do something or to achieve something.

capacity
The necessary requirements to do, or achieve, something. This could include someone who may have the ability (they have worked with children, are suitably qualified and keen) to organise a play group in the church hall, but does not do so because they do not have the capacity (not enough spare time and no other volunteers willing to help).

capillaries
The smallest of the body's **blood** vessels that transport and remove substances and waste products between **veins**, **arteries** and **tissues** of the body. Capillary walls are composed of only a single layer of **cells**.

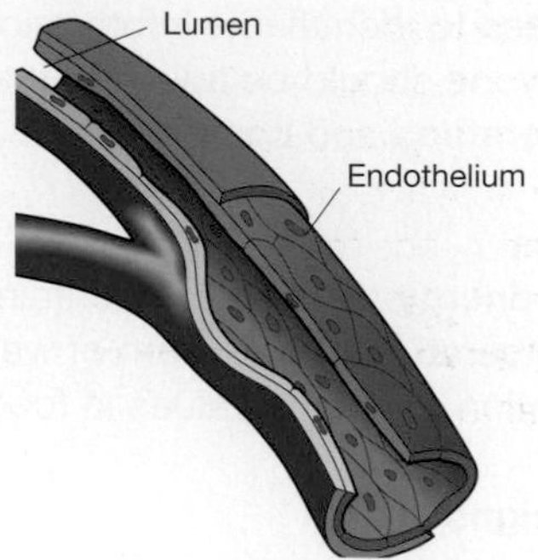

The structure of a capillary.

carbohydrates
Essential macro **nutrients** that provide and store **energy**. Complex carbohydrates should make up about a third of a healthy, balanced **diet** and can be found in starchy **foods** such as bread, potatoes, rice and pasta. Complex carbohydrates slowly release energy over a period of several hours. Simple carbohydrates are found in **sugar**; these are processed much faster by the body so only have a short-term effect on energy, and should be consumed only in small quantities.

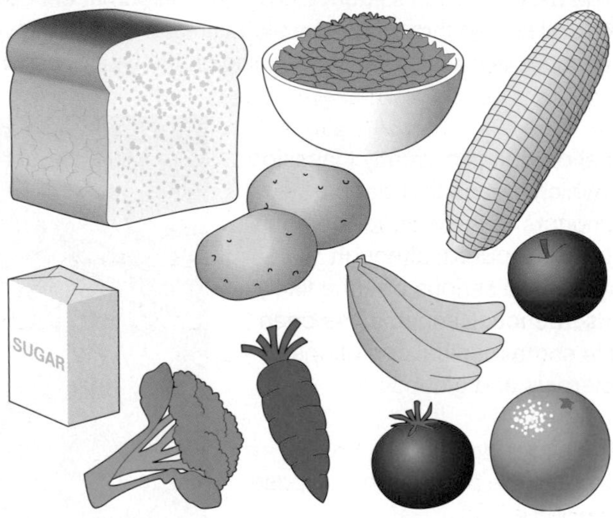

Foods containing carbohydrates.

carbon dioxide
A colourless, odourless waste gas from the **respiration process** of all humans, animals and plants. It is breathed out of the body. It is present in the earth's atmosphere and is a 'greenhouse gas' thought to have an impact on **global warming**.

carbon monoxide
A **toxic**, odourless, tasteless gas. Found in the exhaust fumes from vehicles, it forms during the burning of carbon and burns with a blue flame. Leaks of carbon monoxide from incorrectly functioning gas heaters can kill in a short time.

cardiac arrest
The sudden stopping of all **heart**-pumping activity, resulting in a loss of **circulation.** The heart needs to be restarted within a very short period of time, otherwise there is a risk of **brain** damage.

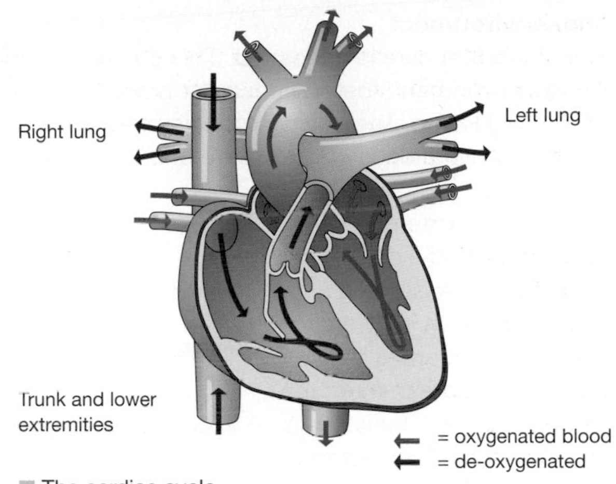

The cardiac cycle.

cardiac cycle
The way **blood** flows from the start of one heartbeat to the start of the next. There are three major stages to a 'beat' of the **heart**: atrial systole, ventricular systole and complete cardiac diastole. 'Systole' refers to contraction or shortening of heart muscle, and 'diastole' refers to relaxation of heart muscle. The chambers fill with blood during diastole.

- Atrial systole: the contraction of the heart **muscle** of the left and right **atria** completes the pushing of blood into the **ventricles**.
- Ventricular systole: the contraction of the muscle of the left and right ventricles pushes blood out of the heart and into the large blood vessels, the aorta and the **pulmonary artery**.
- Atrial diastole: the relaxing of the atrial muscle allows blood to flow into the atria from the **venae cavae** and **pulmonary veins**. This starts while the ventricles are in systole.
- Ventricular diastole: the relaxing of the ventricular muscle enables blood to flow into the ventricles from the atria to start the cycle again.

cardiologist
A **doctor** specialising in **diagnosing** and treating **heart disease**.

cardiorespiratory system
The **heart** and **lungs. Pulse**, **blood pressure** and **respiration** rate are all indicators of the **health** of a person's **cardiorespiratory system**.

cardiovascular system
The **heart** and all the **blood** vessels (**arteries**, **veins** and **capillaries**).

Care Council for Wales
Established under the Care Standards Act 2000 in order to promote high standards of conduct, practice and training among **social care** workers. The Council is also responsible for registering social workers and social care workers in Wales.

A B **C** D E F G H I J K L M N O P Q R S T U V W XYZ

care environment
Anywhere that care is **accessed**. This can be in an individual's home, a **supported living** environment, foster care, adult placement, daycare, **residential care, hospital** or **nursing home**. The **environment** is more than just physical surroundings; it also includes the attitudes of the **carers** and the quality of the care.

care management
The **process** of a care **professional** assessing the **needs** of an individual and **commissioning** a package of care to meet the identified needs. Individuals and their **families** used to be **consulted** as part of the **assessment** process and the needs of the individual were matched to the **services** available. This approach has now been replaced by **person-centred planning, direct payments** and **individual budgets**.

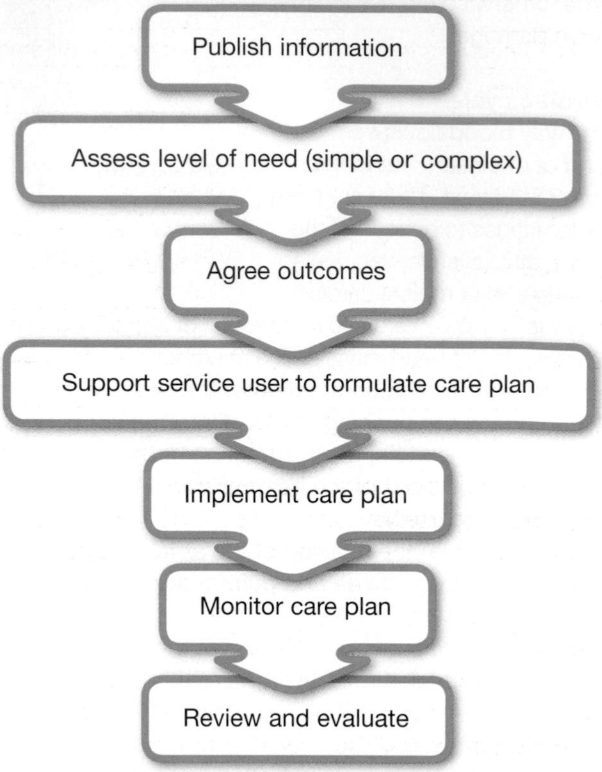

Publish information
↓
Assess level of need (simple or complex)
↓
Agree outcomes
↓
Support service user to formulate care plan
↓
Implement care plan
↓
Monitor care plan
↓
Review and evaluate

The seven steps of care management.

care order
An order made by a court (under Sec 31 of the Children Act 1989) when there is evidence that a child is suffering, or is at risk of, **significant harm**. It places a child in the care of the relevant **local authority** children's services, who then have the **responsibility** to 'look after' the child and to share **parental responsibility**.

care pathway
A way of describing the way services are brought together to meet a person's needs over a period of time.

care plan
A written **record** of the arrangements for a person's care or **treatment**. Care plans contain **information** about the **services** an individual has chosen and the

CARE PLAN REQUIREMENTS

Name Daniel Baker	Date of Birth 21.12.72
Relevant information RTA resulting in open complicated fractures to both legs	
Unit Woodrush Rehab Unit	Date of Plan 08.08.08

Planned Activity	Target Date	Nursing Requirement	Date Achieved
To minimise effects of immobility	08.08.08	1) Assess risk of pressure sores and address any issues arising from the assessment	08.08.08
To safely use crutches to mobilise with support	30.08.08	1) Arrange physiotherapist assessment and input 2) Encourage and support short walks to and from the bathroom	
To safely use crutches to mobilise without support	07.09.08	1) Reduce support whilst observing safety 2) Withdraw physical support giving only verbal support	
To ensure adequate nutrition	01.01.08		

ways in which they are to be delivered. Care plans are developed by the individual where they wish to do so, but may be recorded by a **health** or care **professional**. They can also be jointly developed by individuals, **carers** and professionals.

carer

A person who provides the physical or emotional **support** to enable another individual to participate in daily life. **Families** or friends are the biggest **group** providing care and are sometimes called 'informal carers' or 'family carers'. In the United States the term is 'caregivers', and this is growing in popularity. Carers have the right to have their **needs** identified and **assessed** along with the person they are caring for. Carers can claim some **benefits** depending on their circumstances. **Professional** carers are employed either by the individual or by an **organisation**, and should be trained and qualified to do their job. They should follow professional codes of conduct and **standards**.

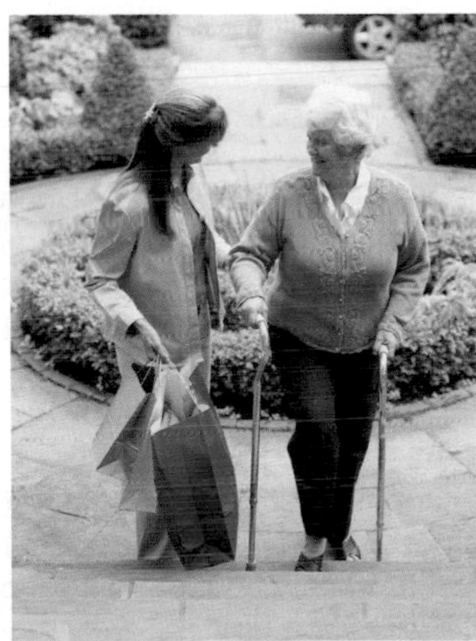

Carers can help individuals with everyday activities.

A B C D E F G H I J K L M N O P Q R S T U V W XYZ

Carers UK
A national charity that represents the interests of people who care for **family** or friends. The organisation lobbies on behalf of carers and provides advice and information. More information can be found at www.carersuk.org.uk

cartilage
Smooth glassy connective tissue which covers bone ends, forms the end of the nose, and intervertebral discs. It forms slightly moveable **joints** between **bones** and reduces friction at synovial joints.

case conference
A meeting of individuals, **carers** and **families** with a **multi-disciplinary team** of relevant **professionals**. It is usually called as the result of a crisis or because of serious issues. The term is most commonly used in **child protection**.

case history
Background **information** about an individual including detailed information about development, **family**, **education**, medical history and **relationships**. Taking a case history is a traditional way of finding out and **recording** information.

case law
The implementation of Acts of **Parliament** by the **courts**. Law that has been decided by precedent, on the basis of previous court decisions.

case study
An example of the particular circumstances of an individual, **family** or **community** that is used to illustrate a specific point or to contribute to **research**. Also known as a scenario.

catheter
A clean, flexible, hollow tube. Urinary catheterisation is a **process** where the tube is inserted into the **bladder**, usually through the **urethra**, in order to release **urine** from the bladder. This may need to be done if the urethra is blocked, or if an individual is very ill or **unconscious**, or if a person is unable to control the emptying of the bladder.

caution
A method of dealing with an arrested person that does not involve **prosecution** for an **offence**. If the offence is minor or it is a first offence, the **police** may decide to issue a caution. A caution is **recorded** against the name of the individual concerned.

cell
The basic unit of all living things. There are millions of cells in the human body in many different shapes and sizes. All have the same basic structure at some stage:

- an outer membrane
- cytoplasm, the fluid that fills the cell and supports cell repair and growth
- **nucleus**, containing the **DNA** and surrounded by a nuclear membrane.

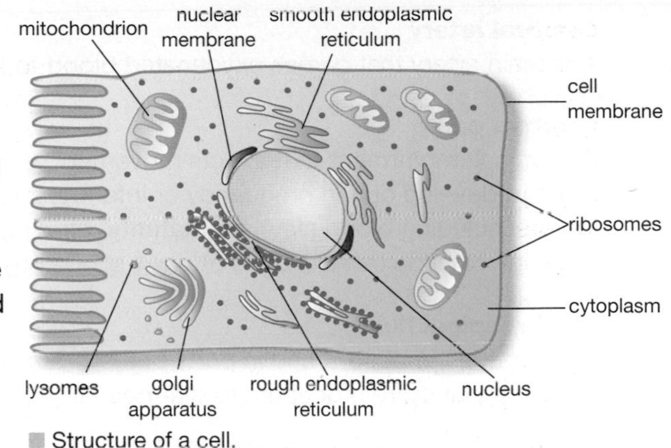

Structure of a cell.

Celsius
The **temperature** scale used in the UK and Europe. On this scale, water freezes at 0 degrees (0°C) and boils at 100 degrees (100°C). Normal human **body temperature** is 37 degrees (37°C). An alternative measurement is Fahrenheit.

census
A **government survey** of the **population** undertaken every ten years. The first census was in 1801. All households have to respond to the **questionnaire** and the results are collated and **analysed** to provide **statistics** about the population of the UK, including **lifestyle** and social developments.

centile charts
Charts that measure the growth and development of **babies** and children and **record** progress against the expected height and weight to ensure that the child is developing healthily.

central nervous system
The control centre for the body, based in the **brain** and the **spinal cord**. It controls all the actions, both voluntary and involuntary, of the body. The brain controls all the functions of the body including movement, speech, creativity and **understanding**. The spinal cord conducts most of the 'messages' from the brain to all parts of the body.

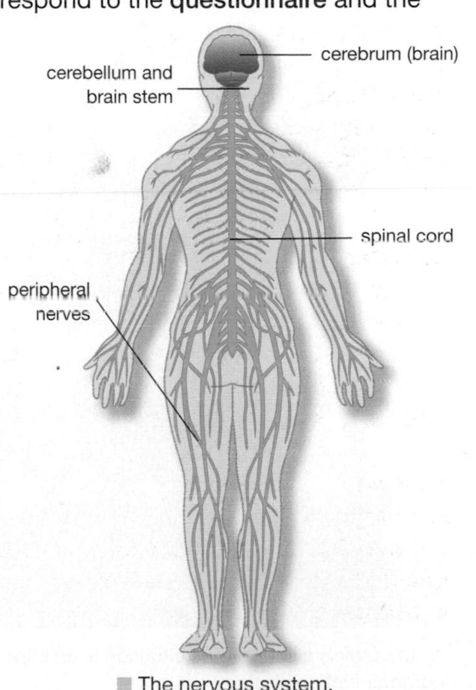

The nervous system.

cerebral artery
The main artery that carries oxygenated blood to the brain.

cerebral palsy
A physical **impairment** that affects movement, caused by a failure of part of the **brain** to develop during **pregnancy** or **infancy**. It can be caused by a range of factors including **blood** clots, **prematurity**, birth **injury** or illness shortly after birth. More information can be found at www.scope.org.uk

cerebrospinal fluid
Fluid in the **spinal cord** and in parts of the **brain**. The fluid can be collected through a **lumbar puncture** procedure to **diagnose infections** of the brain.

cerebrovascular accident (CVA)
A **stroke**, caused by a major loss of **blood** supply to the **brain**. This can occur as the result of a blood clot or burst blood vessel. A stroke results in permanent brain damage of varying degrees, including loss of speech, weakness or **paralysis** in one side of the body, difficulties in **communication** and **understanding**. The extent of recovery is often linked to the speed of **access** to **treatment** when the stroke occurs.

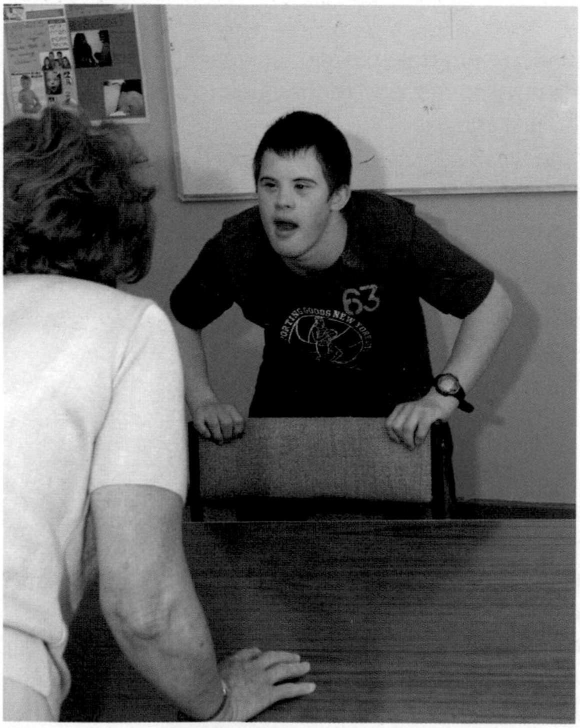

Managing a challenging situation is an important communication strategy.

cervical smear
A screening test for the presence of abnormal **cells** at the neck of the uterus (known as the **cervix**) that could develop into cervical **cancer**. There is a national **screening programme** where women between 20 and 65 are offered the test every five years.

cervix
The neck of the **uterus** which protrudes into the vagina. The cervix, normally closed tightly, opens for the **birth process**.

challenging behaviour
Behaviour that may be unacceptable or difficult to deal with. People who

present challenging behaviour often do so as a means of communicating anger or frustration. An example may be a person ripping their own clothing regularly. It can also be **violent**, **aggressive** or abusive and can pose risks to individuals and test the **skills** of **health**, care and **education professionals**. The reasons for challenging behaviour include **mental health problems**, **learning disabilities**, **personality disorders**, anger, frustration and emotional issues.

change
The **process** of moving to something different. Changes can be split into those that are predictable, such as starting **school**, going through **puberty**, getting a job, or getting married, and those that are unpredictable such as illness or **accident**, being made **redundant**, or being **bereaved** unexpectedly.

charity
An **organisation** that exists in order to benefit a specific cause. Charities are governed by strict **laws** and are overseen by the Charity Commission. Charities can provide **benefits** in **cash** or in kind to their chosen causes, but by law all money raised, after the costs of running the organisation, must be used for the benefit of those for whom the charity was established. Charities raise money through fundraising, donations and bequests. They tender for **contracts** to deliver **services** and grants.
More information can be found at www.charity-commission.gov.uk

chemotherapy
Treatment for various forms of **cancer**. It involves administering highly **toxic** chemicals in order to attack cancerous **cells** and stop them reproducing. In the **process** it also attacks healthy cells and can cause very unpleasant side effects.

chest
The part of the body just above the **abdomen** and protected by the **ribs**. It contains the **heart** and **lungs**. Also known as the thorax.

child abuse
See **abuse**.

Child Benefit
A non means tested state benefit provided to the main carer of each child in the UK. All families are entitled to receive this benefit and is paid from **birth** to the 18th birthday of young people who are no longer in full-time **education**, and the 19th birthday of those still in education.

childcare register
The record, held by Ofsted, of all childcare providers in England.
More information can be found at www.ofsted.gov.uk

child development
The increasing skills and capacities/abilities of **babies** and children. There are six main areas of **learning** and development:
- personal, social and **emotional development**
- **physical development**
- **communication**, language and **literacy**
- **problem solving, reasoning** and **numeracy**
- **knowledge and understanding of the world**
- **creative development**.

Children's development in all these areas should be **monitored** and **recorded** so that any areas where development is not as expected can be identified and **supported**.

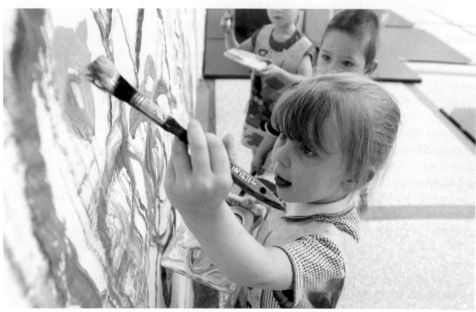

Child development.

Child Health Promotion programme
A national programme available to all children through **GPs**, health visitors and **clinics** that aims to reduce the number of children with illnesses and to ensure that any children who are not progressing as expected are identified and provided with **support**. The core Child Health Promotion programme includes:
- childhood screening including **assessment** checks, hearing tests, 'heel prick' test
- **immunisations** against diseases including diphtheria, whooping cough, **meningitis**, polio, **mumps**, **measles** and **rubella** (**MMR**)
- a **holistic** and systematic **process** to assess the individual child's and family's **needs**
- **early interventions** to address those needs
- delivering universal health-promoting activities.

childhood
Generally accepted as the time between the end of babyhood and the start of adolescence.

childminders
Self-employed childcare businesses where people provide childcare in their own home. Childminders are registered with either the **local authority** or the inspectorate (**Ofsted**) depending on the UK country in which they live.

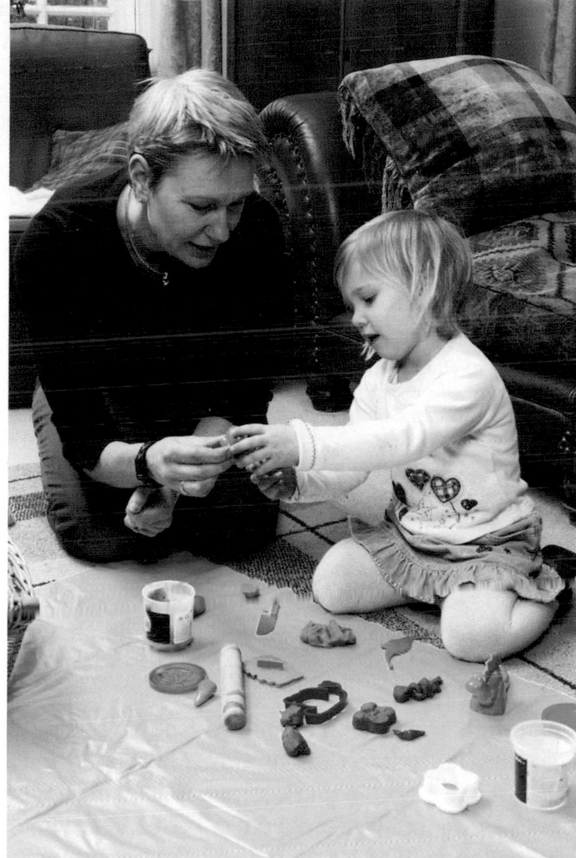

Childminding.

child protection
A key part of **safeguarding** children. Child protection procedures are used when there is evidence or suspicion that a child has suffered, or is at risk of, **significant harm**. **Agencies** such as children's **services**, **police** and **health** services work together with **families** and take joint decisions where possible to ensure that children are protected and made safe. Children can be protected by reaching agreements with families or by using **legislation** and the **courts** in order to keep a child from **harm**.

children and young people
Children and young people from birth to 18 years of age.

children's centres
Integrated centres where services for children and their families are available. The centres are a further development of Sure Start programmes in England.

children's commissioners
People appointed to the role of **promoting** and championing the rights and interests of children and **young people**. Commissioners in Scotland, Wales and

Northern Ireland are responsible for **safeguarding** and defending **children's rights**, whereas in England the commissioner has to raise awareness of children's rights.

Commissioner independence	Wales	Northern Ireland	Scotland	England
Secretary of State can direct Commissioner to carry out an **inquiry**	No	No	No	Yes
Commissioner must **consult** Secretary of State before holding an independent inquiry	No	No	No	Yes
Commissioner's annual **report** goes directly to **Parliament**/Assembly	Yes	Yes	Yes	No
Legislation ties Commissioner to **government** policy	No	No	No	Yes

Children's Plan
A government ten-year plan for children's services in England. The document sets out how the government will achieve its **Every Child Matters** outcomes for children, such as being happy and healthy, staying safe, enjoying and achieving, making a positive contribution and achieving economic well-being.

children's rights
The **human rights** that are recognised as belonging to all children and **young people**. The **United Nations Convention on the Rights of the Child**, agreed in 1989, is a legally binding international instrument covering the full range of human rights – civil, **cultural**, economic, political and social rights. Out the 194 countries of the world, 192 agreed to be legally bound by the Convention. The two which are not are Somalia and the United States.

children's services
A general term used to describe the services that affect children and are provided by a local authority, along with other statutory bodies such as health services and police services. These services include education, children's social care, early years services, youth service, Connexions services and playwork services.

Child Support Agency (CSA)
Responsible for assessing and obtaining financial contributions from absent **parents**. Set up in 1993, the **agency** has been widely criticised for not being effective in collecting and processing payments to **lone parents**. There are plans to replace it with the Child Maintenance and Enforcement Commission with the changeover to take place in stages between 2008–2014.
More information can be found at www.csa.gov.uk

chiropody/podiatry
The care and **treatment** of feet. **Services** are provide through the **NHS** and the **private sector** by qualified **professionals**.

chiropractic
A treatment method involving manipulation of the spine, **pelvis** and other parts of the **skeleton** to relieve painful musculo-skeletal conditions. Similar to **osteopathy**, this **alternative** to traditional medicine is now so commonly used that it is almost mainstream. Chiropractors and osteopaths train for five years before **qualification**.

choice
Selection from among alternatives. One of the key requirements of planning any **provision** of care **services** is that individuals must be able to choose the services they want and the way they want them delivered. **Direct payments** and **individual budgets** have provided real choice for individuals.

cholesterol
A fatty substance present in the human body. Cholesterol is necessary for the body to function, but levels that are too high can cause medical problems such as narrowing of **arteries**, leading to **strokes** and **heart attacks**. Cholesterol is found in **foods** high in fat. **Medication** can be effective in lowering cholesterol levels, as can a **change** of **diet**. High blood cholesterol runs in families.

Chomsky, Noam
An American **psychologist** (born 1928) who believes that children are born with an **understanding** of language structure and grammar. He argues that children will apply logical rules to language; for example, they may assume that the plural of *mouse* is *mouses*. Chomsky maintains that if children only learned from hearing others, they would never say *mouses* because they would never hear the word.

chromosomes
Structures found in the **nucleus** of a **cell**. They contain **DNA**, very tightly packed. There are 23 pairs of chromosomes in every human cell.

chronic condition
An illness or **disease** that is long term and for which there is **treatment**, but no cure. Examples are **asthma**, **diabetes** and **emphysema**.

circulation of blood
The **process** of the **heart** pumping **blood** around the body through the **veins** and **arteries**.

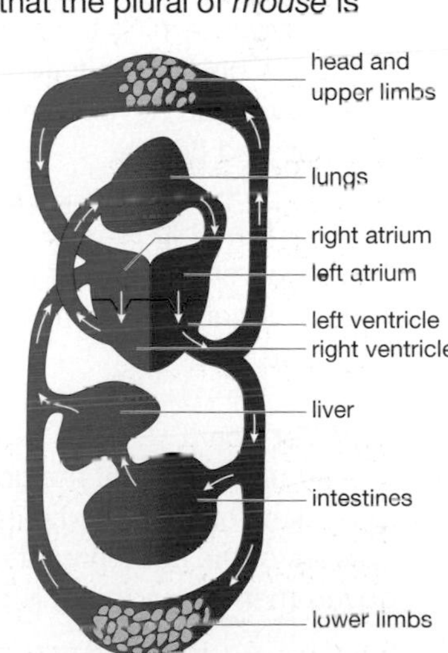

The circulatory system.

circumcision
Removal of the foreskin of the male **penis**. This can be done for cultural or **religious** reasons, medical problems, or for **personal hygiene** preferences. Female circumcision, on the other hand, has been an **offence** in the UK since 1985, but is still carried out in many **cultures**; it involves the removal of the clitoris and the labia around the entrance to the **vagina**.

circumstances
Social, economic, educational and the physical factors which influence individuals, families or carers and their abilities to cope.

Citizens Advice Bureau (CAB)
A national **charity** with over 1,000 local offices across the UK. The bureaux provide advice and **information** about finance, **housing**, **benefits**, managing debt and **access** to legal advice.
More information can be found at www.citizensadvice.org.uk

citizenship
The active participation in, and acceptance of the responsibiliy for, the local or national community. Also refers to the controversial Government policy where other nationalities can apply to gain British Citizenship through tests.

civil law
The set of **laws** governing how individuals and **organisations** must behave and perform. Civil law is not enforced by the **police**, but through the **courts** or sometimes by **regulatory organisations,** for example **environmental health** issues or those concerning the protection of children would be taken to court by the **local authority**; health and **safety** breaches would be pursued by the **Health and Safety Executive.** The Revenue and Customs can act without a court to enforce payment of taxes and duties.

civil partnership
The legal recognition of a partnership between two people of the same **gender.** It is the legal equivalent of a marriage and provides the same legal status for both partners.

Civil Service
The administration of the **government**. In the UK, the Civil Service is permanent regardless of the government in power. It is in charge of making sure that the policies of the government of the day are carried out. Anyone who works in a government department is part of the Civil Service.

civil society

A broad general term covering the process of various groups, organisations and institutions coming together to follow common interests and goals. Civil society often includes organisations such as registered charities, development non-governmental organisations, community groups, women's organisations, faith-based organisations, professional associations, trades unions, self-help groups, social movements, business associations, coalitions and advocacy groups.

classical conditioning

A **learning theory** developed by **Pavlov**, concerned with associations between events such as if a child is scratched by a cat while stroking it, there will be a 'startle response' and the child will back away. This could set up an association in the child's mind between stroking a cat and being scratched, so the child is afraid of all cats even if they don't scratch.

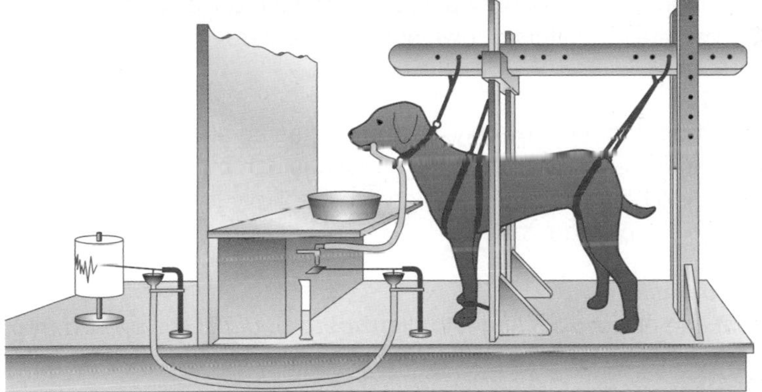

Pavlov's dogs.

clinic

A local **access** point for a range of **primary health care services**, including **GPs**, health visitors, **community nurses**, **immunisation**, **midwifery** services, developmental checks and many **health**-related **groups** and activities. The term can also describe specialist health care in a **hospital** where **patients** attend to access particular types of **treatment**.

clinical audit

The **process** of **reviewing** clinical **performance** in **health care** against agreed **standards**, an important part of **clinical governance**. The process has five stages and is a cycle:

- set standards to form the criteria to measure against
- measure performance against criteria/standards
- identify the extent to which performance meets criteria/standards
- make any necessary **changes** to improve performance
- re-audit to check whether changes have been effective.

clinical governance
A **system** for **monitoring** and improving **standards** of **health care** throughout the **NHS**. It includes **clinical audits**, benchmarking, critical incident **reviews**, **risk management** and **professional development**.

clinical practice
The work of **health professionals** when working in a health setting such as a **hospital**.

clinical trials
See **randomised clinical controlled trial**

closed-circuit television (CCTV)
A surveillance **system** where cameras can film activity in a specific area or building. Whole areas can be **monitored** by watching the recording. It is widely used in **schools** and **hospitals** for **security** purposes, and almost all parts of the UK have many CCTV cameras monitoring town and city centres.

closed question
A **communication** that requires only 'yes' or 'no' as an answer. Also for answering your name, address etc. These types of questions can be useful for finding out **information** quickly and clearly, but otherwise are likely to reduce communication and discourage people from talking.

Clostridium difficile
Bacteria that can cause **vomiting** and **diarrhoea**. *C. difficile* is spread through contact and cannot be removed with **alcohol hand rub**. **Hand washing** is essential to reduce the spread of infection.

cocaine
An addictive illegal drug that provides a stimulating effect. It is derived from the coca plant.

code of conduct
Professional code of behaviour and practice drawn up by a professional body in order to set standards e.g. **General Medical Council**, the **Nursing and Midwifery Council**.

code of practice
A set of **guidelines** for **professional** behaviour that set out clearly the expectations of those who are working in a professional area. Most **health** and **social care** professionals are governed by the codes of practice of the four **regulatory** bodies across the UK: the **General Social Care Council** (England), the **Care Council for Wales**, the **Scottish Social Services Council** and the **Northern Ireland Social Care Council**. Health professionals such as **midwives**, **nurses**, **physiotherapists** and **doctors** have their own codes of conduct.

cognitive behavioural therapy (CBT)
Cognitive behavioural therapy is a way of looking at what people think, how they feel and what they do. It attempts to help people to think about things in a different, more positive way helping to change the way they behave.

cognitive development
See **problem solving** *and* **reasoning**.

co-habitation
Co-habitation is where two people are living together as partners, but without a legal basis for their relationship such as marriage or a civil partnership.

collaboration
Working together with **colleagues**, sharing information and exchanging ideas.

collate
Collect and combine.

colleagues
Other professionals from the same team or **organisation**, or different teams or organisations.

colon
The large **intestine** part of the alimentary canal responsible for forming, storing and expelling waste matter.

colostomy
A surgically created abdominal opening to allow the body to expel **faeces**. This is necessary when the **bowel** is unable to function in the normal way due to disease or surgery. Some colostomies can be reversed and others are permanent.

Commission for Social Care Inspection (CSCI)
A statutory body set up in 2004 to register and inspect all **social care** organisations. A Care Quality Comission will combine the responsibilities of this organisation with those of the Healthcare Commission and the Mental Health Act (2008).

commissioning
The **process** of planning, designing, **contracting** and purchasing **services**. This can be on a large scale, with some **health** projects costing many millions of pounds, or can be an individual deciding which enabling services to commission.

committee
A number of people who work together, like a team, to take responsibility, or make decisions, for a specific purpose. This could be to run a project, to organise a protest

A B C D E F G H I J K L M N O P Q R S T U V W X Y Z

A B C D E F G H I J K L M N O P Q R S T U V W XYZ

or to raise funds. Some committees are formed to investigate issues or problems such as the Police Complaints Committee while others may have a role to check on the work of others such as the Public Accounts Committee in the House of Commons.

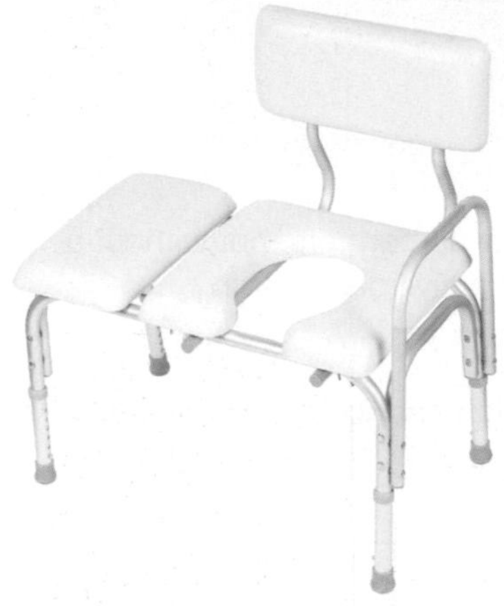

A commode.

commode
A portable chair designed to contain a bedpan. It can be used when people are unable to get to the **toilet** because of illness, confusion or lack of **mobility**.

Common Assessment Framework (CAF)
A process of gathering and evaluating information about a child, or young person, in order to work with them to find out about their needs. The basis for the process is that information is only gathered once and that all professionals involved in working with the child and their family will use the same assessment information. The CAF is only used in England.

communicable disease
A **disease** that can be passed from one person to another through **touch** (in the case of a contagious disease), droplets in air, **food**, water or from contaminated objects (an infectious disease).

communication
The exchange of **information** between people. This can be face to face, by telephone, written or electronic. Information can also be provided through large-scale mass **media**; this is usually a one-way communication such as through television, the **Internet** or the printed word and there is very limited exchange. In face-to-face communication, the spoken word accounts for only about 7 per cent of what is communicated. Most **understanding** of communication comes from non-verbal signals through **body language**. Different types of communication are appropriate for different circumstances and **cultures**. **Barriers** to communication can be differences in spoken or signed language, differences in hearing ability, differences in visual ability or differences in understanding.

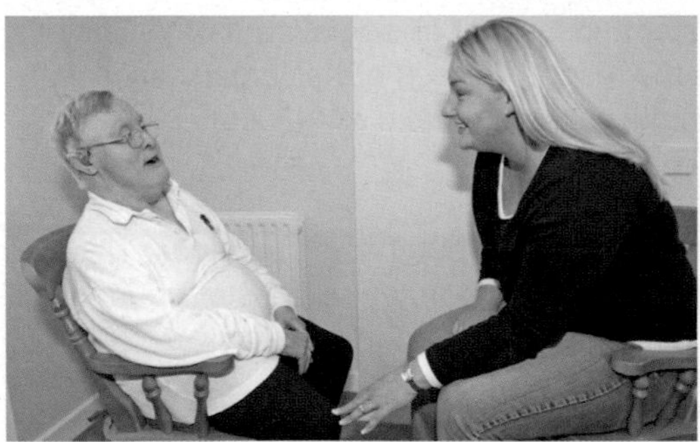

Communication is a key skill in health and social care.

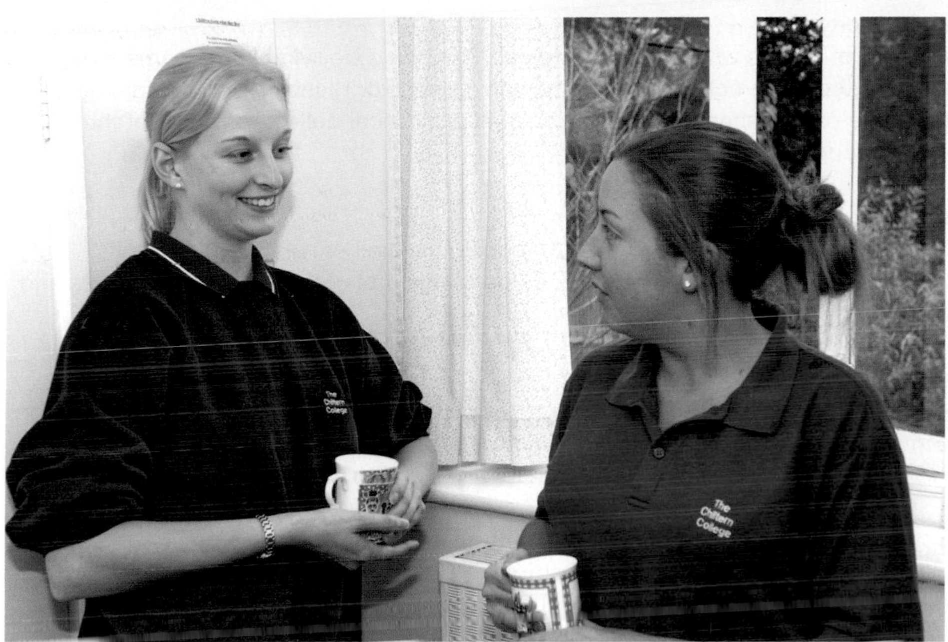

Watching people's body language can help you work out what they are communicating

communication channels
The different routes people may use to communicate.

communication cues
Actions and **behaviour** (verbal or non-verbal) which indicate the communicator's thoughts and **feelings** and help the person receiving the **communication** to understand the message. In terms of technological aids it might be cues that the individual wants to speak, etc.

communication support worker
A trained worker who supports a deaf person in education to access information. They are sometimes called a personal communications assistant. They work according to the needs of the individual but will help with communication between the deaf person, hearing people, the tutor and other students.

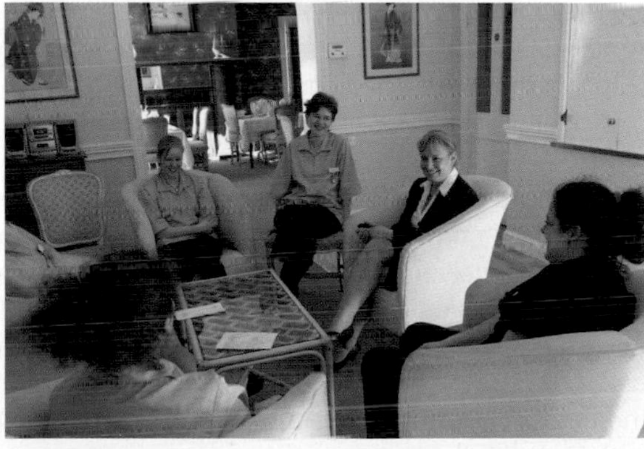

Communication is a way of sharing information.

community
A **group** of people with a shared interest. This could be living in the same area, being at the same **school**, having the same illness or **disability**, campaigning for the same cause, sharing **religious**, cultural or political **beliefs**, or being of the same **racial group**.

community safety
The identification and steps taken to reduce the level of risk in a community. Communities work together to look at the things that make people feel unsafe and look at ways to improve them.

community service order
An order that can be used by the **courts** as an alternative to a fine or custodial (prison) **sentence**. It requires someone to undertake **supervised** activities that will benefit the local **community**. Orders can be made for any length of time from 40 up to 240 hours.

community support officers
Community support officers are employed by police forces to work alongside the police in a supporting role and to provide a visible police presence. They deal with minor disturbances, but do not have full **police** powers.

community work
Working with local **communities** to develop and improve the **quality of life** in a local area. This can be through a range of activities such as **environmental** improvements, **housing** developments, **self-help** and **support groups**, **education** projects, childcare and **play** projects, or community **health facilities**. Community workers will normally have completed a community work **qualification**, either a degree or **S/NVQ**, and can be employed by a **local authority**, **government** project or voluntary **organisation**.

competence
Ability, demonstrated by providing evidence of **performance** and knowledge against a set of **standards**. The achievement of an **S/NVQ** is evidence of competence in a particular field.

complaints procedure
The method people can use to complain if they are not satisfied with the service they have received. All **organisations** providing **health** and **social care services** must have a readily accessible complaints procedure. The procedure must be well advertised, and people using the services must be told about it and enabled to use it. All complaints procedures should state who will deal with any complaint, the timescales for dealing with it, and what complainants can do if they are not satisfied with the response.

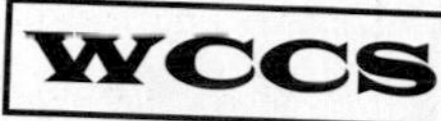

WARMSHIRE COUNTY CARE SERVICES

Complaints Policy

This leaflet outlines the ways you can make a complaint if you are dissatisfied with our services. If you feel that you have a complaint to make about our service or the way you have been treated then follow the simple guidelines shown below.

It Is often simpler to refer your complaint to the member of staff with whom you have been dealing. They may be able to sort the issue out immediately for you.

If you prefer not to speak to the member of staff then please ask to see their supervisor or line manager.

Failing either of these two options you can:

- use the attached form to make a complaint
- write a letter and send it to us
- ask someone else to write the letter on your behalf and send it to us.

Our staff are here to help you and you will not be discriminated against because you have made a complaint.

....

Please return this form to:
Warmshire County Care Services, Heaton Place, Warmshire.

Please state your complaint below and continue on a separate sheet if necessary.

Your complaint will be acknowledged within one week and will be dealt with within 28 days.

Your details:
Name: ....

Address: ....

....

....

Telephone number: ....

An example of a complaints policy.

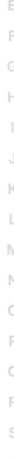

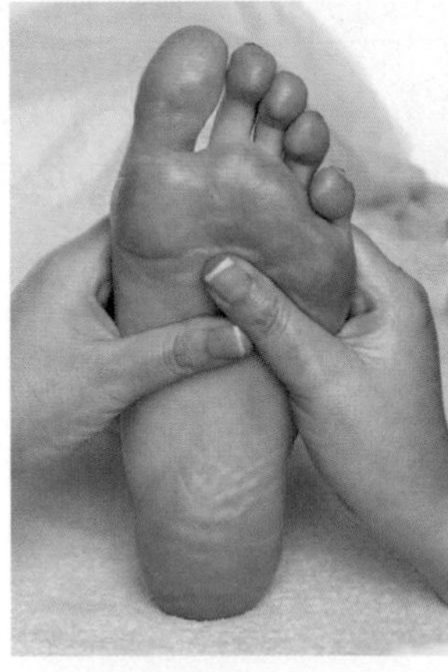

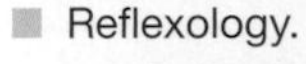

Reflexology.

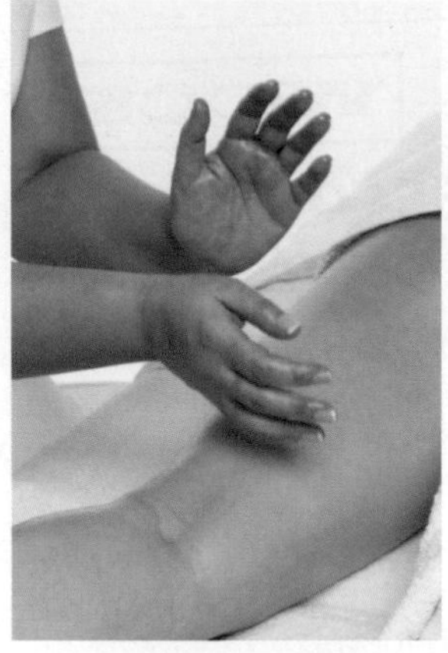

Massage movements.

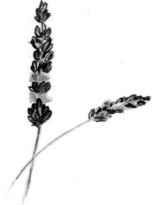

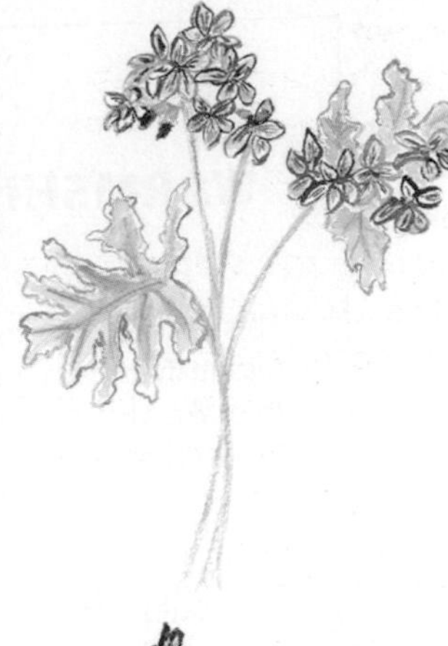

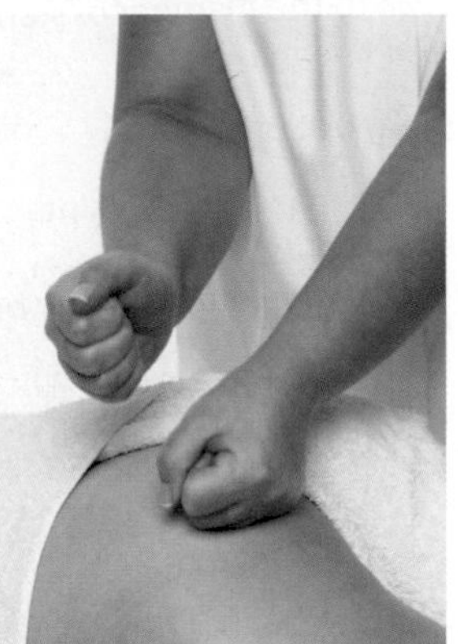

Complementary therapies.

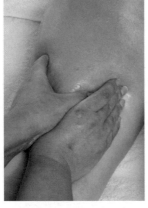

Lavender and geraniums supply the base for aromatherapy oils.

complementary therapies
Treatments that complement and **support** the effects of traditional, mainstream medicine. This can include therapies such as **acupuncture**, **aromatherapy**, **osteopathy**, **chiropractic**, **homeopathy** and **reflexology**.

computed axial tomography (CAT) scan
A scan creating cross-sectional **X-rays** showing the density of body **tissues**. This can help to **diagnose** the presence of **tumours**, growths or other abnormalities.

conception
The **process** of **fertilisation** of a human egg and the **implantation** of the resulting **embryo** in the wall of the **uterus**.

concepts

Ideas that underpin new developments and plans.

condom

A **contraceptive** device made of fine latex rubber that fits over the male **penis** during **sexual intercourse** in order to prevent **semen** from entering the female **vagina**. Condoms are also effective at reducing the transmission of **sexually transmitted diseases**.

confidence

The extent to which individuals feel positive about themselves and have belief in their own abilities.

confidentiality

Keeping **information** private; not sharing information about individuals without their knowledge and agreement, and ensuring that written and electronic information cannot be **accessed** or read by people who have no genuine need for it.

conform

To behave in line with the norms and expectations of society or those of an organisation.

confusion

A state of a person not being aware of all aspects of the world around them and often being anxious, distressed or frustrated because they do not understand.

Weeks 1 and 2

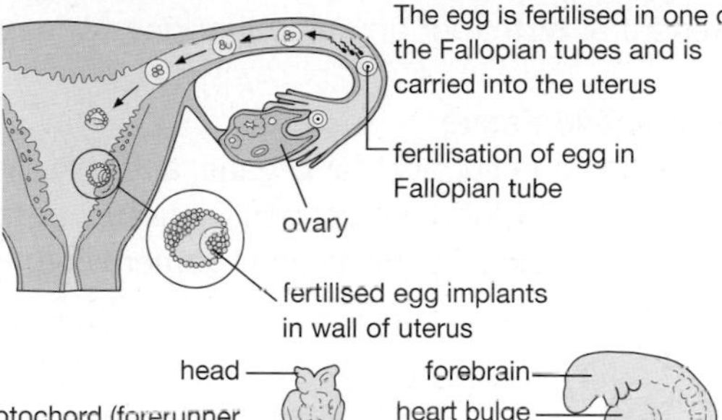

Passage to the uterus
The egg is fertilised in one of the Fallopian tubes and is carried into the uterus

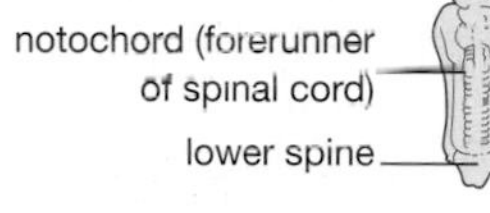

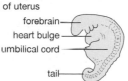

Three weeks
The embryo becomes pear-shaped, with a rounded head, pointed lower spine, and notochord running along its back.

Four weeks
The embryo becomes C-shaped and a tail is visible. The umbilical cord forms and the forebrain enlarges.

Internal organs at five weeks
All the internal organs have begun to form by the fifth week. During this critical stage of development, the embryo is vulnerable to harmful substances consumed by the mother (such as alcohol and drugs), which may cause defects.

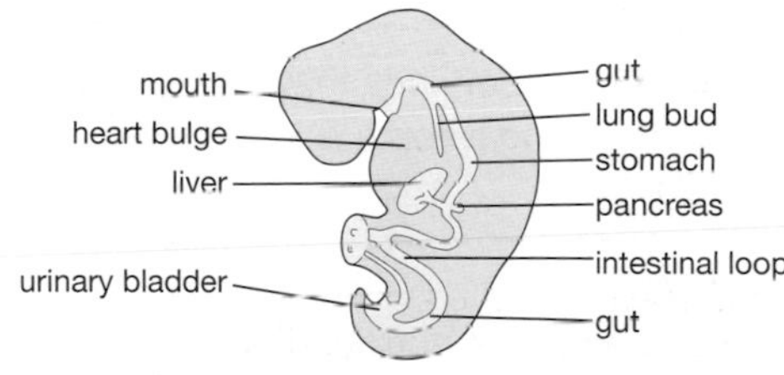

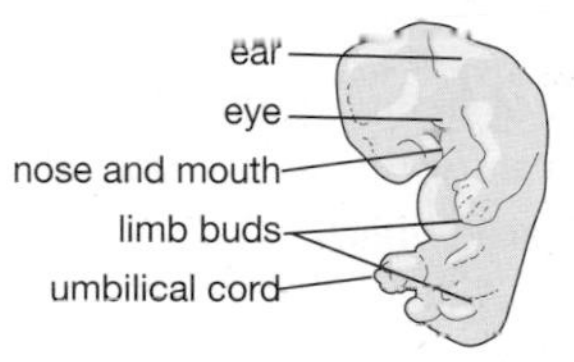

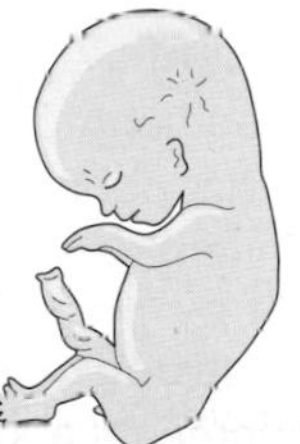

Six weeks
Eyes are visible and the mouth, nose and ears are forming.The limbs grow rapidly from tiny buds.

Eight weeks
The face is more 'human', the head is more upright, and the tail has gone. Limbs become jointed. Fingers and toes appear.

■ Conception and embryo development.

congenital
Present at **birth**; not anything that develops or occurs after birth.

connective tissue
Protection and **support** for **organs**, and links between **tissues** and organs. **Bone, cartilage** and **blood** are connective tissue, as is the **adipose tissue** that lies just beneath the **skin. Tendons** and **ligaments** are types of fibrous connective tissue.

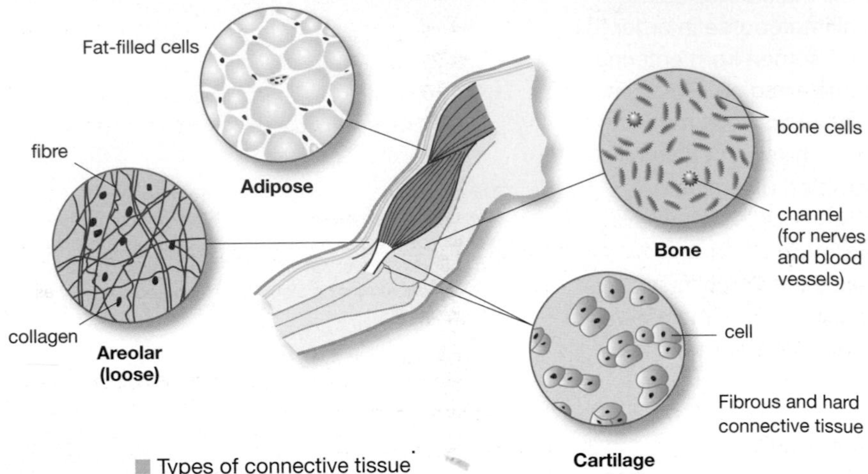

Types of connective tissue

Connexions
Part of children's services that provides advice, practical or emotional support and guidance to young people about careers, employment, training, housing, money or lifestyles.

conscious
Awake and aware of surroundings.

consent
Agreement to a course of action, plan or **treatment. Information** must be provided so that people are able to **understand** what they are agreeing to before their consent can be considered valid.

constructive feedback
Comments about performance that contain information on areas for improvement with helpful suggestions about how to make the improvements.

consultation
The **process** of asking for the views, **feelings** and opinions of those people likely to be affected by any decision, and taking their responses into account when deciding on any actions to be taken.

contact order
An order that can be made under the Children Act 1989 specifying the people with whom a child may or may not have contact, the way the contact should take place (for example, with **supervision**, overnight stays, or visits only), and how frequently contacts should take place.

contagious
Medically it means a **disease** spread by bodily contact rather than by other means of passing on **bacteria**. In everyday terms it is used in the same ways as **infectious**.

contaminated
Any item not considered sterile and potentially tainted by other substances, particularly micro-organisms.

continuing professional development (CPD)
Ongoing development of skills and knowledge of an organisation's staff in order to continue learning and to ensure that practice skills and knowledge are up to date.

contraceptive
A method used to prevent **conception**. These can be barrier methods such as condoms or caps that prevent **sperm** reaching the egg; intra-uterine methods such as the coil that prevents conception by preventing the fertilised egg from **implanting** on the uterine wall; or the contraceptive pill, which prevents **ovulation** and the preparation of the **womb** lining. **Barrier methods** can be purchased in chemists and supermarkets, or, like contraceptive pills and intra-uterine devices, can be obtained through Family Planning Clinics and GPs. Some people choose not to use contraception, but prefer **natural birth control methods** such as: only having sexual intercourse at the times in the menstrual cycle when there is less risk of pregnancy, or by a male withdrawing his penis from the female vagina before ejaculation, thus not placing any sperm into the female. These methods have limited success when used alone.

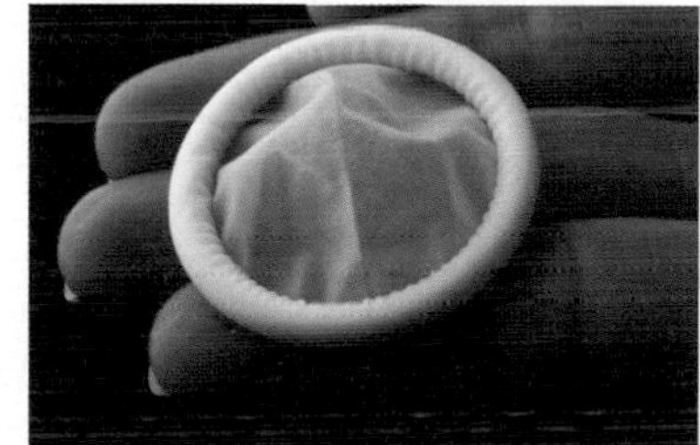
A condom.

contract
A legally binding agreement to provide goods or **services**. Also relates to a written agreement of employment.

contribute
A term used in **National Occupational Standards** and related **S/NVQs** stating a workers role in tasks. It makes it clear that the worker does not have full **responsibility** for the task and would demonstrate their competence by working with colleagues.

Control of Substances Hazardous to Health (COSHH)

Regulations set out by the **Health and Safety Executive** under the umbrella of the Health and Safety at Work Act 1974. Since April 2005 employers have been required to focus on the following eight principles of good **practice** in the control of substances hazardous to health.

Symbol	Abbreviation	Hazard	Description of hazard
	E	explosive	Chemicals that explode
	F	highly flammable	Chemicals that may catch fire in contact with air, only need brief contact with an ignition source, have a very low flash point or evolve highly flammable gases in contact with water
	T (also Carc or Muta)	toxic (also carcinogenic or mutagenic)	Chemicals that at low levels cause damage to health and may cause cancer or induce heritable genetic defects or increase the incidence of these
	Xh or Xi	harmful or irritant	Chemicals that may cause damage to health, especially inflammation to the skin or other mucous membranes
	C	corrosive	Chemicals that may destroy living tissue on contact
	N	dangerous for the environment	Chemicals that may present an immediate or delayed danger to one or more components of the environment

These symbols, which warn you of hazardous substances, are always yellow.

- Design and operate **processes** and activities to minimise emission, release and spread of substances **hazardous** to **health**.
- Take into account all relevant routes of exposure – inhalation, **skin** absorption and **ingestion** – when developing control measures.
- Control exposure by measures that are proportionate to the health risk.
- Choose the most effective and reliable control options which minimise the escape and spread of substances hazardous to health.
- Where adequate control of exposure cannot be achieved by other means, provide, in combination with other control measures, suitable personal protective **equipment**.
- Check and **review** regularly all elements of control measures for their continuing effectiveness.
- Inform and train all employees on the hazards and risks from the substances with which they work and the use of control measures developed to minimise the risks.

- Ensure that the introduction of control measures does not increase the overall risk to health and **safety**.

More information can be found at www.hse.gov.uk/coshh

controlled drug
A substance regulated under the Misuse of Drugs Act 1971. These include cocaine, diamorphine, **methadone**, levorphanol, **morphine**, opium, pethidine, amphetamine, dexamphetamine, dihydrocodeine injection, mephentermine and methylphenidate. These drugs must be prescribed by registered **medical practitioners** and **dentists**, and **records** of their use must be maintained.

co-operation
Working together towards a common goal.

cornea
The front of the eye where much of light is focused on to the **retina**. A transparent cornea is essential for clear vision; if **disease** or **injury** damages the cornea, it can result in severe **visual impairment**. It is possible to **transplant** clear, healthy corneas to replace damaged ones.

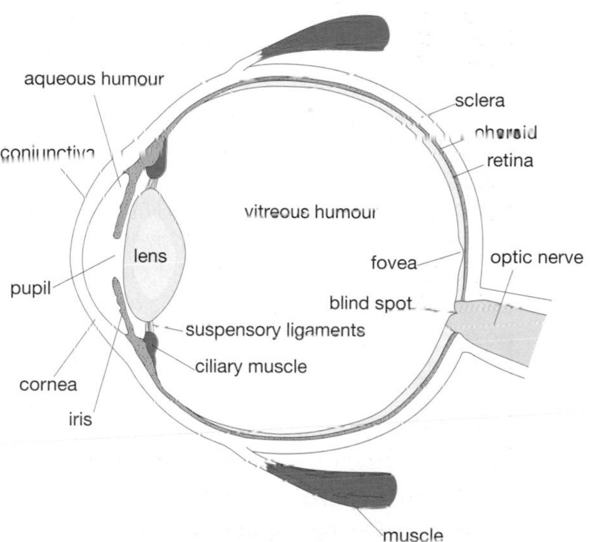

The structure of the human eye.

coronary arteries
Arteries that carry **oxygenated blood** to the **heart muscle**.

coronary heart disease
A condition where the **coronary arteries** become narrowed or blocked, thus preventing or reducing the flow of **blood** to the **heart**. This can result in a **heart attack** (**myocardial infarction**).

coroner
A public official, qualified as either a **doctor** or a lawyer, who investigates any sudden or unexpected **death** by holding an inquest.

corporal punishment
The physical punishment, usually of children, by **smacking** or hitting with implements such as canes, rulers, ropes or sticks. This has been **illegal** in all **nurseries** and **schools** in the UK since 1986 in the state sector, and since 1999 in the **private sector**.

A B C D E F G H I J K L M N O P Q R S T U V W X Y Z

cot death
See **sudden infant death syndrome**.

councillor
An elected member of a **local authority**.

council tax
A local property tax raised by the **local authority** and used to provide public services.

counselling
Counselling helps to explore and clarify problems an individual may be facing. Counselling is not only about feelings, it can offer an opportunity for the person to get to know him/herself better in a safe secure environment, and develop as a person. 'Counselling may be concerned with developmental issues, addressing and resolving specific problems, making decisions, coping with a crisis, developing personal insight and knowledge, and working through feelings or inner conflict or improving relationships with others.' (British Association for Counselling and Psychotherapy)

counsellor
A person who provides counselling through two way interaction with the aim of enabling someone to identify how to resolve his or her difficulties. Whilst not telling a person what to do, a Counsellor can help him or her explore the options so a greater understanding can develop. This may give clients a greater sense of choice and power to exercise new ways of being in the world and developing relationships.

court
The **access** point for the **justice system**; the place where **law** and order is enforced. There are courts at different levels and for different purposes. The majority of **criminal** cases are heard in the Magistrates Courts, or Justice of the Peace (JP) Courts in Scotland. These courts can deal with offences carrying penalties of up to six months in prison or fines of up to £5,000. More serious criminal cases are heard in the Crown Court, or the Sheriff Court in Scotland. **Civil** cases, dealing with disputes between individuals or companies, are heard in the County Courts or the High Court and the Court of Sessions in Scotland. In Scotland the supreme court is the High Court of Justiciary. Elsewhere in the UK it is the Appeal Court and ultimately the House of Lords. Defendants who want to appeal against conviction can do so in a court at a higher level than the one in which they were sentenced. The House of Lords is due to be replaced as the final court of appeal in 2009 when the new Supreme Court is introduced.

crack
A rapidly addictive form of the **controlled drug** cocaine mixed with **heroin**.

cream
A medium for dispensing medication that needs to be applied to the skin.

creative development
The development of a child's **imagination** and exploring **skills.** Children learn how they can build and develop objects, about how different things feel and what they can be used for. Children will **experiment** by using materials and techniques as their fine **motor control** develops.

credit card
A plastic card with an electronic chip that gives **access** to amounts of money, up to an agreed limit, from a bank. The money is effectively a loan; it attracts interest charges and can be paid back over a period of time.

criminal
Someone who has been tried in a court and convicted of an offence.

criminal justice system
The **administration** and implementation of **law** and order. This includes the **police**, prosecutors, judges, magistrates, **probation service**, **youth justice system** and the **courts**.

Criminal Records Bureau (CRB)
A government **organisation** that has **access** to all criminal **records**. Employers are required to request the CRB to check all employees who are to work with children or **vulnerable adults** to ensure that they do not have a record of having committed an **offence** that would make them unsuitable for the role.
More information can be found at www.crb.gov.uk

critical incident reviews
A no-blame review of situations where something went wrong or could have gone wrong. It is an important part of learning and taking action to identify what caused the problem and how to change systems so it does not happen again. The reviews do not apportion blame; they identify the system failure that allowed the problem to arise.

cross-infection
The process of transferring **infection**, bacteria or disease from one person or object to another.

Crown Prosecution Service (CPS)
A government **organisation** independent of the **police** that considers the evidence in a case where someone has been arrested, and decides whether the person should be **prosecuted** for the **offence**. In Scotland the Procurator Fiscal has a similar role.
More information can be found at www.cps.gov.uk

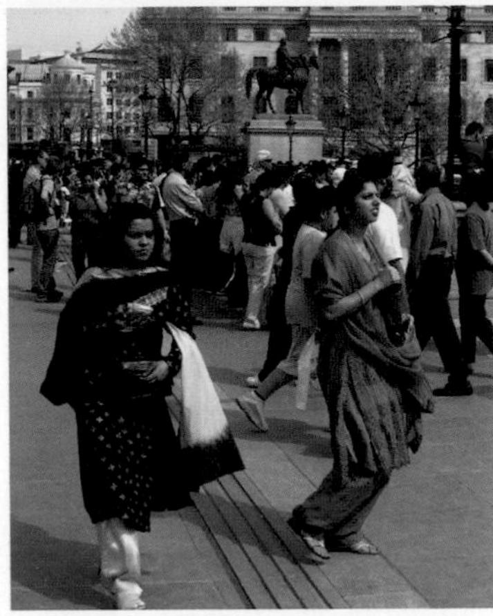

An individual's culture can affect their choice of what to wear.

culture

Shared aspects held in common among a **group** of people. These can include:

- **beliefs**
- **values**
- **language**
- **customs**
- rituals and ceremonies
- **social norms**
- dress.

curfew

A curfew is a requirement to be indoors by a certain time each evening. This can be a requirement of an **Anti-Social Behaviour Order** or **other** court orders.

curriculum

The specification detailing what must be included in children's **education**.

curriculum vitae

A record of experience, **education** and employment that is presented to potential employers when applyng for a job.

custodial sentence

This is a sentence given by the **court** where the criminal is locked up in either a prison or, for young offenders, a secure training centre, a secure children's home or a young offender institution.

customs

Rituals, **beliefs** and ways of behaving that are specific to racial or cultural groups. There are customs around important life events such as **birth**, **marriage** and **death**. There are also customs associated with moving through life stages, such as the move from childhood into adolescence and then into adulthood. Customs can also be associated with behaviour and expectations, for example the complex expectations around hospitality in many Arab cultures and the custom of giving gifts that is common in Japanese and other Asian cultures.

cyst

A small cavity that forms a closed sac (pouch) containing fluid, semi-solid matter or air. Cysts can occur anywhere in the body and may be single or multiple. Some common cysts include sebaceous cysts (in the skin and filled with keratin), ovarian cysts (fluid-filled cysts in the ovary), ganglions (fluid-filled cysts connected to a joint) and popliteal cysts (behind the knee).

Personal profile

Name:	Sarah Smith	Telephone number	0110 390189
Address:	20 Pickle Street, Smallville, Hampshire PO2 2OP	DOB: Mobile: Age:	9 November 1991 0797 8695949 17 years

Friendly, good humoured, quick to learn, with good listening and communication skills. Experience in customer services and dealing with customer complaints. Hard working with a good college attendance record.

Qualifications

2008	BTEC First Diploma in Health and Care (equivalent to 4 GCSEs A-C) including communication and individual rights, individual needs, vocational experience, anatomy and physiology, cultural diversity and life span development Key Skills, Communication, Application of Number and IT all at level 2. First Aid at Work Certificate
2007	3 GCSE passes in English, Science, History

Occupational Skills

Customer services: Welcoming and serving customers while maintaining a friendly, appropriate manner in the 'Fit for life leisure centre'. Taking bookings, planning children's activities and dealing with customer complaints.

Child care: collecting two 6-year-old children from school, preparing them a meal and supervising play and coordinating their after school activities.

Organising child activities: Extensive experience helping to organise Saturday clubs, after school fun days and Brownie revels.

Employment and work experience

2007 to date	Receptionist at 'Fit for life leisure centre' (part time)
2008 January	Two weeks' work experience at Neverland day nursery for pre-school children
2008 March	Two weeks' work experience at Rainbow centre for children with disabilities
2006	Baby sitting twins for Mr and Mrs Bold. After-school care

Education

2007–2008	South Downs College, Portsmouth
2003–2007	Westergate Community School, Bognor Regis

Interests and other skills

I have been a helper at a Brownie unit for 3 years and have taken the Brownies on several pack holidays, as well as organising weekly activities for them. I am also a keen reptile keeper and have developed a successful breeding programme for snakes.

Referees

Mr. D. Ruby, Course manager, BTEC First Diploma in Health and Care, South Downs College, Portsmouth PO3 1ZZ
Ms F. Itness, Manager 'Fit for life leisure centre', Smallville, Hampshire PO2 3PP

Example of a good CV.

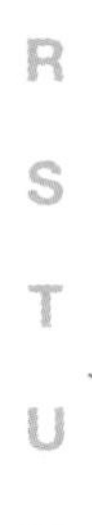

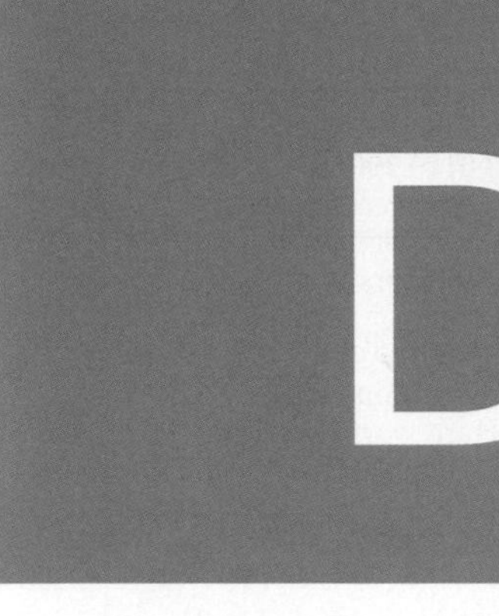

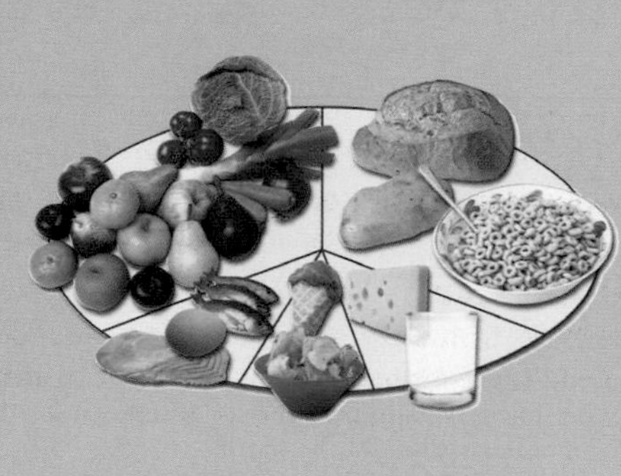

daily living programmes
The day-to-day living activities of children and young people who are looked after in residential settings.

daily living tasks
The normal day-to-day activities that people include in their everyday life.

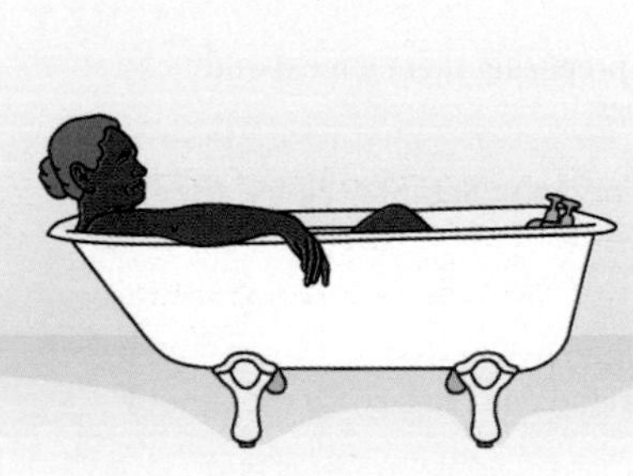

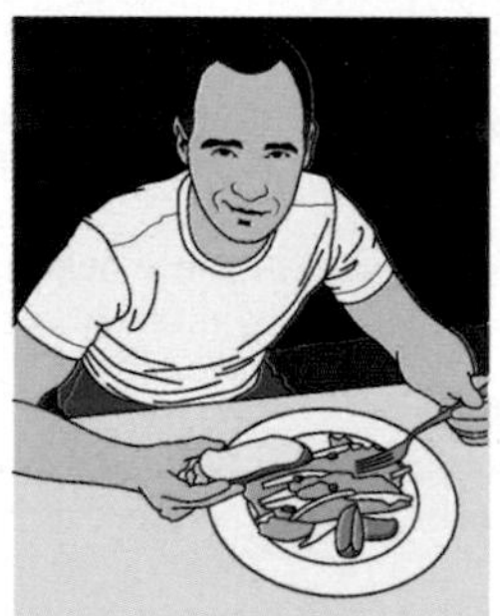

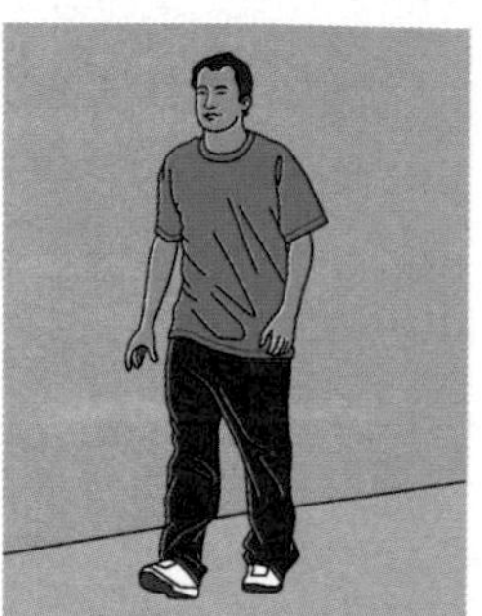

■ Daily living tasks.

danger
The possibility that something may happen that will cause harm.

dangerous occurrence
A near-miss **accident** in a **workplace** that did not result in a reportable **injury**, but could have done. Reporting of injuries, **diseases** and dangerous occurrences is required by **RIDDOR** regulations.

data
Information collected for any purpose, such as a piece of **research** or a project **evaluation**. Depending on the purpose for which the information has been collected, it can be **quantitative** (numbers, **statistics**) or it can be **qualitative** (opinions, views, **feelings**).

data analysis

The **process** and methods of examining all the collected **data** and reaching some conclusions about what has been found.

data protection

Ensuring that **data** are collected and stored securely and in compliance with the Data Protection Act 1998, which requires data to be:

- **processed** fairly and lawfully
- obtained and used only for specified and lawful purposes
- adequate, relevant and not excessive
- accurate, and where necessary, kept up to date
- kept for no longer than necessary
- processed in accordance with the individual's rights
- kept secure
- transferred only to countries that offer adequate data protection.

Data Protection Act (1998)

A law to ensure the safety of data held. A business must comply with this Act, which regulates how personal information is used and provides protection from misuse of personal details.

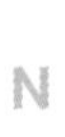

day care

Services provided away from home, during the day. The term can be used to describe **early years education** for children in **nurseries**, or various types of day care that offer different **facilities** for **older people**, people with **mental health problems** or people with **learning disabilities**.

deaf

The effect of having a **hearing impairment**. Deafness can be permanent or temporary. People who have **total hearing loss** are **profoundly deaf**; people who can hear some sounds or can hear with a hearing aid are partially deaf.

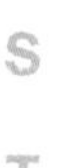

death

The point at which all the **systems** of the human body cease to function and cannot be revived.

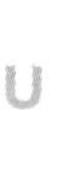

death rate

The number of **deaths** each year per thousand of the **population**. All deaths in the UK are **recorded** and the figures are produced by the Office of National Statistics.

debilitating
A condition that reduces the level of a person's physical health or energy and making certain tasks, or activities, difficult or impossible. **Anaemia**, for example, can make people very tired and have little energy.

debriefing
Discussions following a critical incident, or a difficult or emotional situation. The aim of a debrief is to examine the incident and the actions taken, ensure that all **information** is known and understood, and identify what can be learned.

debt
Money owed to another person, an organisation or company.

debt management
The **process** of **prioritising** and organising debts and negotiating affordable repayments. Priority debts are mortgage/**rent**, bills for heat and light, and taxes.

decision makers
The people and the process of saying what will happen. In any organisation the ability to make decisions is greater, the higher up the organisation a person works.

decision-making
Most organisations have a clear decision-making process involving research, reviewing evidence and reaching a decision.

decision-making forums
Decision-making forums are reviews, or meetings, where decisions can be discussed and agreed. These can be formal conferences or reviews, or meetings called especially to discuss particular decisions with the person involved and their family/carers.

decubitus ulcers
Pressure sores or bedsores. These are caused when **skin** is in poor condition because of illness or poor **diet** and breaks down under the pressure of lying or sitting in one position for a long time usually due to an interference with local **circulation**.

defecation
The **process** of evacuating **faeces** as body waste. Faeces are stored in the **rectum** and pushed out of the body through the **anus**.

defence mechanism
A way in which people attempt to protect themselves emotionally from threatening, unpleasant or painful experiences. These mechanisms can include:
- **aggressive behaviour**
- **denial**
- inappropriate humour
- blaming others.

defendant
The accused person in a **court** case. In British law a defendant is innocent until proven guilty. The defendant is not required to prove their innocence, the prosecutor is required to prove guilt.

deficiency
In **diet**, the lack of an essential **nutrient**. The lack of essential **vitamins**, **minerals** or any nutrient can cause illness and **diseases**. Lack of vitamin C can result in **scurvy**, and lack of vitamin D can result in **rickets**.

degenerative disease
A continually progressing **disease** that cannot be cured and causes the condition of the human body to deteriorate over a period of time. Examples are **multiple sclerosis** and **motor neurone disease**.

dehydration
A condition where there are insufficient fluids in the body. It is brought about by:
- not drinking enough
- excessive alcohol intake
- exposure to hot, dry conditions with insufficient water intake
- illness with high **temperature**
- illness with severe **vomiting** or **diarrhoea**.

Fluids must be replaced as soon as possible, if necessary through a **drip**. Prolonged or severe dehydration can result in **death**.

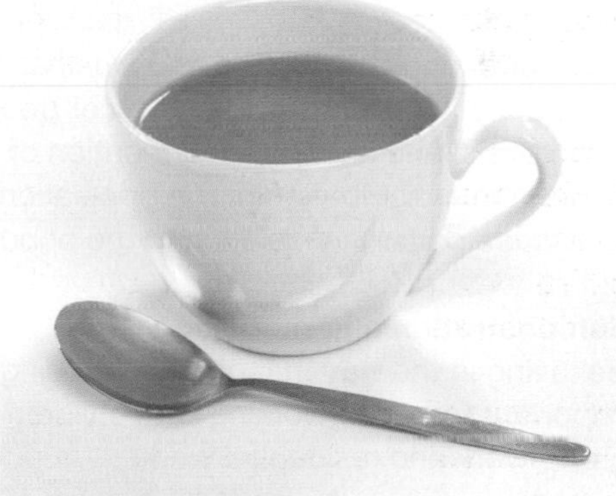

It is important to drink plenty of fluids to avoid dehydration.

delinquent behaviour
Behaviour that is outside the accepted norms and laws of society. Usually used to describe the behaviour of young people rather than adults.

A B C D E F G H I J K L M N O P Q R S T U V W X Y Z

dementia

A loss of brain function and ability. This can be caused by **degenerative**, irreversible illnesses such as **Alzheimer's disease**, **Dementia with Lewy bodies** or **vascular dementia**. All types of dementia result in increasing confusion, memory loss, disorientation and communication difficulties. Dementia develops at different rates for different people, but progress is usually over a period of years ultimately resulting in the need for significant care. Reversible dementia can be the result of treatable conditions such as brain **tumour**, **deficiency** of vitamin B12, **thyroid** conditions or **infections**.

Dementia with Lewy bodies (DLB)

A form of dementia that has symptoms of both **Alzheimer's disease** and Parkinson's disease. Lewy bodies are minute, spherical deposits from proteins that are found in nerve cells. This prevents the action of chemical messengers and interrupts the normal functioning of the brain. People with DLB will experience the shuffling, muscle tremors and stiffness seen in Parkinson's disease and also the memory loss and disorientation of Alzheimer's disease.

demographic trends

Information about a country's current and future **population** resulting from study and research. **Data** is gathered in order to help the **government** planning **process**. Trends will show:

- where the population is living and which parts of the country have more people
- whether there are changes and people are moving from one part of the country to another
- the **birth** and **death rates** and whether the age profile of the population is resulting in concentrations of **older people** or children in any particular area
- the social and economic distribution of the population
- the **ethnic** distribution of the population
- **disease** patterns in relation to the population.

demonstration and modelling

Behaving in the way that others are being encouraged to behave. The technique is important for those working with children and young people and is used mostly in group work and residential work.

denial

A **defence mechanism** where a person will refuse to believe or recognise events that he or she finds threatening, unpleasant or unacceptable. Some people, for example, may refuse to acknowledge serious debt problems; even though they receive letters and court judgements, they simply do not open letters and refuse to take any action to try to resolve the issues.

dentist
A **health professional** specialising in **teeth**, gums and **mouth care**. Dentists train for five years, and when qualified will either work in the **community** providing dental care for a locality, or may specialise in straightening teeth through **orthodontics**, or oral **surgery** dealing with **accidents** or abnormalities of the teeth, mouth and jaw.

deoxyribonucleic acid (DNA)
An acid found in the **chromosomes** of **cells**. Its makeup is unique to each individual. Sections of DNA correspond to genes. **Samples** of any **tissue** or body fluid can be **analysed** and compared to determine links to a particular individual. DNA can be used to show hereditary links, confirm **family relationships**, and assess the likelihood of developing **inherited** illnesses.

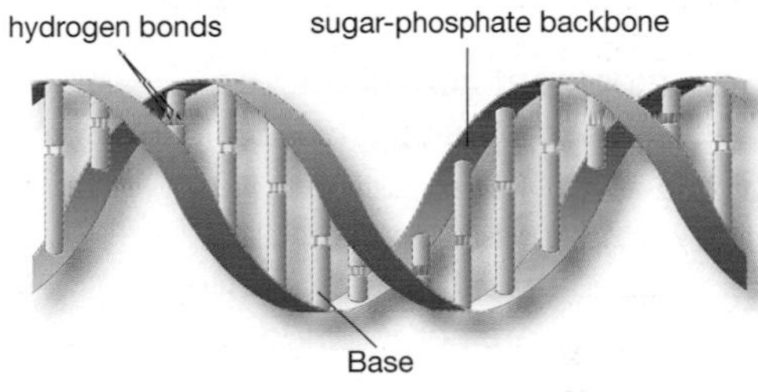

■ The structure of DNA.

Department of Health
The department of government that is responsible for health care and the **National Health Service**. It is headed by the Secretary of State for Health, a cabinet minister.

dependent
Reliant on another person for **support**, either financial, physical or emotional. A person who is dependent on alcohol, tobacco or drugs is unable to cope without these substances.

depression
A **mental disorder** often referred to as 'clinical depression' to differentiate it from feeling unhappy or miserable. It can be a **chronic condition** (endogenous depression) or a short-term one related to life circumstances (reactive depression). Depression following childbirth is called **puerperal** or **post-natal depression**, and is a mental disorder that requires **treatment**; it is much more severe than the '**baby** blues' experienced by most women shortly after giving **birth**. People with depression are unable to cope with day-to-day life and experience **feelings** of worthlessness, and may have **suicidal** thoughts.

deprivation
Deprivation can be a lack of something important. It could be physical as in lack of money, shelter or clothing or it can be emotional as in lack of loving, nurturing and caring.

dermis
The second of the three **skin** layers; it contains connective, fibrous **tissue, sweat glands** and hair follicles. *See* **skin** for diagram.

development
The process of changing, progressing and growing. It can be used to describe the growth process of a child, or to describe how someone improves their knowledge and skills to progress their career.

development activities
Activities that enable individuals to improve, retain and regain their skills and abilities.

developmental norms
Expected **milestones** that children usually reach within certain periods of time. If milestones are not reached, it is a useful **trigger** for further developmental tests to find whether there is a need for any **support**.

developmental scale
The guidelines for expected rates or growth and **development** for all **children**. They can be a useful indication that a child is not progressing as expected and there may be a cause for concern.

development programme
Treatment or activities designed for individuals to improve and make progress towards agreed **goals**, for example following a **stroke** someone may have a programme of **exercises** to strengthen the affected side of the body, along with speech exercises.

deviance
Behaviour that does not comply with the expectations of a particular **group** or **society**. Often used to refer to criminal behaviour, the term can also describe the behaviour of someone who does not conform to what is expected within a group, for example, deliberately turning up to a formal black-tie event in jeans.

diabetes mellitus
A condition where the production of **insulin** is insufficient to control **glucose** levels in the body. Insulin is a **hormone** produced by the **pancreas**. There are two types of diabetes.

- Type 1 commonly occurs in younger people. Insulin production is stopped and has to be replaced by insulin injections taken regularly. This is known as 'insulin-dependent' diabetes.
- Type 2 commonly occurs in people over 50 who are overweight and take little **exercise**. Insulin production is reduced, but if a healthy **diet** is followed, this will usually be sufficient. The condition does sometimes require additional **medication**. This is known as 'non-insulin dependent' diabetes.

Untreated diabetes results in a higher likelihood of **heart disease** and **stroke**, eye disease and poor **circulation**.

Diabetes UK
A national charity that represents the interests of people who have diabetes. The organisation lobbies on behalf of people with diabetes and provides advice and information. It also commissions research into the causes and treatments of the disease. More information can be found at www.diabetes.org.uk

diagnosis
The **process** of investigating the **symptoms** of an illness and using the evidence to reach a conclusion about the nature of the problem.

dialysis
The removal of waste products and toxic substances from the blood by dialysis as a substitute for the normal function of the kidney.

diamorphine
An opium-based pain reliever used for severe **pain**. It works with the pain receptors in the **brain** to reduce the sensation of pain. It is often used for people in the final stages of **cancer**.

diaphragm
The sheet of **muscle** anchored to the lower ribs that separates the **chest** from the **abdomen**.

diarrhoea
Frequent passing of watery **faeces** due to waste passing too quickly through the large intestine. This can be a **symptom** of **infection** or **disease**. In very young **babies** or people who are already ill or frail, it can lead to **dehydration**.

diastolic
The phase of circulation when the **heart ventricles** are filling with **blood** and so the pressure of the blood against the artery walls is at its lowest.

diet
The **food** and drink intake of an individual. The requirements of a healthy, balanced diet include a range of **nutrients**, **vitamins** and **minerals** needed for the body to be healthy and to function properly. A diet should contain the right proportions of: fruit and vegetables; bread, rice and potatoes and other starchy **foods**; meat, fish, eggs, beans and other non-dairy sources of **protein**; milk and dairy foods; and a small amount of food and drink high in **fat** and **sugar**. The right balance for food intake is approximately:

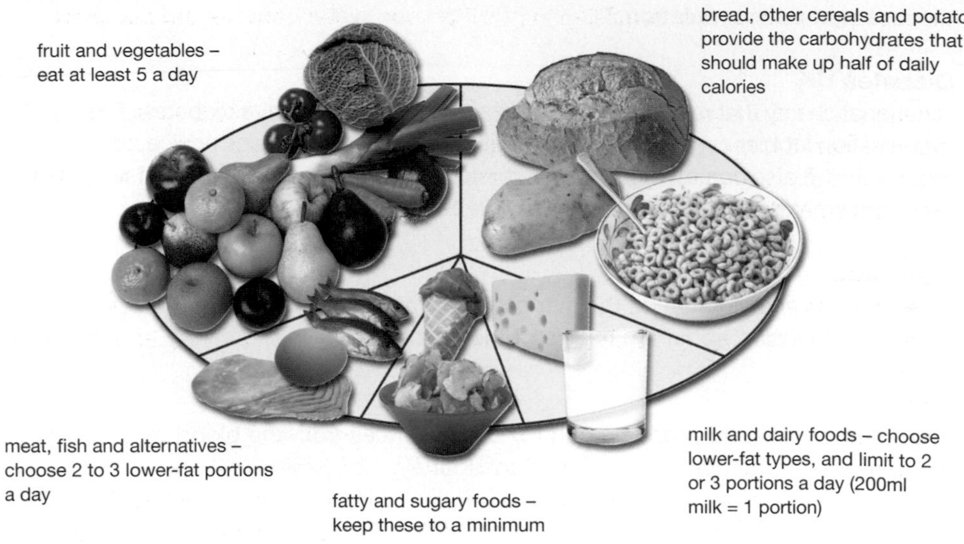
fruit and vegetables – eat at least 5 a day
bread, other cereals and potatoes provide the carbohydrates that should make up half of daily calories
meat, fish and alternatives – choose 2 to 3 lower-fat portions a day
fatty and sugary foods – keep these to a minimum
milk and dairy foods – choose lower-fat types, and limit to 2 or 3 portions a day (200ml milk = 1 portion)

Recommended daily proportions of food.

- one third fruit and vegetables
- one third bread, rice and potatoes
- the remaining third mainly meat, fish and other protein, along with dairy foods and a small amount of high-fat and sugary foods.

Some medical conditions require special diets such as:

- People with diabetes (Type 1 or Type 2) need to follow a **healthy balanced diet** and to ensure that the intake of **carbohydrates** is spread throughout the day so that there is no surge in blood glucose.
- People with coeliac disease will have to follow a gluten-free diet. Gluten is contained in wheat, so the diet must be free of cereals, flour, bread, cakes, biscuits and pasta and any other food such as sauces that may contain flour.
- Some people are lactose intolerant because they lack an **enzyme** that breaks down the lactose, a sugar found in all animal (including human) milk. This diet must also exclude all milk-related products such as cheese, butter and yoghurt.
- **Obesity** requires the management of people who are obese which require a balanced diet, but which reduces the calorie intake below the number of **calories** spent in activity each day. This way weight will gradually be reduced.
- Babies and children under 5 years should not be given a diet that is considered healthy for adults, i.e. one that is high in fibre and low in fat. Babies, once they are weaned, and children, need full fat milk, yoghurt and foods packed with **protein** such as meat and fish. They should not be given bulky high-fibre foods such as wholemeal rice and pasta.

dietician
A **health professional** specialising in **nutrition** and dietary advice and planning.

diffusion
An important process responsible for the movement of many molecules into, and out of, cells. It is the movement of molecules form a high concentration to a low concentration. Gaseous exchange and the absorption of nutrients into the blood after enzyme digestion are two examples of diffusion.

diet industry
The multi-million-pound business selling various 'diets' and products to people attempting to lose weight. Many of these do not comply with the requirements of a balanced diet.

digestion
The processing of **food** so that it can be used by the body for **energy**, repair and growth. Digestion reduces large complex food molecules into simple soluble molecules capable of passing through the walls of the small intestine into the blood. Food taken in through the mouth is processed through various parts of the body by **enzymes**, acids and the physical **process** of being pushed along by the **muscle** contractions called **peristalsis**. The body absorbs the **nutrients** it requires from food and the waste is expelled from the body as **faeces** through the **anus**.

digestive system
The system of organs that are involved in the process of **digestion** that begins with the mouth and ends with the **anus**. Food is chewed into a bolus in the mouth and **swallowed**, then passes down the **oesophagus** into the **stomach**, moved along by muscular contractions called **peristalsis**. In the stomach, food is churned and mixed with acid and **enzymes** and then moves into the first part of the small intestine, the duodenum. Further enzymes and digestive

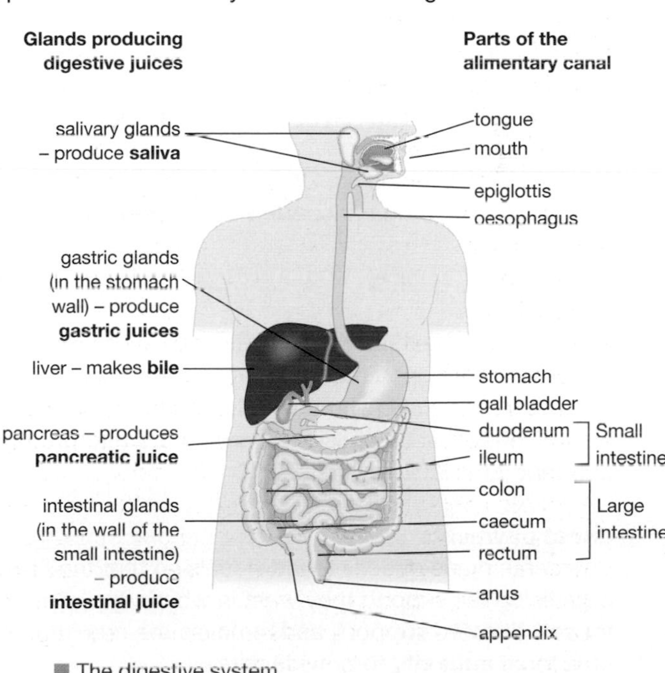

■ The digestive system.

juices from the **pancreas** and **liver** continue to break down food as it passes into the ileum, where final breakdown and enzyme activity takes place. Nutrients are absorbed into the body through the wall of the **ileum**, the remainder passing into the colon (large intestine), where most of the water is absorbed into the body and the remaining **faeces** pass into the **rectum**, where they are stored before being **excreted** through the anus.

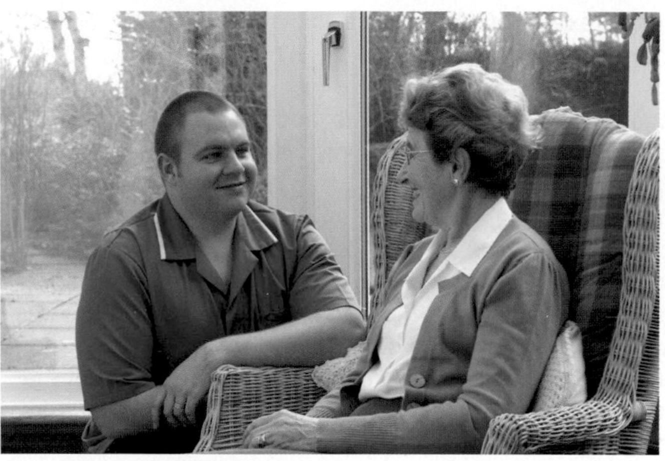

■ Dignity and self-esteem.

dignity
The quality or state of being worthy of esteem and respect. Everyone who receives **health** or **social care** has the right to dignity; that is, to be treated with **respect** and to have his or her **self-esteem** supported.

Dignity Guardians
Groups of representatives including Help the Aged, Action on Elder Abuse and Which? consumer group who focus on the regulation of social care in respect of the dignity of service users.

dilate
Enlargement or widening. Occurs in **blood vessels** when body temperature rises allowing blood to be transported to the **skin** and so heat is lost allowing the body to cool down.

dimensions
This refers to the three dimensions used in the Assessment Framework. These are the child's developmental needs, the capacity of their **parents** to care for them and the **family** and environmental factors. The aim is that by assessing all these dimensions it will be possible to safeguard and promote the welfare of the child and their best interests.

direct payments
Payments made directly to individuals so that they take on the **responsibility** for organising the support they want in whatever way suits them best. This is the basis for self-directed **support**, and removes the requirement for people to be dependent on a **local authority** to provide care.

disability
The problem that occurs when a person's ability and the **environment** do not match. A disability can be a long-term, permanent **impairment** of **mobility**, **understanding**, vision, hearing or **mental capacity** that may not be compensated for by the environment in which an individual lives or **works**.

disabled facilities grant
A **local authority** grant to make adaptations to enable a disabled person to access day-to-day living essentials such as a bathroom or access to the outside.

disabled person
Someone whose abilities are not catered for by the **environment** he or she lives or **works** in. Examples could include a **workplace** with narrow doorways disables a person who would like to work there but uses a wheelchair, and a college that only delivers spoken **lectures** disables a **deaf** person who would like to **learn** there.

disadvantage
The effects of negative influences such as **poverty**, **unemployment**, poor **housing**, poor **education** and **ill health**.

discipline
The enforcement of the **boundaries** of acceptable and expected behaviour. Discipline can be used in a positive way where desired behaviour is rewarded, or it can punish unwanted behaviour. It is important for children's development that they have clear boundaries and are rewarded and recognised for behaviour within the boundaries.

disclosure
Where a survivor of **abuse** tells someone about the abuse he or she has experienced. When people disclose abuse they do so because they want it to stop; any disclosure of abuse must be **reported** and the correct procedures followed. Also relates to the Public Disclosure Act where staff are protected whilst disclosing poor practice at work if they follow correct procedures.

discrimination
Treatment of one **group** or individual in a less or more favourable way than another on the basis of **race**, **ethnicity**, **gender**, **sexuality**, age or other **prejudice**. It is important to recognise that discrimination can be indirect, and therefore less obvious, as well as direct. Direct discrimination is, for example, where someone is refused a job because she uses a wheelchair. Indirect discrimination would be where she is told she can have the job but the work must be carried out on the first floor and there is no lift.

disease
A state where the whole parts of the body are not functioning correctly and causing **ill health**. Diseases can be treated with **medication** or sometimes **surgery**. They are caused in various ways including **bacterial infection**, **heredity** and **viral infection**.

disinfection
The **process** of removing **micro-organisms** that can cause **infection**. This is done by using chemicals known to kill bacteria, or by heating to a **temperature** known to kill bacteria.

disorder
A malfunction of an organ or system.

district nurse
A qualified **nurse** who visits people at home to undertake medical and nursing procedures, such as changing **dressings** and administering **medication**.

diversity
The differences between individuals and **groups** in **ethnicity**, **culture**, **gender**, ability, **sexuality** and age. It is important to recognise the **value** of the differences.

divorce
The legal ending of a marriage.

doctor
A qualified **medical practitioner** who **diagnoses** and prescribes **treatment**. Following **qualification**, doctors can specialise in particular areas of medicine. Training takes five years. Doctors can work in the **community** or be **hospital**-based.

domestic abuse
Abuse or exploitation within a domestic **relationship**. Abuse can take various forms, but it is often accompanied by **violence**. The majority of reported cases are attacks on females but males can also be victims. Domestic violence has a profound impact on any children.
More information can be found at www.refuge.org.uk, www.mankind.org.uk/domesticabuse.html

domiciliary care
Social care services provided in the home of an individual.

doula
A non-medical assistant who provides emotional and practical **support** for women during **pregnancy** and childbirth.

Down's syndrome
A **congenital** condition caused by an additional **chromosome.** Children with Down's syndrome have similar physical features and will share some degree of **learning disability**, but the degree varies in individual children.

dressing
A covering to protect **wounds**, sores or broken **skin**; there are many different types.

drip
A means of providing fluid and/or **medication** directly into a **vein**. Medication can be absorbed into the body more rapidly by this method, and in larger amounts than taking tablets orally. A flexible bag containing the liquid is hung on a stand, and a tube is attached to the bag and into a vein using a fine **needle**. The contents of the bag are then set to 'drip' at a specific rate into the vein.

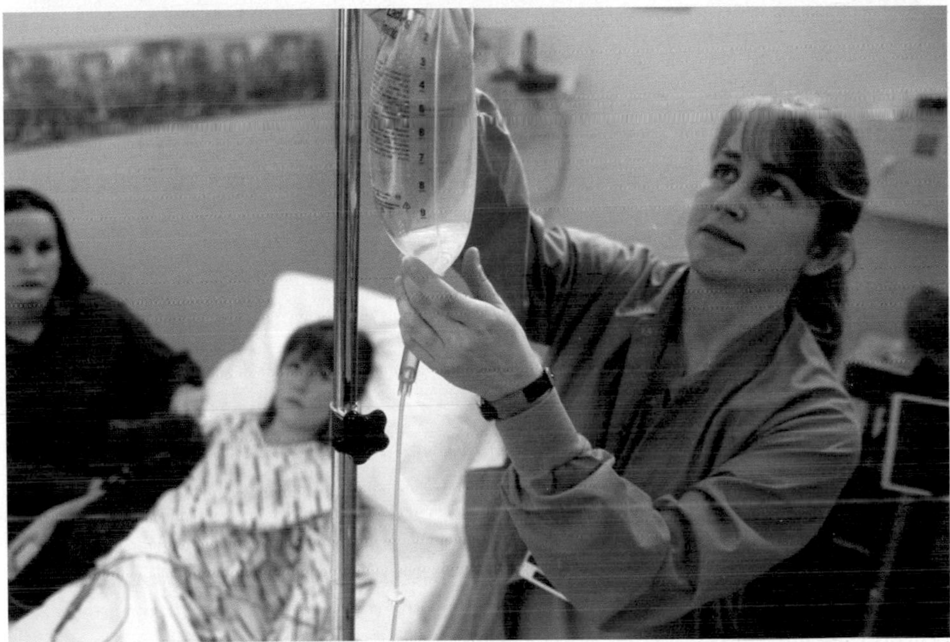

A drip stand with bag in use.

drop-in centre
An informal **service** where people can come to a centre without having to make arrangements in advance. The services provided will be dependent on the **needs** of the people who go. They are available most commonly for **older people**, people with **mental health problems**, **mothers and babies**, substance abusers and **young people**.

droplet infection
The spread of **infection** through someone sneezing, coughing or just breathing minute drops of liquid containing micro-organisms into the air. These are then breathed in by others and the infection may spread.

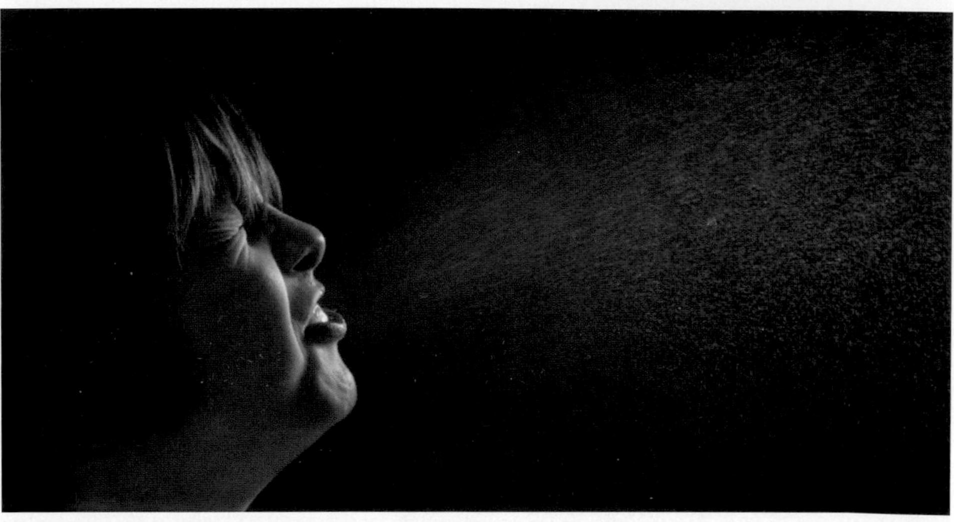

■ Infection can be transmitted through sneezing.

drug(s)
Refers to both medicines in any form and substances that are illegal that change the state of a person.

drug abuse/misuse
Using **medication** for non-medical reasons. Most drugs that are abused are **illegal**. Some may be available on **prescription** only.

drug action teams
Multi-disciplinary partnerships that deliver the National Drugs Strategy at local level. The partnerships include representatives from education, social services, housing, health, probation, the prison service and the voluntary sector.

drug addiction/dependency
A situation where the use of drugs interferes with everyday life and the individual's main concern is how to ensure the next supply of the drug.

drug rehabilitation
The supportive process to assist people who are recovering from an addiction to drugs.

duodenum
The upper part of the small **intestine** leading from the **stomach** to the ileum.

duty of care
The requirement that all **health** and **social care professionals**, and **organisations** providing health or care **services**, must put the interests of people who use their services first. They also have to do everything in their **power** to keep people safe from **harm**.

dying
The physical **process** of approaching **death**. Support to the person, and their family, at this time is referred to as End of Life care.

dysfunction
Where the physical or emotional aspects of an activity, capability or **relationship** are not working as expected.

dyslexia
A specific **learning** difficulty with **processing** language or numbers. This can impact on reading, spelling, calculating or writing.

dyspraxia
A **neurological** condition causing problems with motor co-ordination, poor concentration and poor **memory**.

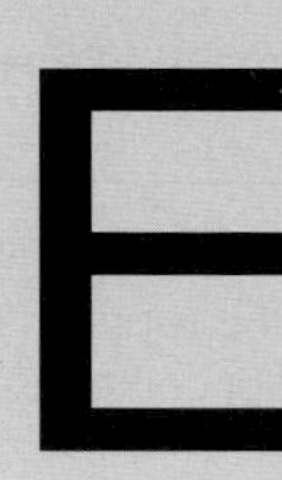

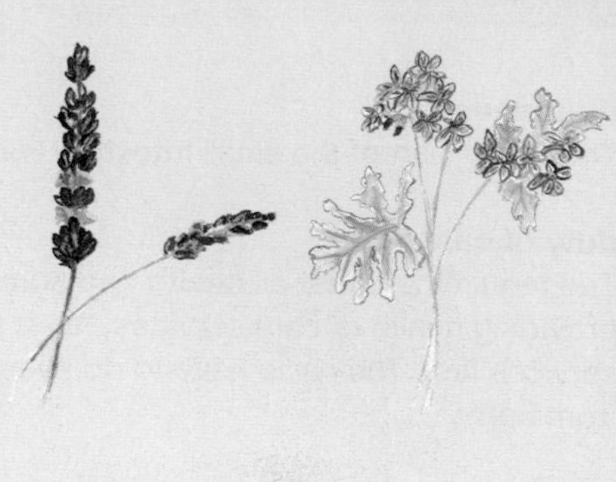

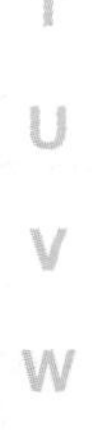

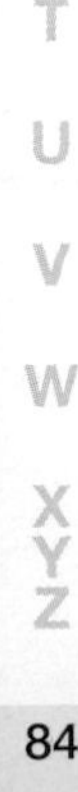

E numbers
Additives placed in **food** by manufacturers to provide flavour, colour or texture. The serial numbers show that the additive has been tested by the **European Union** and placed on a list of those safe for human consumption. There is a growing movement of people who prefer not to eat food that contains additives, and there appears to be some evidence that children's behaviour is calmer and less **aggressive** if they are not given food containing additives.

early adulthood
A life stage between 20 and 40 years. Legally adolescents reach adulthood at 18 years.

early intervention
An approach used across most areas of **health** and **social care**, but particularly with children, that takes action at the first sign of difficulty, issues or challenges. This more proactive approach has been found to be more effective that waiting until problems and difficulties are more established and thus harder to resolve.

early years education
The **learning** and development of young children before entering formal schooling. This can take place in **nurseries**, **playgroups** or with **childminders**. Early years education is inspected by **Ofsted** and is structured through a formal curriculum framework.

early years foundation stage
The framework that identifies the **learning** and development requirements for settings delivering **early years education**. It includes areas of learning and early learning **goals** for children, and the process for **assessment** of progress.

early years services
All **services** relating to pre-**school** children aiming to provide the **Every Child Matters** outcomes.

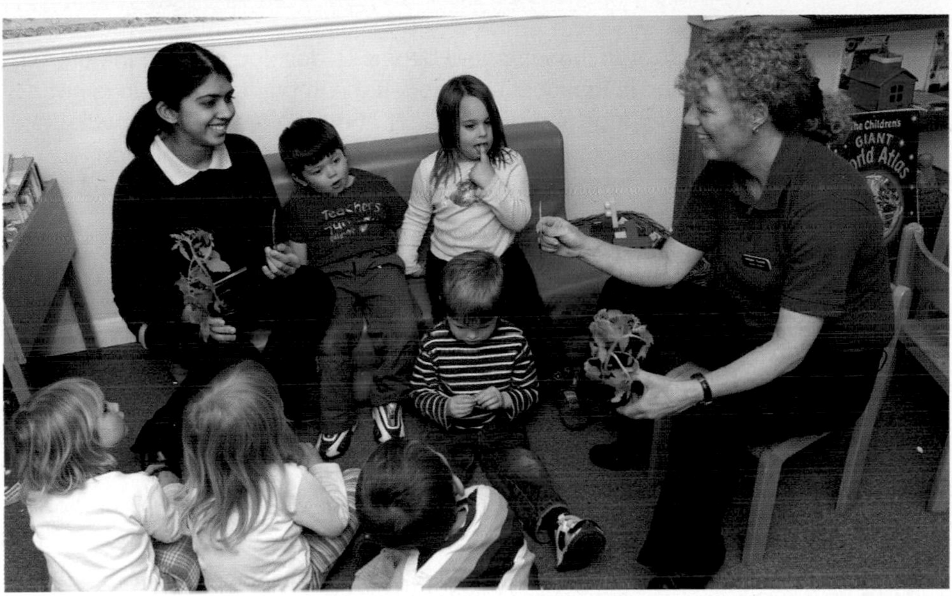

Nursery workers are a key contact for children in early years education.

eating disorder
A damaged or inappropriate **relationship** with **food**. This can result in a failure to eat healthily to the extent where serious **harm** can result, such as in **anorexia nervosa**. Other eating disorders include **bulimia nervosa**, which involves binge eating followed by **vomiting**. The conditions are essentially emotional and psychological in origin, although the consequences can have a serious impact on **physical heath** and **well-being**.

echocardiograph
A **diagnostic ultrasound** study of the movements of the **heart**. Ultrasound studies can be helpful in identifying structural heart problems.

economies
Reductions made in the costs of delivering **services**. Sometimes these can be achieved through **commissioning** services in a different way, or by negotiating lower costs, or by redesigning services to be more efficient.

ecstasy
An **illegal** stimulant, often taken by young people in dance clubs and raves. It produces a feeling of euphoria and **energy**, and people can become seriously **dehydrated** as the result of prolonged dancing in very hot conditions. There have been several **deaths** caused by ecstasy.

A
B
C
D
E
F
G
H
I
J
K
L
M
N
O
P
Q
R
S
T
U
V
W
X
Y
Z

ectopic pregnancy
A pregnancy where an **embryo implants** and begins to develop outside the uterus, although the **fallopian tube** is the most common. If the implanted embryo is not detected early, the fallopian tube can rupture after about six weeks of growth. This is a serious medical emergency that requires immediate **hospital** admission.

eczema
A condition causing dry, flaky, cracked and very itchy **skin**, commonly found in **babies** and young children. Patches of itchy dry skin are also found in adults. Eczema in children is often associated with **asthma**, and appears to be hereditary.

education
The experience of **learning** and developing. Formal education is provided in **schools**, colleges and universities, but human beings learn from all life experience, making education about much more than formal learning.

education welfare
A system providing **social work support** to children and **families** where there are **education**-related concerns such as **school phobia**, attendance issues or **bullying**.

educational psychologist
A **professional** who tests and assesses children's educational **needs** and works with children and **families** and other professionals to provide ongoing **assessment** and **support**. The educational psychologist is part of an integrated **team** of professionals working together in the interests of the child.

effective
When something produces the intended or expected result.

ejaculation
The expelling of **semen** from the male **urethra** through the **penis**. If this occurs during **sexual intercourse**, the **sperm** in the semen will enter the female **vagina** with the potential to fertilise an egg if the conditions are right.

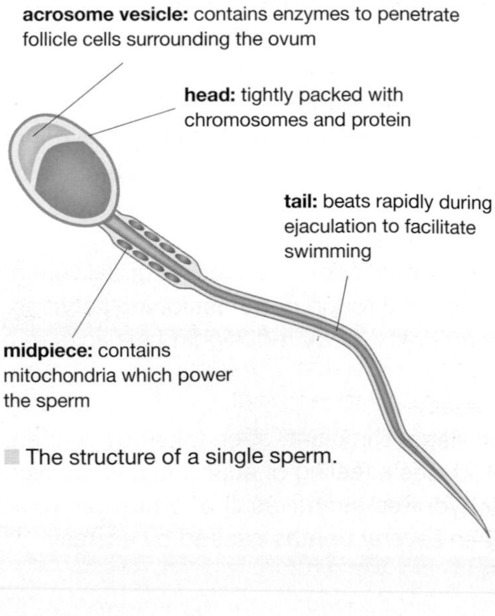

elder abuse
The **harming**, **neglecting** or exploiting of **older people**. Abuse can take several forms:

acrosome vesicle: contains enzymes to penetrate follicle cells surrounding the ovum
head: tightly packed with chromosomes and protein
tail: beats rapidly during ejaculation to facilitate swimming
midpiece: contains mitochondria which power the sperm

The structure of a single sperm.

- physical abuse
- emotional abuse
- sexual abuse
- financial abuse
- neglect.

Traditionally, there has been less publicity about the abuse of older people or other **vulnerable adults** because of a focus on abuse of children, but now that there are **guidelines** and **legislation** about Safeguarding Vulnerable Adults, the issue is better recognised.

More information can be found at www.elderabuse.org.uk (Protection of Vulnerable Adults (PoVA))

electrocardiogram (ECG)

A procedure where electrodes detect the electrical activity of the **heart** and **record** it on an electrocardiograph. The record is a tracing of the activity of the heart in waves; this helps to **diagnose** any irregular or unusual activity.

electroencephalogram (EEG)

A procedure where electrodes detect the electrical activity of the **brain** and **record** it on an electroencephalograph. The record shows the activity of the brain in waves and can be used to **diagnose** any unusual electrical activity that may indicate a problem or an illness, such as **epilepsy**.

eligibility criteria

The means used by **local authorities** to decide which people are allowed to **access services** and at which level. Some services are universal, such as **education**; but others, such as **domiciliary care**, are targeted for use by people who need them most, so eligibility criteria are used to identify them.

email

An electronic means of instant written **communication**. Useful for making quick contact and for sharing **information** rapidly, it is not secure, and highly sensitive or confidential information is not suitable for communication by this method.

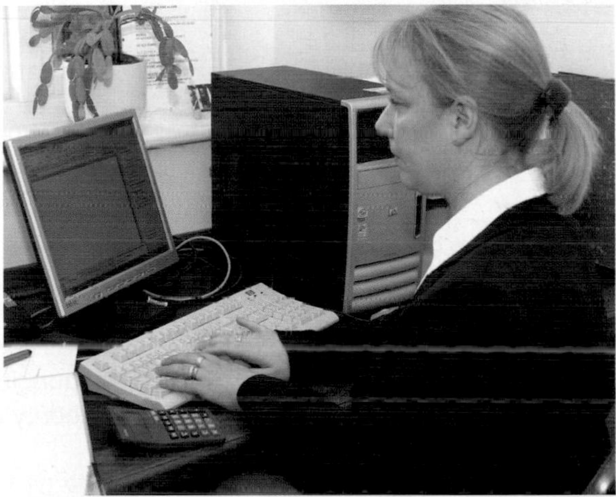

Email is a means of communication within and between workplaces.

embolism
A **blood** clot that forms, then can move through the bloodstream and can lodge in an **artery**. Depending on where it lodges it can have different consequences:
- an embolism in the cerebral artery in the **brain** can result in a **stroke** (**cerebrovascular accident**)
- an embolism in the **pulmonary artery** in the **lung** can cause respiratory failure
- an embolism in the **coronary artery** can cause a **heart attack** (**myocardial infarction**).

embryo
A fertilised egg that has travelled into the **uterus** and implanted in the uterus wall. It is an embryo for a few weeks after **implantation** and after about six weeks of development, when it is about the size of a baked bean, it becomes a **foetus**.

emergency
Immediate and threatening danger to individuals and others. A sudden unforeseen crisis (usually involving danger) that requires immediate action.

emergency duty team (EDT)
Out-of-hours emergency **service provision** for **local authority social services** and children's services. **Teams** normally deal with **statutory** emergencies that cannot wait until the next working day; this can mean **child protection**, **mental health** emergency admissions, emergency provision for **older people**, acting as an 'appropriate adult' for **young people** in the **justice system**, and providing accommodation for children and young people needing placements.

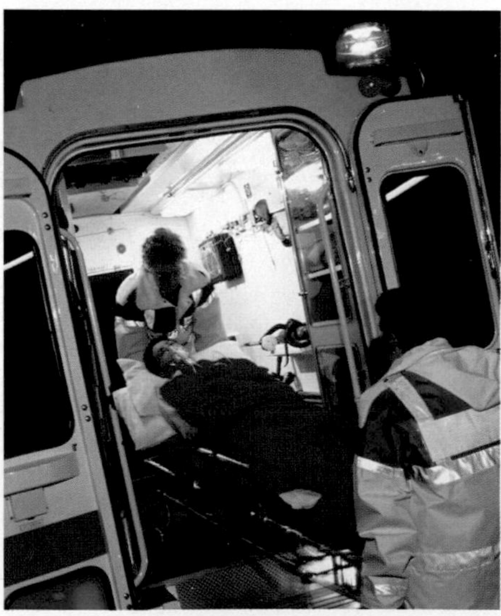

Ambulance emergency services.

emergency protection order (EPO)
A **provision** of the Children Act 1989 where a **magistrate** can make an order for the immediate removal of a child if there is cause to believe that the child is at risk of **significant harm**. The application to the magistrate is usually made by a **local authority social worker**. The order is in force for 8 days, after which time the local authority must go to court and provide evidence as to why the child needs continued protection. **Parental responsibility** is transferred to the local authority under the order.

emergency services
The fire service, **police**, ambulance and HM Coastguard are the **statutory** emergency

services. Mountain and cave rescue teams also provide emergency services in some parts of the country. The lifeboat service is called out by HM Coastguard if required. All emergency services are contacted by telephone, by dialling 999.

emotion
A feeling, or aroused mental state, which is usually evident in a person's behaviour and psychological changes. See **emotional development**.

emotional abuse
Bullying, threatening, taunting or any sort of behaviour that is likely to damage someone's feelings, confidence and self-esteem.

emotional development
The growth and **understanding** of **feelings**. All people need to be able to give and receive love, care and affection and to feel **secure** and positive about themselves. People who have not been able to develop emotionally in a warm, safe and secure **environment** where they have been loved are likely to experience difficulty in giving love and affection and caring for others, and may also lack **confidence** and have low **self-esteem**.

emotional harm
The results of emotional abuse which can include very low self-esteem, an inability to trust others and difficulty in making relationships with others.

empathy
The ability to share and **understand** the emotions of another, to 'walk a mile in their shoes', and to share the sadness, happiness or **anxiety** that someone is experiencing.

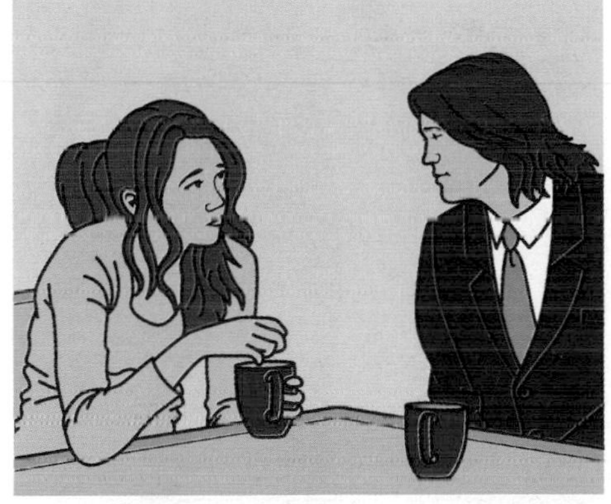

Empathy.

emphysema
A **chronic lung disease** that makes breathing difficult. It is caused by **environmental** factors such as **smoking** or working in **hazardous** conditions such as coal mines, engine rooms, and dusty manufacturing plants.

employment
Being paid for providing labour on an agreed, **contractual** basis. The terms and conditions of employment are governed by **legislation** to protect the employee (the person providing the labour) and the employer (the person paying).

employment tribunal
An informal court that hears disputes to do with employment.

empowerment
The **process** that enables people who had previously depended on others to make decisions and take control of their own lives. People can be empowered through finding **access** to **information** and knowledge, or through growing and developing **confidence** in their own abilities.

enable/enabling
Removing the barriers that stops someone doing something.

enabling environment
An environment that is adapted to ensure that everyone is able to participate in day-to-day life and work on an equal basis. This may include making physical changes and also changing attitudes.

endocrine system
The system in the body made up of **hormone**-producing **glands** such as the **thyroid**, **hypothalamus**, **pituitary**, adrenal, **pancreas** and **gonads**. The hormones are carried around the body in the bloodstream and are required to maintain the proper functioning of various **organs**.

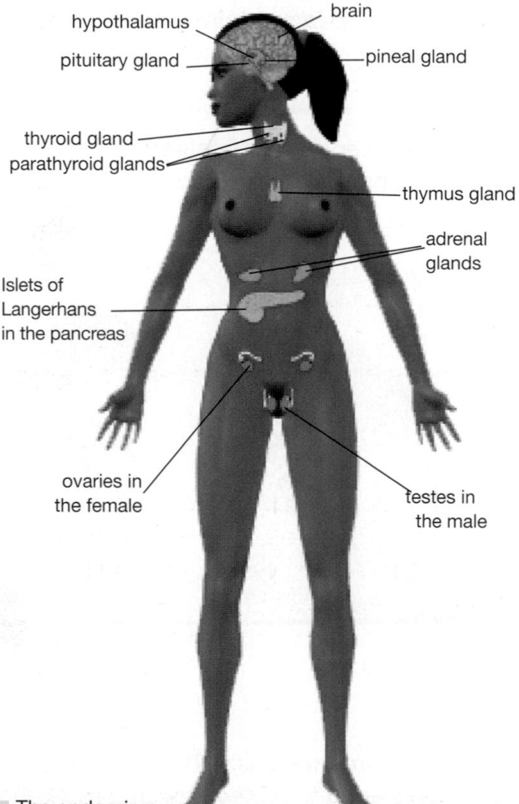

The endocrine system.

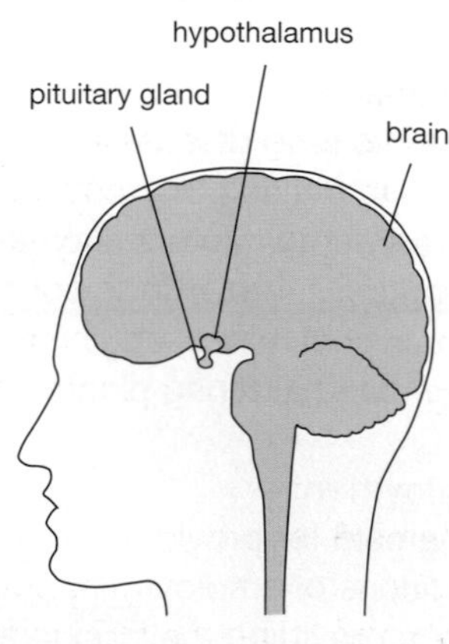

endothelial layer
The single layer of epithelial tissue which lines the interior, or lumen, of blood vessels.

energy
The ability of a **system** (such as the human body) to do work or perform activity. Human energy comes from **food** intake and the conversion of the food into substances that the body can use in order to function.

environment
The physical, social and emotional surroundings and circumstances of a person's life. It includes living and educational or working environments. Many different factors will have an impact on an individual's environment, for example, **housing**, **health**, economic circumstances and **education**. Local, national and international **communities** also exist within environments and there is overall concern about the global environment and the impact of human activities upon it.

environmental health service
A **local authority service** responsible for **monitoring** and maintaining safe **standards** of **food** production, service and sale. It is also responsible for investigating and dealing with **pollution**, whether of water, land, or by noise.

environmentalist
Someone who is concerned with the protection and positive development of the environment.

enzymes
Essential chemicals within the body that perform key functions in many of the **processes** within the body, such as **digestion**. Internal enzymes control all activities inside cells. Enzymes alter the rate of chemical reactions and are likened to biological catalysts.

epidemic
Widespread **incidence** of an **infectious disease**. An epidemic can be among a local **population** or can be over a wider area, among people who are in vulnerable **groups**. There could be an epidemic of **meningitis** among young adults, influenza among older and ill people, or whooping cough among **babies**. Epidemics can also occur when there is reduced immunity to a particular disease, for example as a result of the reduction in the number of children being **immunised** against **measles**, **mumps** and **rubella**.

epidemiology
The study of **diseases**, including how common they are and how widely they are distributed and the factors influencing such distribution.

A B C D E F G H I J K L M N O P Q R S T U V W XYZ

epidermis
The outermost layer of skin, above the dermis. It contains no blood vessels and consists of five layers and provides protective outer covering. The stratum corneum is a layer of dead keratinised cells, which forms a waterproof barrier against invasion by micro-organisms.

epidural anaesthetic
A **spinal anaesthetic** administered by inserting a **needle** into the lower back. It is commonly used in **labour**, and for performing **caesarean sections** so that the **mother** can remain awake throughout the delivery. It can also be used for other lower-body surgical procedures.

epiglottis
A cartilaginous flap which covers the entrance to the trachea during swallowing of food.

epilepsy
A disorder where there is abnormal electrical activity in the **brain**. The electrical discharges in the brain can cause epileptic **seizures** or fits. Depending on the type of epilepsy, these can cause people to fall, lose **consciousness**, have **muscle** spasms and possibly foam around the mouth ('grand mal' epilepsy). Alternatively, seizures can be for a few seconds and appear to be just a momentary loss of concentration, perhaps with minor confusion and **memory** loss for a short time. People may just lose track of what they were saying, or look blank or confused for a moment. They then resume whatever they were doing and there do not appear to be any lasting effects. (This is called 'petit mal' epilepsy.)

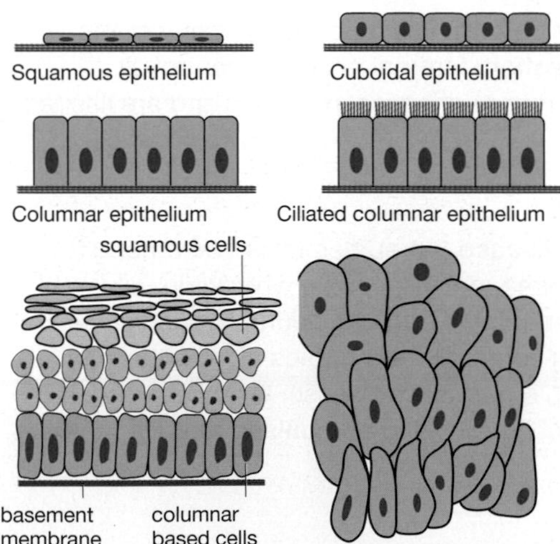

Types of epithelial tissue.

epithelial tissues
Cells that form the covering of **organs**, or are found in linings of passages or organs. The mucous membranes lining the mouth and part of the rectum, the lining of the lungs and the outer part of the cornea are all made of different types of epithelial tissue.

equal opportunities
Providing the circumstances for everyone to have the same chances as everyone else to achieve. It may require treating people differently in order for this to happen.

equality
The availability of the same rights, **access** and opportunities to everyone regardless of **gender**, **race**, ability, age, **sexual orientation** or **religious belief**.

Equality and Human Rights Commission
Formed in October 2007, the commission brings together the work of the three previous equality commissions: the Equal Opportunities Commission, the Commission for Racial Equality and the Disability Rights Commission. It also has **responsibility** for equality relating to age, **sexual orientation** and **religious belief** as well as **human rights**. More information can be found at www.equalityhumanrights.com

equipment
In **health** and **social care**, objects, machines and tools used to assist people in everyday living and **mobility**. Equipment may be used by **professional** staff in order to lift and move people, or by individuals in order to accomplish daily living tasks.

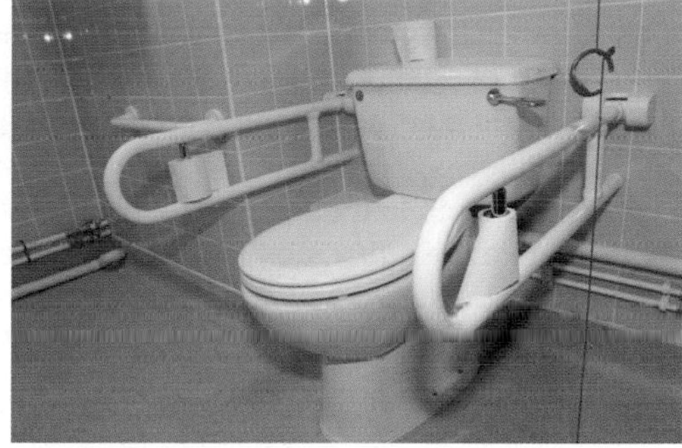
Toilet facilities may be specially designed to make access easier.

equity
Fairness and transparent dealings.

erection
Usually occurs in response to sexual stimulation when the male penis becomes erect and hard as a result of blood filling the small vessels in the tissues of the penis.

erythrocytes
See **red blood cells**.

Escherichia coli (E. coli)
Bacteria that live in the large **intestine**. Most strains are harmless but problems arise if the bacteria are carried outside the human body, usually on **faeces**, and then contaminate **food** or water. Food or water contaminated with *E. coli* through failure to wash hands before handling food, or through sewage getting into the supply of drinking water, can cause serious **infections** such as gastro-enteritis or even dysentery.

essay
A written explanation, description or discussion that demonstrates knowledge. It is important for an essay to have structure with an introduction, body of argument and a conclusion. An essay is usually undertaken by students.

essential nutrient
A nutrient which must be present in the diet and cannot be made from other raw materials by the body.

essential oils
The fragrant essences of plants, herbs, flowers, leaves, berries, fruits, bark, resin, seeds, wood, roots, grasses, etc. used in **aromatherapy**. They are extracted for therapeutic use and for their perfume. They are classified as top, middle and base notes. Top notes are light and fresh, middle notes provide the heart of a fragrance and base notes are rich and heavy in aroma.

ethics
Moral codes that **professionals** in **health** and **social care** must adhere to when working. Ethical working includes respecting the basic **values and principles** that underpin **practice**, but ethics also involves facing moral questions such as whether to prolong life against the wishes of a **terminally ill patient**, or the provision of painful or degrading **treatment** in order to prolong life rather than to bring about a cure. Research projects involving people usually have to be agreed by an ethics committee in order to make sure that there is no part of the research or experiments that can harm, exploit, disadvantage or degrade the people taking part. There are ethics committees for professional issues and in many **NHS Trusts**. Some hospitals are now employing people qualified in ethics to provide advice to medical staff in difficult situations.

ethnicity
The elements of **culture**, **religion**, language, appearance, traditions and heritage that define the **group** to which an individual can identify himself or herself as belonging.

ethnic minorities
A term previously used to describe **cultural** or **racial communities** of people who are living in a country where another cultural or racial group is in the majority. Minority cultures are an important part of the **diversity** of any **society**, but sometimes such communities are **marginalised** and **excluded** rather than **valued**. The term now used is **minority ethnic**.

euphoria
A state of extreme happiness and excitement. This may be as the result of joyful events or it may sometimes be the result of **mental health problems** that can cause a state of euphoria that is not related to real events.

European Convention on Human Rights
The European Convention of Human Rights passed by the Council of Europe in 1950, it identifies the rights that the Council believed everyone in Europe should have. The Convention is the basis of the Human Rights Act 1998 in the UK.

European Court of Human Rights
A court system set up in 1998 to deal with disputes relating to the European Convention on Human Rights. The courts can require countries that are

members of the **European Union** to change **laws** if they are judged to contravene **human rights**.
More information can be found at www.echr.coe.int/echr/

European Union (EU)
A political and economic union of 27 member states, including the UK. The EU consists of the following key bodies:
- the Council of Ministers – the political leaders of each of the member states
- the European **Parliament** – with members (MEPs) elected by each of the member states
- the European Commission – the executive or **civil service** that implements the decisions of the Council of Ministers and Parliament, issues **guidelines** and regulations, and runs the EU on a day-to-day basis.

euthanasia
The deliberate ending of a person's life, usually at his or her own request, and with the intention of following the person's best interests. It is **illegal** in the UK, although not in all countries. It may be requested when a person is **terminally ill** and in great pain and no longer wishes to continue life, or it may be requested by relatives of someone who has little or no **quality of life**, but has no ability to **communicate** his or her own wishes. It is an **ethical** issue and presents **moral** difficulties for many **professionals** in **health** and in **social care**.

evaluation
The **process** of gathering and **reviewing** evidence, then reaching a judgement. It can be carried out for **services**, **treatment** or **development programmes**, new **initiatives** or projects; or the **learning** or **performance** of individuals, **teams** or **organisations** against set **goals** and **targets**.

Every Child Matters (ECM)
The government programme to improve services for **children** in England. The programme identified five outcomes that must be achieved for children:
- be healthy
- stay safe
- enjoy and achieve
- make a positive contribution
- achieve economic well-being.

See **Children's Plan**.
More information can be found at www.everychildmatters.co.uk

eviction
The removal of a person or **family** from their home. This could be because of failure to maintain **rent** or mortgage payments, because of **anti-social behaviour**, or because the owner of the property wants it to be vacated.

evidence
Proof, or confirmation, that events or actions have taken place or that something is known or understood. In the legal system this is something that is provided to the courts to establish the guilt, or innocence, of an accused person, and can be provided by witnesses, forensic evidence, documents or objects. In learning, it is the confirmation that performance, knowledge and understanding is in place at the level required. Evidence can be provided by witnesses, through direct observation or through written documents.

examination
A check carried out by a **doctor** or other **health professional** to assist with **diagnosis**. In education, an examination is a test of knowledge through written or **oral questioning**.

exclusion
The process of someone becoming isolated from society as a result of barriers to participation not being challenged and overcome.

excretion
Removal of the waste products of **metabolism** from the body, such as **carbon dioxide** from the **lungs**; **urea**, water and salts through the **kidneys** and urinary system.

exercise
Physical activity that requires **energy**, uses **muscles** and raises the **heart** and **breathing** rate. This is beneficial for the human body and **promotes** good **health**.

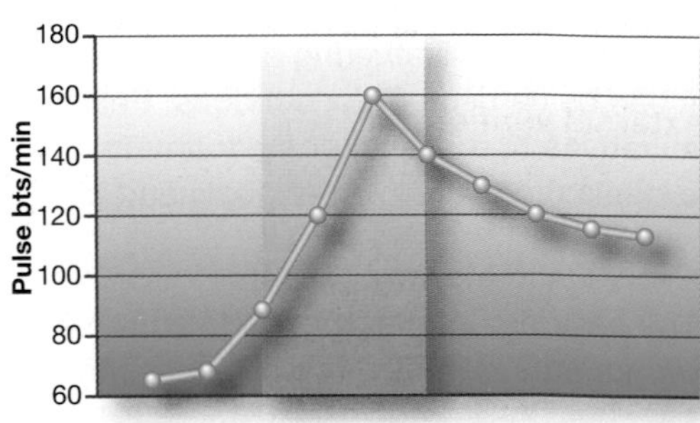

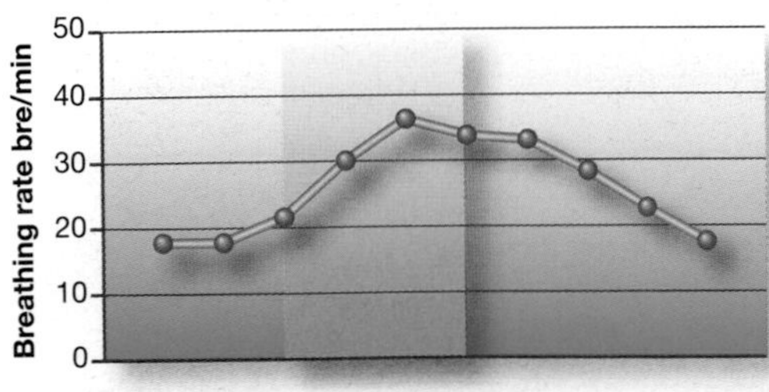

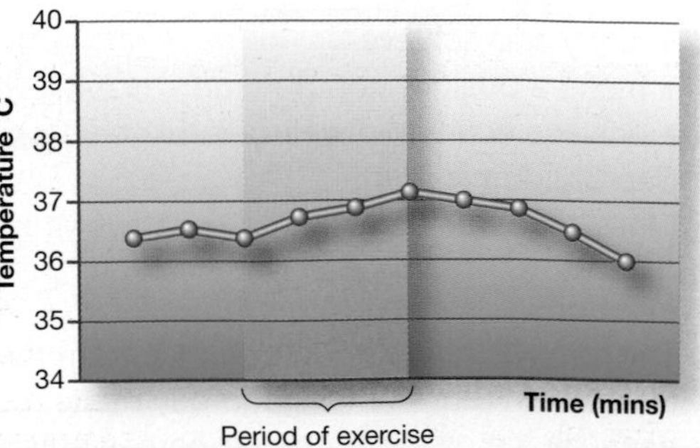

How pulse, breathing rates and body temperature vary with exercise.

expectations
With regard to behaviour refers to agreed boundaries of behaviour in a range of social contexts and in relation to different activities in which the individual may engage. Boundaries may include statutory requirements and limitations.

expenditure
Spending to cover costs and payments. Individuals and **organisations** try to balance expenditure with **income.**

experiment
A test of something new, or a new procedure, where the **outcome** is not known beforehand.

expertise
Skill and ability in a particular area of **practice**.

exploitative behaviour
Behaviour that deliberately takes advantage of another person who may be a more vulnerable adult, or a child.

extended family
The wider network of relatives (cousins, aunties, uncles, grandparents) who may have a key role in the care and support of family members. The role of the extended family varies between cultural groups.

external verifier
A person who carries out checks on the quality of the assessment of **S/NVQs** and other **vocational qualifications** on behalf of the awarding bodies.

eye contact
Where people in an **interaction** look each other in the eye. This is an important part of **non-verbal communication**, because looking directly at the person speaking is an essential way to show interest and concern. Eyes also show the emotions someone is feeling, so looking into a person's eyes can provide **information** about real **feelings**, regardless of what may be said.

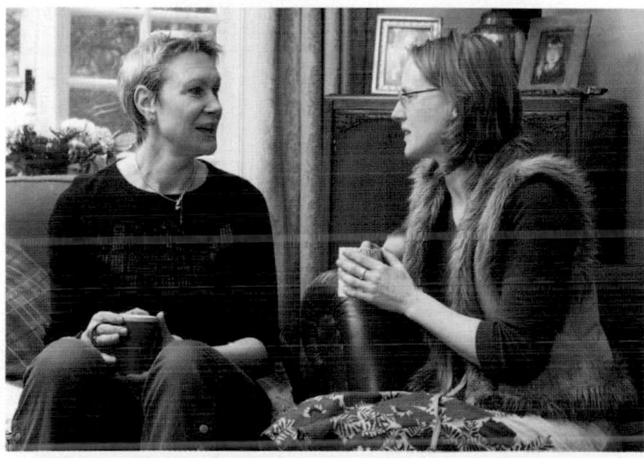

Eye contact is an important part of non-verbal communication.

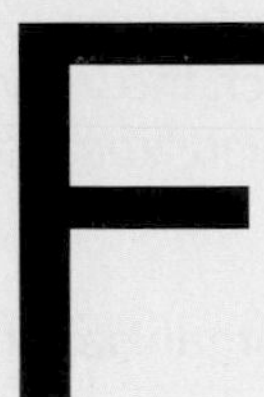

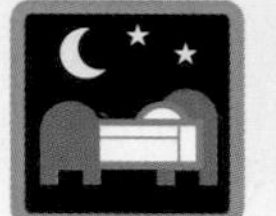
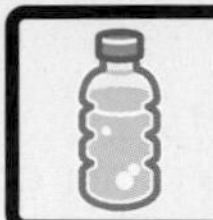

facial expression

The way all the different part of the face appear; a clear indicator of the way someone is feeling. Facial expression is one of the most important aspects of **non-verbal communication**. It is possible to judge how someone is feeling, and whether he or she is receptive to **communication**, by looking at the face. It is so easy to express **feelings** by facial expressions that everyone recognises even very simple, basic drawings of them, such as those used in electronic messages to share feelings.

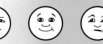

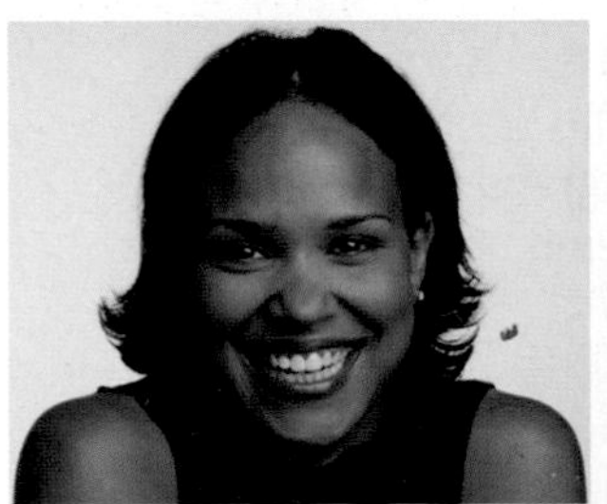
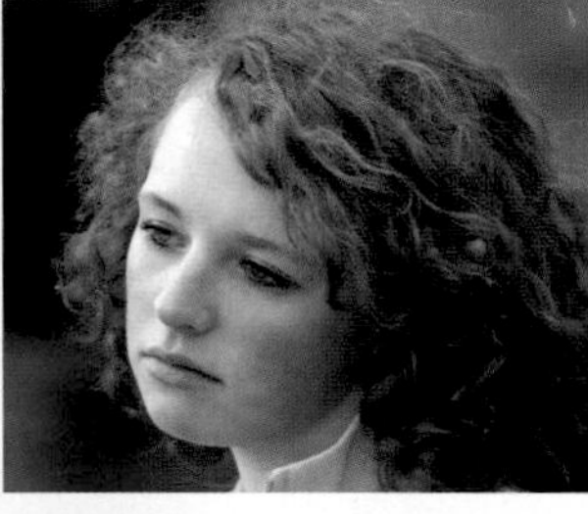
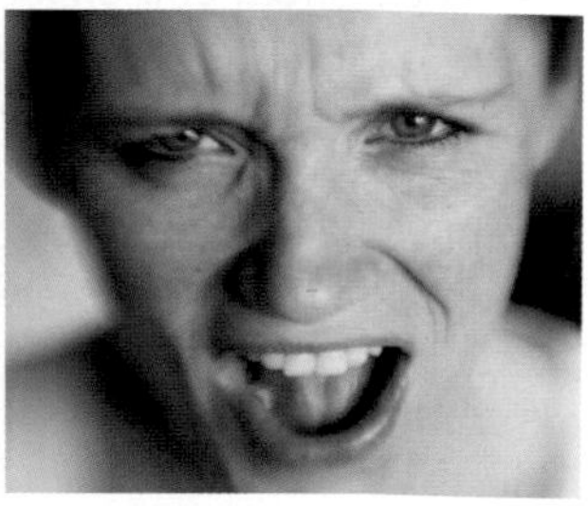
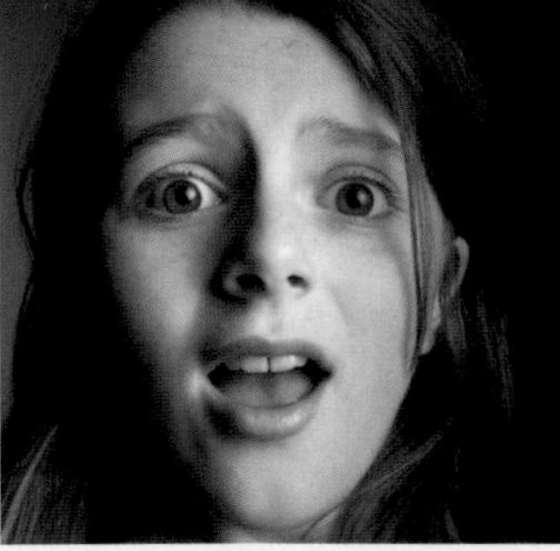

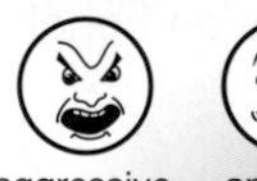
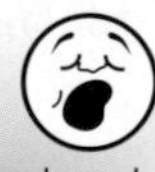
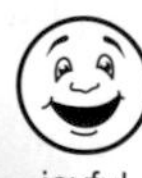
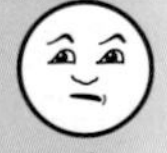
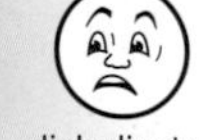
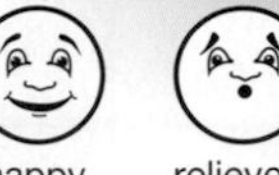
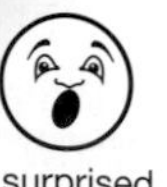

Facial expressions can say many things.

facilities

Places, **provision** or **equipment** that people need or want to **access** for **support**, **services**, **treatment**, enjoyment, **work**, **education**, **leisure** or **relaxation**. This can include anything from libraries to cinemas or from **Internet** cafés to hairdressers.

factor
Something that contributes to, or affects, something else.

facts
Things which are known to be true or can be proved to be correct.

faecal incontinence
The inability to control when faeces are expelled from the anus. This can result from injury, neurological disease or dementia.

faeces
Bodily waste remaining from the **digestive process**, passed from the body through the **anus**.

failure to thrive
A condition where a **baby** or child is not developing at the expected rate given the **genetic** make-up of the **family**. This can be the result of:

- **physical illness** or **allergy** – **food** may not be absorbed, or may be rejected by the child's body
- incorrect **feeding** – the child may not be provided with adequate or appropriate foods
- **environmental factors** – the **carers** may not understand the need to provide love, warmth, affection and stimulation in order to **promote** growth and development.

fallopian tube
Part of the female **reproductive system** that links the **ovaries** and the **uterus**. An egg will emerge from the ovary and move down the fallopian tube towards the uterus where it will either **implant** if it has been **fertilised** or be discarded along with the uterus lining during **menstruation**.

family
Kinship **groups** across generations, which people define through **genetic** or **blood** ties, legal steps (marriage, **adoption** or civil partnership) or simply by **choice**. The role of the family varies in different **cultures**, but it is the legal and social structure for bringing up children in the UK and the developed world, as opposed to a few cultures where children are the **responsibility** of a whole **community**. Families can take different forms and have different structures – *see* **nuclear family**, **re-constituted family** and **extended family**.

family courts
Courts that deal with all **family**-related issues including:

- **adoption**
- **divorce**
- custody of children
- contact and **access** arrangements for children.

The proceedings of these courts are heard in private; the press and public are not allowed access in order to protect the identities of the children involved.

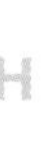

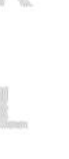

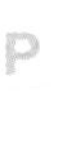
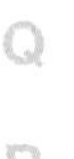
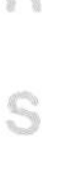

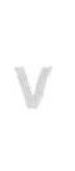

Family Planning
Provides sexual and reproductive health information including **contraception** to avoid unplanned **pregnancies**. Access to family planning advice and contraception can be through **GPs** or through **family planning clinics** (both NHS and private). More information can be found at www.familyplanning.org.uk

Family Planning clinics
Clinics offering contraceptive and sexual health advice and treatment. Family planning services are available through voluntary organisations such as the Family Planning Association and Brook Advisory Centres, or through GPs and Health Centres.

fats
Also known as **lipids**, fats provide **energy**, protection for vital **organs** and heat insulation for the body. They enable the absorption of **vitamins** A, D, E and K which are not **soluble** in water, but are soluble in fats. An excess of fatty layers in the body can be a contributing factor in several **diseases** such as type 2 **diabetes**, **heart disease**, osteo-**arthritis** and **stroke**.

fear
A natural response to **threat** or danger. The body will prepare for 'fight or flight' by increasing the supply of the **hormone adrenaline**, increasing **heart** and **breathing** rate and possibly sweating. Sometimes fears can become out of control to the extent where a **phobia** develops, which can interfere with people's day-to-day lives.

Have there been any changes in your health since the last report? If so, please say what.	*Not really - much the same*
Have there been any changes in your circumstances since the last report? If so, please say what.	*My sister has come to live a few streets away*
Are the services you receive still giving the support you need?	*Yes, still very good, but don't need day centre on Thursdays now as my sister takes me out every Thursday*
How would you like the services to change what you receive?	*Cancel Thursday at the day centre, but everything else is fine*

A feedback form from an individual in care.

feed
Nutritional or fluid intake prescribed or ordered for an individual by a professional, such as a dietician, nurse or doctor, e.g. PEG feeding.

feedback
Views and opinions given about **performance**, quality or effectiveness. Ideally feedback should be constructive and offer suggestions about how to improve. As part of **reflective practice**, **health** and **social care professionals** need to seek feedback from managers, colleagues and people who use their **services**.

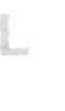

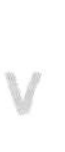

feeding (PEG)
Providing **food** for **babies**, or **supporting percutaneous endoscopic gastrostomy** (PEG feeding) through a tube directly into the **stomach**. Older children, **young people** or adults who are conscious and taking food by mouth may need assistance to eat, but the term 'feeding', which implies that they do not have an active role, is not appropriate in these cases.

feelings
Emotions and their effect on mood, **well-being** and responses to events and other people. They include sadness, despair, joy, delight, happiness, anger, rage and jealousy. Feelings influence behaviour.

female reproductive system
See **reproductive systems**.

feminist
Modern term for someone who campaigns for women to be treated equally with men in all aspects of life. Historically, women campaigning for the vote in the UK were called 'suffragists'; those who took militant action and broke the **law** were called 'suffragettes'. A feminist approach recognises the continued power inbalances in society that favour men.

fertilisation
The **process** of a **sperm** penetrating the outer membrane of an egg (ovum) and its nucleus, fusing with the **nucleus** of the egg to form a **zygote**. As the zygote moves down the **fallopian tube** towards the **uterus**, it divides into two, then doubles, then doubles again so that by the time it **implants** in the uterus it is a **group** of **cells** called an **embryo**.

fertility rate
The number of live **births** in a specific **population** divided by the number of women of childbearing age (15–49 years) in that population. See **birth rate**.

fever
A condition, usually as the result of an **infection**, involving a high **temperature** and sometimes delirium.

fibre
Also known as **roughage**, fibre is found in vegetables and fruits and is an important part of a healthy diet. Fibre is not digested but assists the digestive process by adding bulk as food moves through the system.

financial abuse
The exploitation of a vulnerable person by dishonestly obtaining money, **property** or **resources** from the person through deception or **threats.**

fine motor skills
Control of the smaller muscles, such as those in the fingers (e.g. holding a pencil). These skills are more difficult to acquire than gross motor skills and develop later.

fire exit
A special door to be used in emergencies such as fire. It is an outward-opening door with an easy-to-open crash bar and exit signs leading to it. Fire exits should never be blocked or jammed open. Also known as emergency exit.

fire extinguisher
A portable, manually operated container filled with carbon dioxide, foam, dry powder or water that can be sprayed in a steady stream to put out a small fire. Each type has a coloured panel indicating the contents: black (carbon dioxide); cream (foam); blue (powder); and red (water).

Extinguisher type and patch colour	Use for	Danger points	How to use	How it works
Red Water	Wood, cloth, paper, plastics, coal, etc. Fires involving solids.	Do not use on burning fat or oil, or on electrical appliances.	Point the jet at the base of the flames and keep it moving across the area of the fire. Ensure that all areas of the fire are out.	Mainly by cooling burning material.
Blue Multi-purpose dry powder	Wood, cloth, paper, plastics, coal, etc. Fires involving solids. Liquids such as grease, fats, oil, paint, petrol, etc. but **not** on chip or fat pan fires.	Safe on live electrical equipment, although the fire may re-ignite because this type of extinguisher does not cool the fire very well. Do **not** use on chip or fat pan fires.	Point the jet or discharge horn at the base of the flames and, with a rapid sweeping motion, drive the fire towards the far edge until all the flames are out.	Knocks down flames and, on burning solids, melts to form a skin smothering the fire. Provides some cooling effect.
Blue Standard dry powder	Liquids such as grease, fats, oil, paint, petrol, etc. but **not** on chip or fat pan fires.	Safe on live electrical equipment, although does not penetrate the spaces in equipment easily and the fire may re-ignite. This type of extinguisher does not cool the fire very well. Do **not** use on chip or fat pan fires.	Point the jet or discharge horn at the base of the flames and, with a rapid sweeping motion, drive the fire towards the far edge until all the flames are out.	Knocks down flames.

Cream AFFF (Aqueous film-forming foam) (multi-purpose)	Wood, cloth, paper, plastics, coal, etc. Fires involving solids. Liquids such as grease, fats, oil, paint, petrol, etc. but **not** on chip or fat pan fires.	Do **not** use on chip or fat pan fires.	For fires involving solids, point the jet at the base of the flames and keep it moving across the area of the fire. Ensure that all areas of the fire are out. For fires involving liquids, do not aim the jet straight into the liquid. Where the liquid on fire is in a container, point the jet at the inside edge of the container or on a nearby surface above the burning liquid. Allow the foam to build up and flow across the liquid.	Forms a fire-extinguishing film on the surface of a burning liquid. Has a cooling action with a wider extinguishing application than water on solid combustible materials.
Cream Foam	Limited number of liquid fires.	Do **not** use on chip or fat pan fires. Check manufacturer's instructions for suitability of use on other fires involving liquids.	Do not aim jet straight into the liquid. Where the liquid on fire is in a container, point the jet at the inside edge of the container or on a nearby surface above the burning liquid. Allow the foam to build up and flow across the liquid.	
Black Carbon dioxide CO2	Liquids such as grease, fats, oil, paint, petrol, etc. but **not** on chip or fat pan fires.	Do **not** use on chip or fat pan fires. This type of extinguisher does not cool the fire very well. Fumes from CO2 extinguishers can be harmful if used in confined spaces: ventilate the area as soon as the fire has been controlled.	Direct the discharge horn at the base of the flames and keep the jet moving across the area of the fire.	Vaporising liquid gas smothers the flames by displacing oxygen in the air.
Fire blanket	Fires involving both solids and liquids. Particularly good for small fires in clothing and for chip and fat pan fires provided the blanket **completely** covers the fire.	If the blanket does not completely cover the fire, it will not be extinguished.	Place carefully over the fire. Keep your hands shielded from the fire. Take care not to waft the fire towards you.	Smothers the fire.

Types of fire extinguishers.

fire safety

Precautionary steps that can reduce risks in the event of a fire, such as:

- knowing how to raise the alarm
- knowing what the fire alarm sounds like
- practising ways to leave the building safely
- if the fire can be tackled safely, knowing which extinguisher to use
- knowing how to safely evacuate all those in your care
- keeping up to date with fire safety procedures and fire precautions.

A B C D E **F** G H I J K L M N O P Q R S T U V W XYZ

first aid
Initial **treatment** for a person who has had an **accident** or is suffering an acute condition. Its purpose is to preserve life and to minimise the consequences of the accident or condition. Many people undertake training in first aid and every **workplace** is required to have a trained first aider in place. First aid should only be attempted by people trained to do so, as it is possible to cause further **harm** through incorrect treatment. Those who are not trained in first aid but who are present at a medical emergency should ensure the casualty is not at risk of any further **injury**, raise the alarm, contact the **emergency services** immediately and provide calm reassurance to the casualty until help arrives.

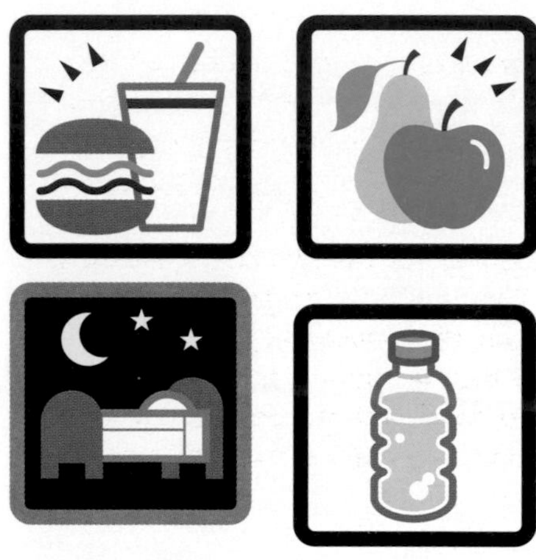

Flash cards can help people with speech difficulties to communicate.

flash cards
Cards used to **communicate** with people who have difficulty using speech. Pictures on the cards can be used to convey simple messages.

fluid balance chart
A **record** of the volume of fluid taken into a person's body, either by mouth or **intravenously**, and the volume of fluid **lost in urine** or **vomit**.

fluoride
A chemical with proven positive effects in reducing tooth decay in children. It is added to the water supply in some areas, and water companies must fluoridate the water if asked to do by the **strategic health authority**, the Scottish **Parliament** or the Welsh Assembly.

focus group
A **group** formed for a specific purpose, usually to produce views, opinions or **feedback** on particular topics.

foetal alcohol syndrome (FAS)
A condition in **newborn babies** that results from excessive alcohol consumption by the **mother** during **pregnancy**. The visible characteristics of foetal alcohol syndrome are:
- low **birth** weight
- small head circumference
- small eye openings
- smooth, wide philtrum (the groove between nose and upper lip)
- thin upper lip.

Babies with FAS can also be irritable, have trouble eating and **sleeping**, are sensitive to sensory stimulation, and have a strong startle **reflex**. Some **infants** may have **heart** defects or suffer abnormalities of the ears, eyes, **liver** or **joints**.

foetal development
Babies take anywhere from 37 to 43 weeks from the time of **fertilisation** to reach full maturity and **birth**. Any birth before 37 weeks is regarded as **premature**. Advances in medicine mean that some babies can survive from 24 weeks' gestation.

- 0–14 weeks: development is from a fertilised egg (**zygote**) to a collection of around 100 **cells** that **implants** into the uterus wall (**embryo**). During the first few weeks the cells continue to divide and **organs**, limbs, **brain**, **heart** and spine continue to develop. By about 8 weeks the **foetus** is about 20 mm long, about the size of a baked bean. By 14 weeks all the organs are formed and require only time to reach maturity, and the foetus is about 60–85 mm long.
- 14–22 weeks: the foetus grows rapidly. Hair, nails, eyebrows and eyelashes develop and fingerprints are fully formed. The foetus will begin to move around and this can be felt by the **mother** from about 18–20 weeks.
- 22–40 weeks: the foetus continues to grow and develops a fat layer under the **skin**; the eyes open and organs mature. The heartbeat can be heard using a **stethoscope**. By about 36 weeks, the foetus has usually turned to lie head downwards in the **uterus** ready for birth.

foetus
An unborn **baby** while it is growing and developing in the **uterus**. After about 7–8 weeks, the embryo is called a foetus.

folic acid
A vitamin that belongs to the B group of vitamins. Very important for the development of a healthy foetus. Women planning to become pregnant are advised to take folic acid prior to becoming pregnant, and then for the first twelve weeks of pregnancy.

follicle
A small cavity (space), sac (pouch) or gland in the skin, generally having a secretory (discharging a substance) function. Examples include hair follicles, ovarian follicles, lymph follicles and thyroid follicles.

follicle stimulating hormone (FSH)
A hormone secreted (released) by the anterior pituitary gland that promotes the formation of ova (eggs) in the female and spermatoza in the male.

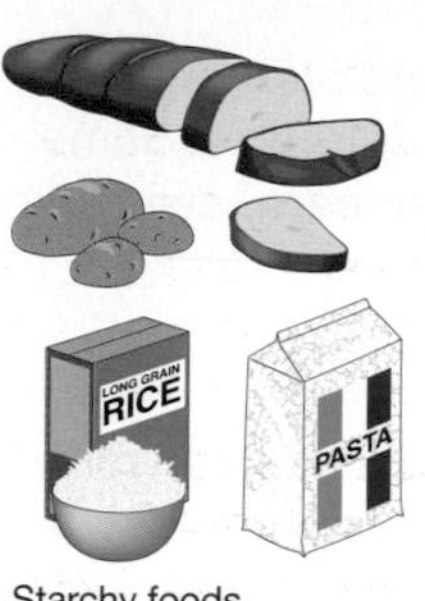

Starchy foods

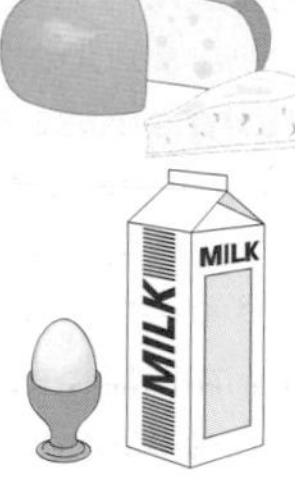

Dairy products

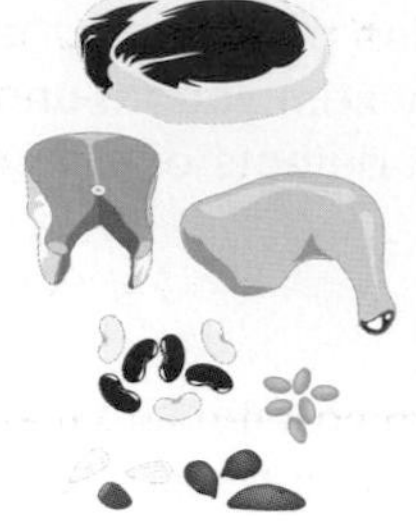
Meat, poultry, fish and alternatives

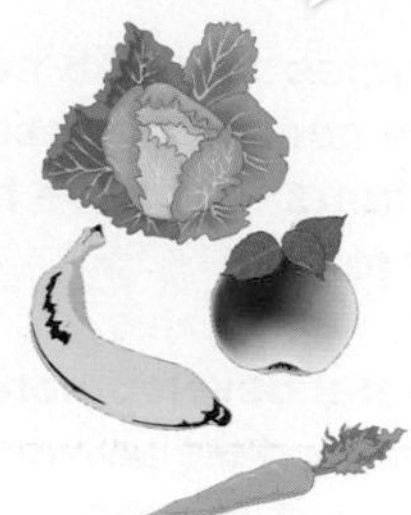
Vegetables and fruit

The four main food groups.

food
Substances that are essential for the **health** and survival of the human body. These are eaten and processed into forms that can be absorbed and used by the body through the **process** of **digestion**. *See* **diet**.

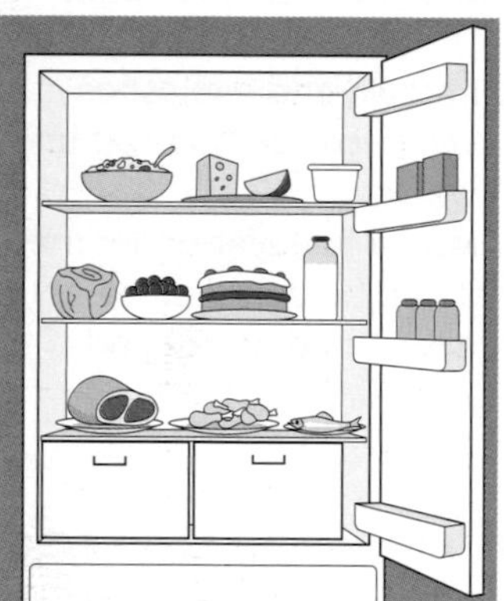
Food must be stored correctly and use-by dates must be adhered to.

food hygiene
The **process** of ensuring that **food** is not contaminated by **bacteria** and that all storage **facilities**, utensils, surfaces and preparation areas are kept clean and follow the required procedures. People who prepare food must also follow strict **guidelines** in order to maintain their **personal hygiene** and cleanliness.

food poisoning
Illness caused through eating **food** contaminated by **bacteria**, other organisms or chemicals. Depending on the bacteria, the consequences can be simply unpleasant, and include **vomiting**, **diarrhoea** and abdominal pain, or can be extremely serious and lead to **dehydration**, **fever**, **unconsciousness** and even **death**. See **Clostridium difficile** and **salmonella**.

forceps
Surgical instrument used for lifting, dissecting or compressing. May be used to assist the birth of a baby.

forum
A meeting or series of meetings that gives the opportunity for people to ask questions, find out **information** and share views and opinions with experts or **accountable** people.

fostering
A way of caring for children and **young people** who are looked after by a **local authority**, where children are cared for in the **family** home of adults who have been

selected and trained, and who are paid an allowance. This approach is favoured for many children who are in the looked-after **system** as it offers an opportunity to experience family life. However, it is not right for all children and some, particularly older children, are more comfortable in a residential setting with other young people. The legal **status** and role of the foster **carer** is always that of a temporary carer, and no **parental responsibilities** for the child are transferred to the foster carer. Some foster carers will work with children and their birth families to enable them to return home, and others will provide long-term foster care until young people are able to become **independent**. Some family arrangements are known as private fostering: the Government want these to be regulated for the well-being of the children concerned.

fracture
A broken or cracked **bone**, usually **diagnosed** by **X-ray**. Broken bones are normally supported by a plaster cast or splint while they heal, but some fractures may require the bone to be fixed in placed with titanium plates, screws and pins.

free play
A form of **play** where there is no direction from adults, and children are able to devise and direct their own activities. The role of adults is to ensure **safety** and to **support** children's play through the **provision** of **equipment** and **resources**, but not to intervene or direct children's activities. This is the ethos of **playworkers**.

Freud, Sigmund (1856–1939)
A **psychologist** who developed a new approach to understanding human behaviour. He was the creator of psychoanalysis, and developed the theory that humans have an unconscious mind where sexual and aggressive impulses are controlled by defences which are stronger in some people than in others. He was convinced that experiences of early childhood were the key to adult behaviour. He is widely regarded as one of the most significant contributors to understanding human behaviour, but there are varying views about the validity of his theories.

funding
The **process** of financing **service provision** for **health** and **social care**. Some finance is from central **government** programmes, some from **local authorities**, and some from the **charitable** and **voluntary sector**. The process depends on the nature of the service and the source of finance. Sometimes there will be an allocation or grant, and at other times a bid or proposal will have to be submitted to the funding body.

fungus
A type of simple organism including yeast, moulds and mushrooms. Certain types of fungi are responsible for infections that may occur anywhere on the body. They usually affect the skin because they live on keratin, the protein that makes up **skin**, hair and nails.

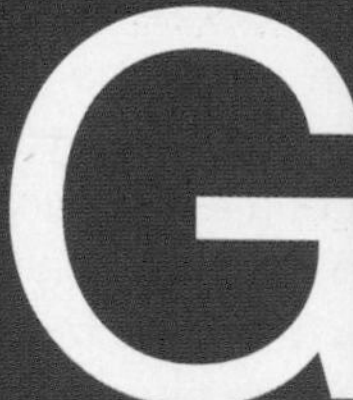

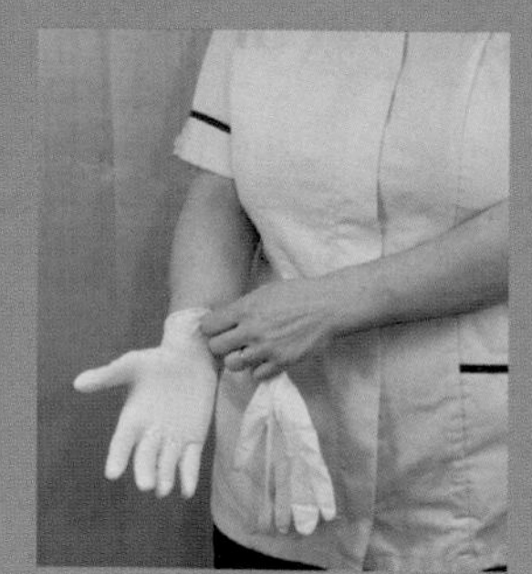

gall bladder

An organ that stores bile and concentrates bile and is part of the **digestive system**. Hard particles, or balls, can form within the gall bladder; these are gall stones. **Bile** is released under hormonal influence into the duodenum.

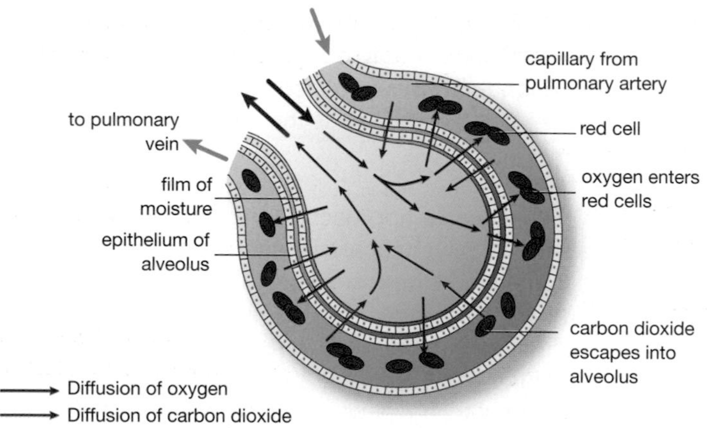

■ Gaseous exchange in the alveolus.

gaseous exchange

The **process** that takes place during **respiration**. The **lungs** fill with **oxygenated** air through breathing in, and **oxygen** enters the bloodstream by being absorbed through the walls of the lungs. **Carbon dioxide** passes in the reverse direction from the **blood** into the lungs and is expelled from the body by breathing out. Both these gases are dissolved in water and pass by diffusion.

gastric juices

A digestive juice produced in the **stomach** by gastric glands. The **enzymes** contained in gastric juices break down **protein** and clot milk **food** into a paste to be released into the duodenum at intervals.

A B C D E F G H I J K L M N O P Q R S T U V W XYZ

gay
Homosexual. The term can be used to describe an individual or a **community**.

gender
The social definition of the biological terms male or female.

gender stereotypes
Assumptions about how people will act and what they will do based on whether they are male or female. **Stereotypes** are based on traditional roles and portray men as being strong, unemotional, better able to undertake physical tasks and more **intelligent**; women are portrayed as caring, nurturing, in need of protection and better at domestic tasks. Stereotyping is still common in expectations about job roles; for example, nursing and childcare are still seen as 'feminine' occupations, and road building and engineering are still considered 'male' jobs.

gene therapy
A controversial way of treating **disease** by changing a person's **genes** through the introduction of alternative **DNA** in order to replace, change, or add to a gene that is causing disease by not functioning correctly, or because it is missing. This is a new way of treating some diseases and is still in its infancy.

general practitioner (GP)
A **doctor** working in the local **community** and based in a **health centre** or **surgery**. GPs deliver primary care and are responsible for initial **diagnosis** and **treatment**, or **referral** to a specialist.

General Medical Council (GMC)
The regulator of medical practitioners in the UK. The GMC is responsible for the code of conduct and maintaining the register of those suitable qualified to practise medicine.

General Social Care Council
The **regulator** of **social work** and **social care** in England. The council is responsible for a code of conduct and maintains the register of those suitably qualified to practise in social work and social care.
More information can be found at www.gscc.org.uk

genes
The part of the **DNA** that contains the pattern for every individual, which is **inherited** by each **generation**. There are millions of genes in human **chromosomes** and each influence different characteristics of growth, development and appearance.

genetic counselling
Advice, guidance and **information** given where there is the potential for couples to conceive a child who will be affected by a **genetic disorder**.

genetic disorder
A disorder present at **birth** as the result of **chromosome**-related abnormalities. This can include damaged chromosomes, the wrong number of chromosomes and defective, abnormal or faulty genes. **Down's syndrome** is a genetic disorder where there is an extra chromosome. **Haemophilia** is a genetic disorder resulting from defective genes.

genetics
Research into and study of **genes** and **inheritance**.

geriatric medicine
The specialist area of medicine working with illnesses and **diseases** affecting **older people**.

gestation
The period of growth and development from fertilisation of the ovum until birth.

gestures
Movements and changes of position of parts of the body, particularly hands and arms. They are an important part of **non-verbal communication**.

girth
The **measurement** around the middle of someone's body, approximately the waist.

glands
Two different types of **organs**, both providing substances needed by the **processes** of the human body. **Endocrine** glands produce **hormones** that pass directly into the bloodstream through **blood** vessels in the glands. Exocrine glands provide substances such as juices directly into body **systems** through tubes or ducts.

glaucoma
Common cause of blindness in older people caused by increased pressure of the fluid inside the eyeball.

global warming
The gradual increase in the surface **temperature** of the earth. This has the potential to be disastrous for large parts of the planet as melting ice causes sea levels to rise in some areas, and higher temperatures result in deserts forming in others. It is likely that this warming is being caused by human activity and is particularly associated with a rise in carbon dioxide levels in the atmosphere.

gloves

Gloves are disposable and should always be worn when undertaking any **personal care** or clinical activity and should be thrown away after use for one activity only.

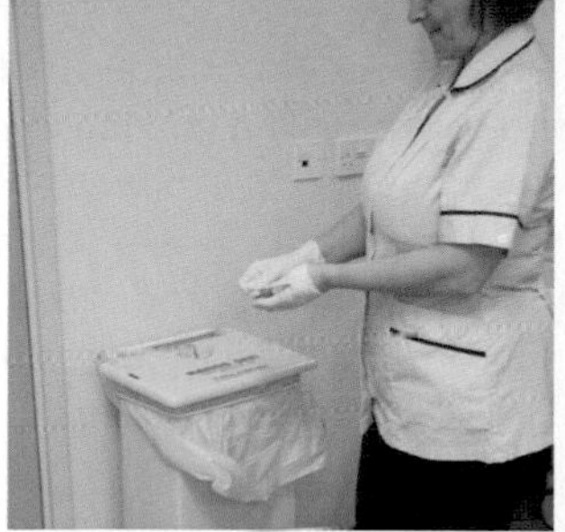
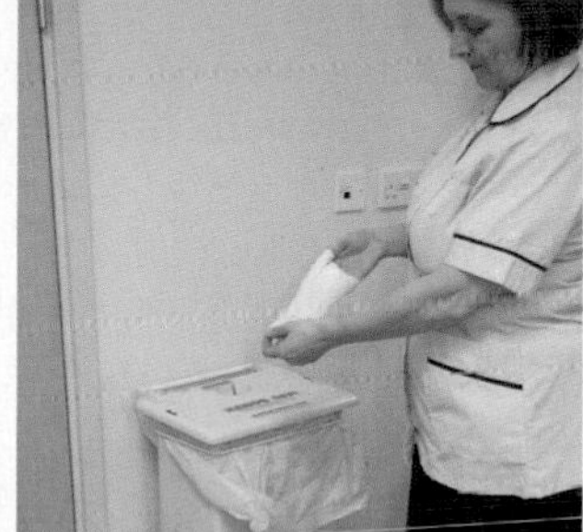
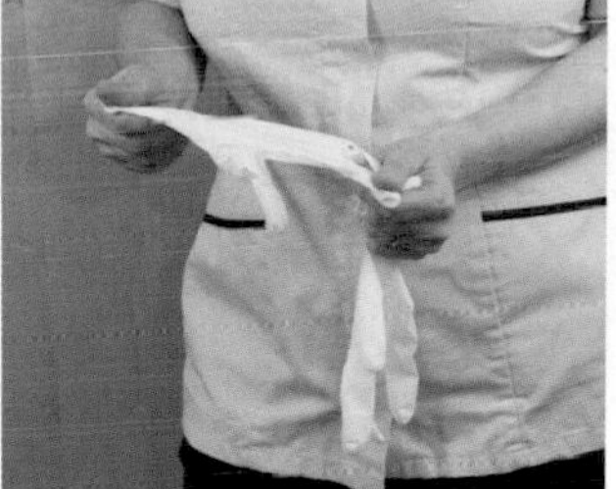
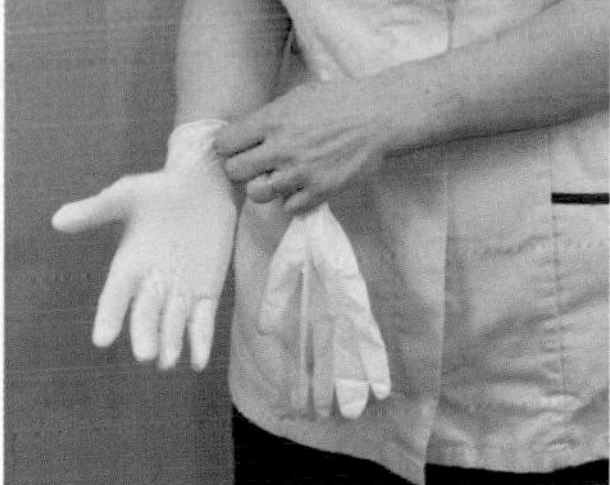
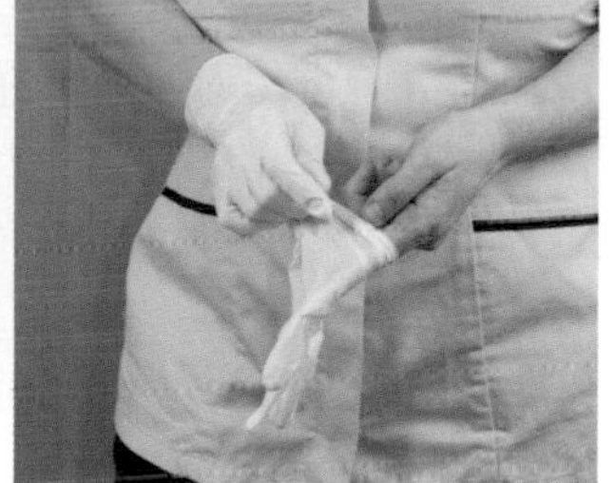

Disposable gloves.

glucose

A simple carbohydrate found in blood. Also an end product of carbohydrate digestion in the alimentary canal which is absorbed in the ileum and carried to the liver. Is also a component of blood plasma available for cells tissue in respiration to produce energy for work.

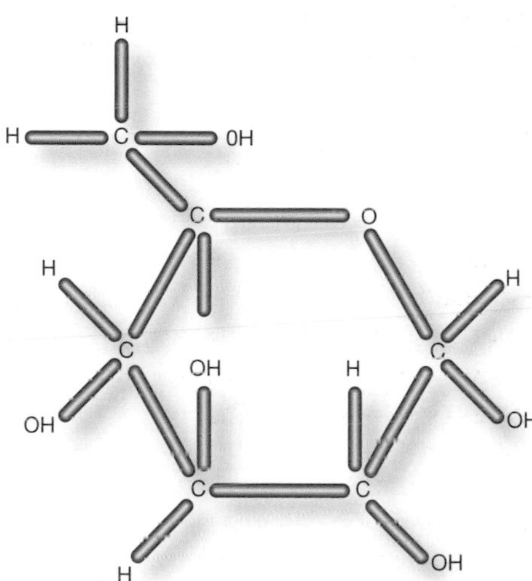

$C_6 H_{12} O_6$

Note the position of the single oxygen atom and the 'extra' C atom added on.

The structure of glucose.

glycogen

Glucose is stored in liver and muscles by conversion into a complex carbohydrate called glycogen. Liver glycogen can be converted back to glucose in times of need by the hormones glucagon and adrenaline. Muscle glycogen tends to be used by muscles for energy.

glycolysis

Reactions within **cells** that provide **energy**. **Glucose** (sugar) is taken up by the cells and broken down in respiration to produce energy in a form the body can use.

goal
A **target** that is set as part of a plan for development. Goals and targets are important as they maintain **motivation** and give people a chance to reflect on their own **practice**.

gonads
Name for both **reproductive organs**. Male reproductive organs are the **testes** and female are the **ovaries**. See **reproductive systems** for diagram.

gonorrhoea
A **sexually transmitted infection**, passed on by sexual contact. It is among the most common sexually transmitted **diseases** in the UK. **Symptoms** are painful urination and a yellow discharge from the **urethra**. **Treatment** is with antibiotics, and it can be prevented by practising safe sex and using a condom.

governance
The arrangements for how an organisation is run and exactly how decisions are made and what people are accountable for.

government
The **administration**, **law**, control, direction and regulation of **society**, and the collection of bodies such as ministries that are responsible for providing these.

graph
A visual **presentation** of **data**, which can be drawn as lines, or using blocks, or as circles – the latter are called '**pie charts**'.

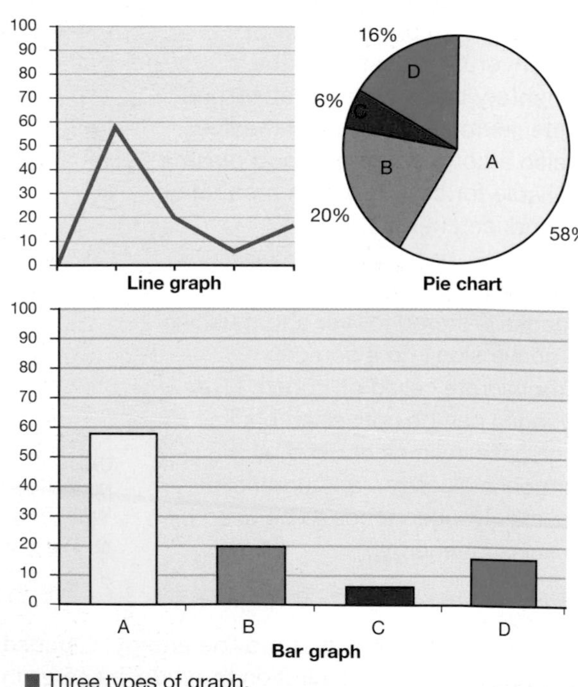

■ Three types of graph.

Green Paper
A government document setting out ideas regarding policy or proposals in a particular area. Successful discussion may progress it to a White Paper.

grief
The normal **reaction** to **bereavement** or loss. Everyone reacts differently and copes with grief in their own way. People grieve over many

losses, not just when someone dies. People who lose a limb will grieve, as will some people who lose a job or a home. Grieving can continue for many years or can be forgotten in a matter of days or weeks.

grooming

Taking care of physical appearance and cleanliness, including that of the face, hair, clothes and shoes. *See* also **personal hygiene**. Also is when an adult paedophile prepares a potential child victim for abuse and exploitation by developing a relationship with them.

Teeth: Prevent bad breath by cleaning your teeth. Remember that smoking can make your breath smell. Drink plenty of water to help to keep your mouth fresh.

Hair: Keep hair neat and tidy. Tie long hair up away from your face. If a service user was confused they could pull your hair.

Clothes: Wear a clean uniform each day. Trousers are more practical for moving and handling. Wear a coat over your uniform when you travel to work.

Jewellery: Keep jewellery to a minimum. Necklaces and dangly earrings are very dangerous because they can get caught in things.

Hands: Keep your hands and nails clean. It is best not to wear rings because you may hurt the service users and germs can get underneath.

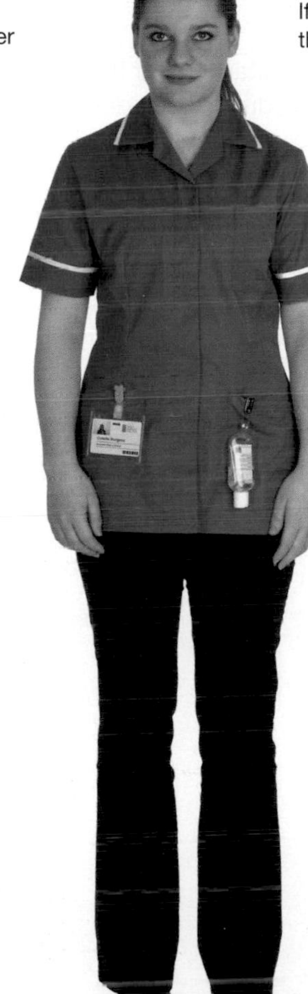

Feet: You can be on your feet for several hours. Make sure that you have well-fitting, comfortable, flat shoes that grip well.

■ Grooming.

gross motor skills
Control of the larger muscles, typically those in the arms and legs (e.g. kicking a ball). These skills develop before fine motor skills and are less sophisticated.

ground rules
General agreements on behaviour that are set at the beginning of a **group** or individual therapy or **support relationship**.

group
A number of people who are together. There may or may not be a shared interest, focus or purpose among the group. Behaviour in groups will usually follow a similar pattern.

growth hormone
A substance developed in the **pituitary gland** that controls the rate of growth of a child and the ultimate size of an adult. A lack of the hormone can mean children fail to grow at the expected rate, and an excess of it can lead to children growing exceptionally large or tall.

guardian *ad litem*
A court-appointed person (usually an experienced and qualified **social worker**) who is responsible for a child and **promoting** his or her interests during a period of **change** or **transition**.

guidelines
Policies or **procedures** that **support** the implementation and **practice** of **laws** or regulations.

gut
A common word for the alimentary canal.

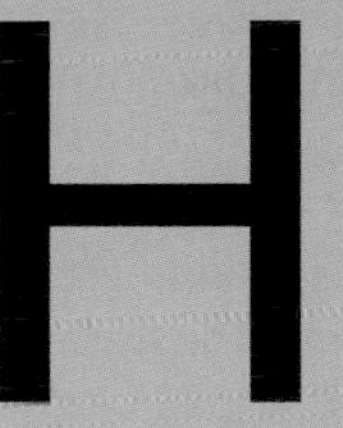

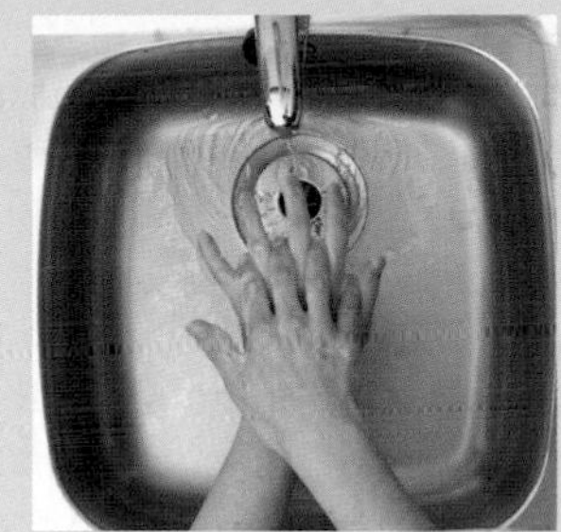

haematology
A medical specialism concerned with the **diagnosis** and **treatment** of **blood** disorders. Blood **samples** can provide significant amounts of **information** about an individual's **health** and the presence of **disease**.

haemoglobin
A respiratory pigment that contains iron, found in **red blood cells** (erythrocytes). It carries **oxygen** in the **blood** as oxyhaemoglobin, and can also combine instead with **carbon monoxide** if exposed to form carboxyhaemoglobin, a major poison for the **respiratory system**. The normal range of haemoglobin levels for a man are between 13.5–17.5 g/dl (grams per decilitre) and between 11.5–15.5 g/dl for a woman.

haemophilia
A **genetic disease**, usually found in males but passed on by females. Sufferers lack a clotting factor in the **blood**, so that any bleeding through **injury** or illness is very difficult to stop and can be life-threatening.

halal food
Food, especially meat, that has been slaughtered and prepared in a way acceptable to Islamic **laws**. This means that animals must be slaughtered by a Muslim in the correct way, and all **blood** must be drained. Pork is not permitted, and animals cannot be slaughtered in a place where pigs have been slaughtered.

hallucinations
Distorted or altered perceptions of reality. People suffering from hallucinations see images, feel emotions and hear sounds that do not exist except within their **consciousness**. Hallucinations can be the result of drug use, a psychotic mental illness or a **physical illness**.

hallucinogen
A drug that can cause people to have **hallucinations**. This includes drugs such as LSD (lysergic acid diethylamide) or 'magic' (psilocybe) mushrooms.

hand washing
Cleaning the hands with soap and water – an essential **hygiene** procedure to reduce the spread of **infection**. Studies have shown that hands are the single most important way in which infection is spread in **health** and **social care** settings. The way in which hands are washed is important in order to ensure that they are as clean as possible.

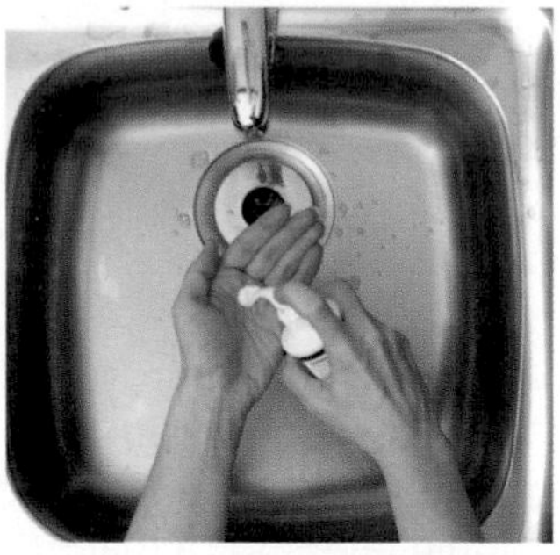

1 Wet hands and squirt liquid.

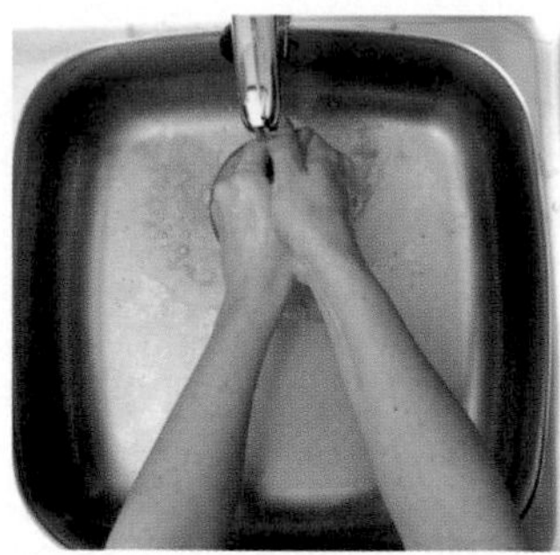

2 Rub hands together and make a lather.

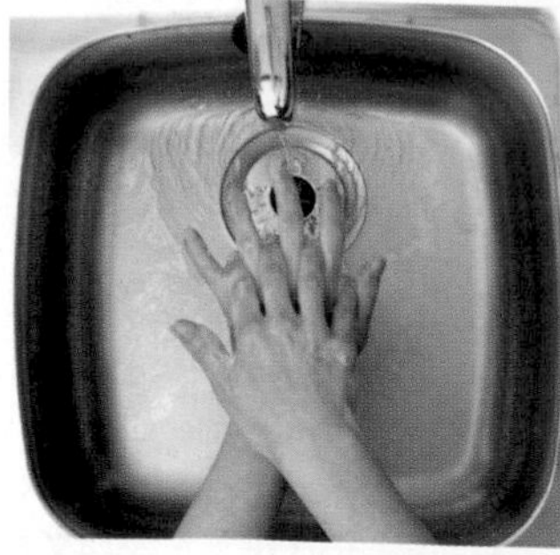

3 Rub palm of one hand along the back of the other.

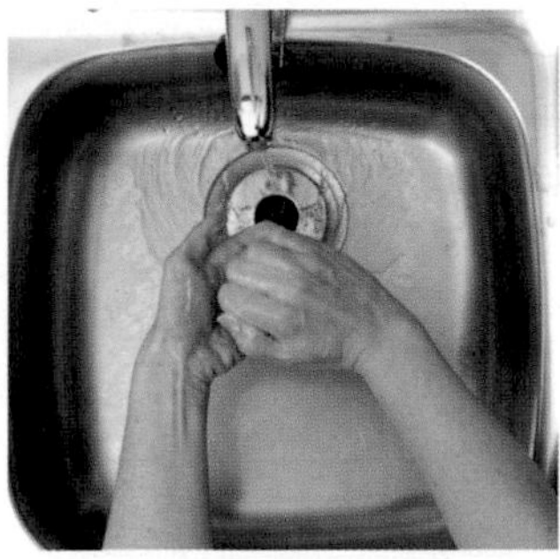

4 Rub in between your fingers and thumbs on both hands.

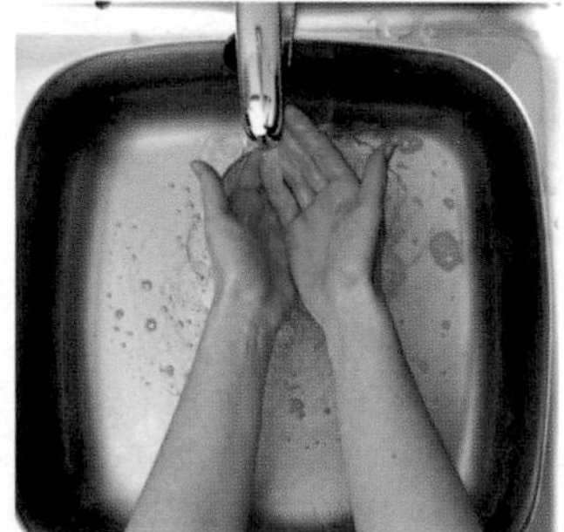

5 Rinse off soap with clean water.

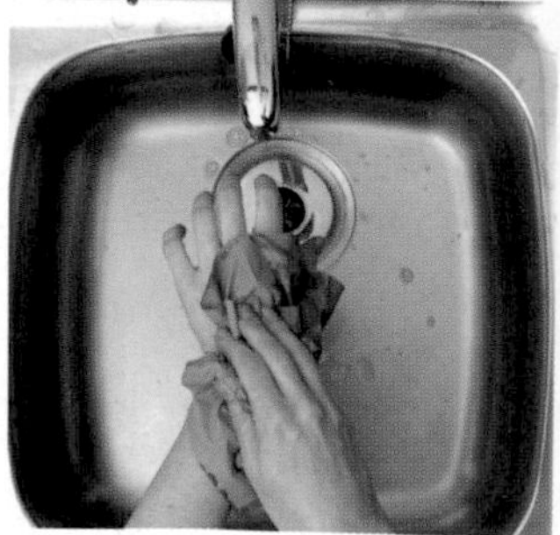

6 Dry hands thoroughly on a disposable towel.

Hand washing.

hand-eye co-ordination
A fine motor **skill** where the movement of the hands responds to a visual signal to the **brain**. This is an almost instantaneous response and enables people to carry out most day-to-day tasks. The speed of the response varies between individuals; for example, people who are very good at racquet sports will have exceptionally fast **reactions** and good hand–eye co-ordination.

handling belt
A belt that provides a means of **supporting** people who are unsteady when walking. The belt fits around the waist and has handles for the **carer** to hold to prevent falls or loss of balance.

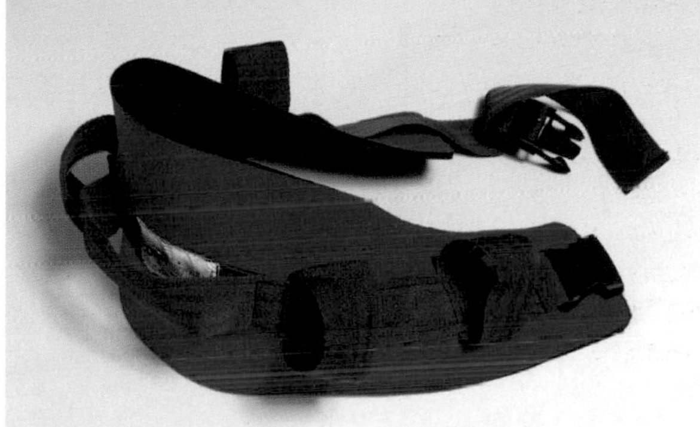
Handling belts prevent harm to the individual.

handouts
Notes given out to accompany **learning**. Handouts may be notes to accompany a **lecture**, a copy of a **presentation**, or related **information**.

harassment
Threatening, bullying or nuisance behaviour, which has a negative effect on the person it is directed against and continues after a request to stop. The unwanted behaviour can be physical or verbal.

harm
Physical or emotional damage as the result of a deliberate act, or **neglect** or **negligence**. **Health** and **social care professionals** have a duty to **safeguard** children and adults from harm.

Harvard referencing system
The most widely used method of **referencing** the books and **research** that are used to inform essays and other academic writing. The system, also known as author-date referencing, requires a short reference to the book or research to be used in the text by giving just the author's name and the date of publication. The full details, including name of author(s), title of the research or book, publisher and date are then shown either as a footnote at the bottom of the page or at the end of a piece of work, ordered alphabetically by authors' surnames. An example of an entry for a book is: Nolan, Y. (2008) NVQ Level 2 Health and Social Care (Revised edition), Oxford: Pearson Education.

hate crime
A criminal act, usually involving **violence** against people or **property**, where the **motivation** is **prejudice** and dislike of an individual or his or her **cultural**, **racial** or **religious** background or **sexual orientation**.

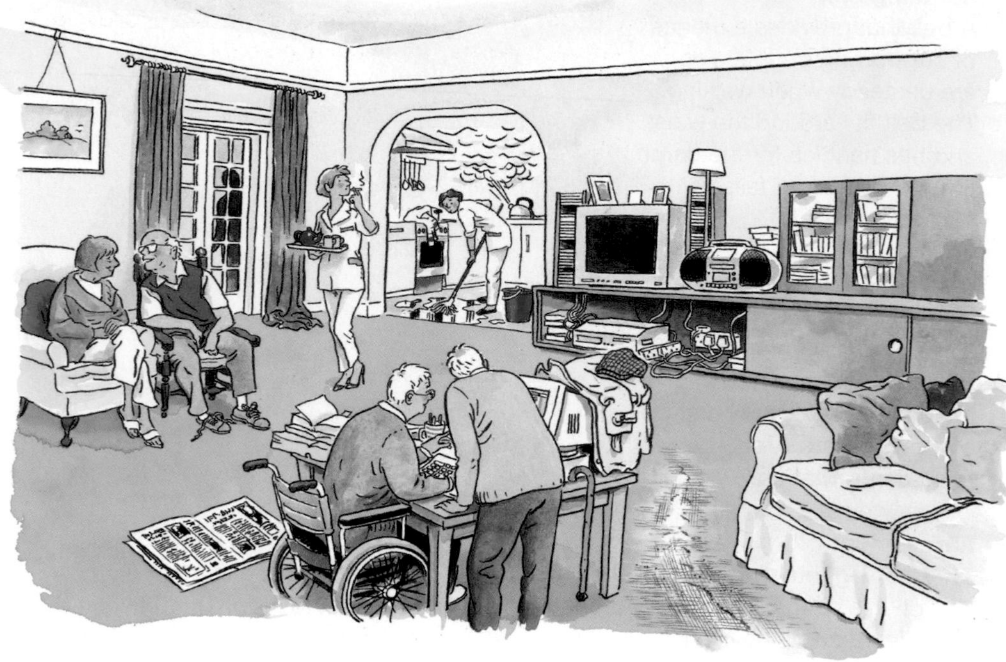

■ How many possible hazards and risks can you find in this picture?

hazard
Anything that has the potential to cause **harm**. It is important to identify hazards in the **workplace** and in a **health** or **social care environment**. Hazards could include where a floor has been mopped and is still wet or a rug with a worn edge that is curled up and easy to trip over.

hazardous waste
Waste that may present a risk to others. This includes body fluids such as **blood**, **urine**, **vomit** or **sputum**, and also **faeces**. Soiled **dressings**, bed linen and **protective clothing** can also be hazardous, as are all sharps such as **syringes**, **needles** and cannulae, tubes and **drips**. Hazardous waste must be collected and disposed of following strict regulations.

health
Defined by the **World Health Organization** in 1948 as a state of complete physical, mental and social **well-being**. This is a very positive definition and identifies health as much more than simply not being ill. The World Health Organization identifies clearly that the concept of health is also about feeling content and fulfilled, and about being confident and able to develop good relationships with others.

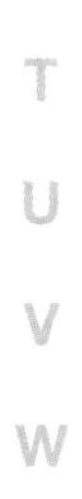

Health and Safety Executive (HSE)

The body responsible for ensuring that **health** and **safety** regulations are followed in nuclear installations, mines, factories, farms, **hospitals** and **schools**, offshore gas and oil installations, the gas supply grid and the movement of dangerous goods and substances. The HSE employs **inspectors** who visit **workplaces** and ensure that they comply with legal requirements. It also investigates any **accidents** or health and safety-related incidents.
More information can be found at www.hse.gov.uk

health authorities

See **strategic health authorities**

health benefits

The **services** provided free through the **National Health Service** for people on **low incomes**. These include eye care, dental care, **chiropody**, and **prescriptions** for **medication** and **vitamins**.

health care

Services provided through the **National Health Service**, either directly or **commissioned** from **providers** in the **private** or **voluntary sectors**. These include:

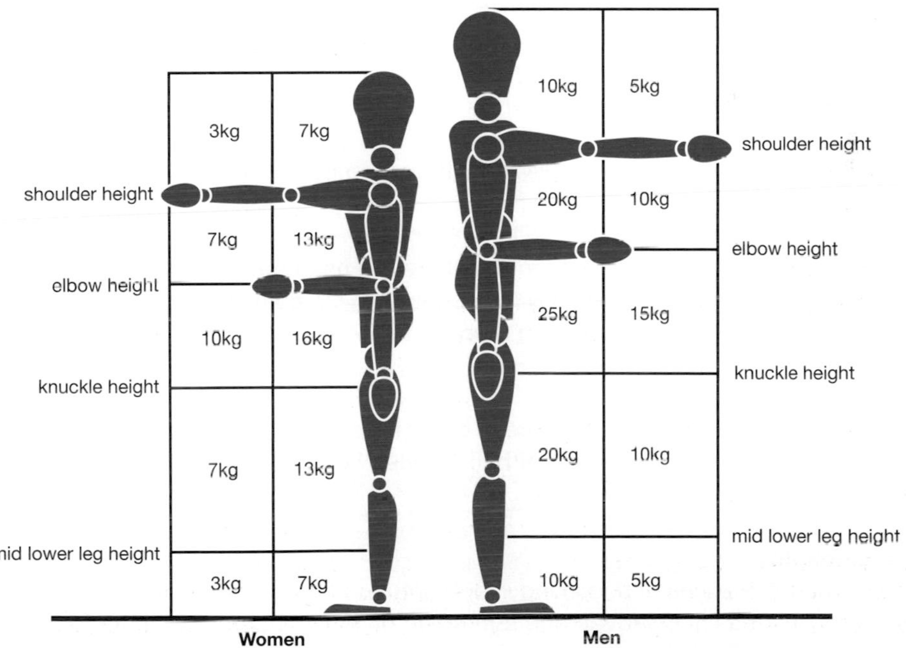

HSE guidelines about weights that can be lifted safely.

A B C D E F G H I J K L M N O P Q R S T U V W XYZ

- primary care – **health** services in the **community**, such as **midwifery**, community nursing, **GPs**, minor procedures, community **mental health services** for **adolescents** and adults, and **dentists**
- secondary care – health services in **hospitals**, including emergency and acute services, **chronic** services, outpatient **clinics** and day and in-patient **treatment**
- **tertiary care** – health services provided in specialist **resources**, such as **oncology** units, spinal injury rehabilitation units and **neurology** units. Most specialist units are regionally or even nationally based.

health care assistant
A **professional** who is trained and usually qualified to work with individuals receiving either health or care **services**. They provide a range of services, including **recording** body **measurements**, helping people to eat, assisting with **personal care**, **supporting** development activities and **promoting** health and **well-being**.

Healthcare Commission
An **independent** body set up by the Health and Social Care (Community Health and Standards) Act 2003 in order to **promote** and drive improvement in the quality of **health provision** in England (and some parts of provision in Wales). The commission inspects all **hospitals** for quality and value for money, and gives them an annual **performance** rating. It also undertakes in-depth studies on various aspects of **health care** and provides **information** for **patients** and the public. It also has a role in promoting improvements to health care **services**.
More information can be found at www.healthcarecommission.org.uk

health centre
A multi-**agency**, **community**-based facility where **teams** of **health professionals** are available under one roof. This may include **midwives**, community nurses, **occupational therapists**, **GPs**, **speech therapists** and **counsellors**.

health education
The provision of **information** and advice in order to raise awareness and encourage positive attitudes towards making **healthy lifestyle choices** for individuals and their **families**. *See* **health promotion**.

health inequality
The fact that the chances of becoming ill or being less healthy are greater for people living in areas of **disadvantage** and those on **lower incomes** than for people on higher incomes living in more prosperous areas. Inequality has been identified by two separate **reports** in the past 30 years. The **Black Report** in 1980 was the

first to link social deprivation with poor health, higher **infant mortality**, levels of **disease** and **access** to **health care**. This was followed in 1998 by the **Acheson Report**, which reached very similar conclusions.
Clear **targets** have been set by the government to reduce health inequalities by 2010.

health professional
A trained and qualified person who provides **health services**; this includes **nurses**, **midwives**, **physiotherapists**, **occupational therapists**, **doctors**, **radiographers**, **chiropodists** and **dentists**.

health promotion
The **process** of enabling people to take control of the factors that determine **health** and **well-being**. This includes making people aware of the factors affecting the **incidence** and **treatment** of **disease**, and involves considering the **choices** that **communities** and **governments** can make to improve opportunities to make positive health and well-being more widely accessible. Examples could be a decision by a **local authority** to make **access** to local swimming pools free in order to encourage the local **population** to take **exercise**, or a local community centre opening a café providing healthy choices of **food**. *See* **health education**.

health visitor
A qualified and registered **nurse** or **midwife** who works in the community to monitor the development of **babies** and **children** and to support the **health** needs of the local **community**.

healthy lifestyle choices
Ways of living that include options that benefit **health**, such as taking regular **exercise**, eating a healthy, balanced **diet**, not **smoking** and limiting **alcohol** intake. The recommended intake of alcohol is no more than 2–3 units of alcohol per day for women and 3–4 units for men, but it is also recommended that people should have 2–3 alcohol free days each week. A unit of alcohol is considered to be 8g of alcohol. This translates as 1 small glass of wine, 1 pub measure of spirits or a half pint of beer. The strength of the alcohol should be taken into account, so is not as straightforward as it may seem.

hearing impairment
Reduced hearing, or total loss of hearing. Some types of hearing impairment can be improved through the use of hearing **aids** or through cochlear implants. Other forms of hearing impairment cannot be improved and people may choose to use alternative means of **communication** such as signing. *See* **British Sign Language**.

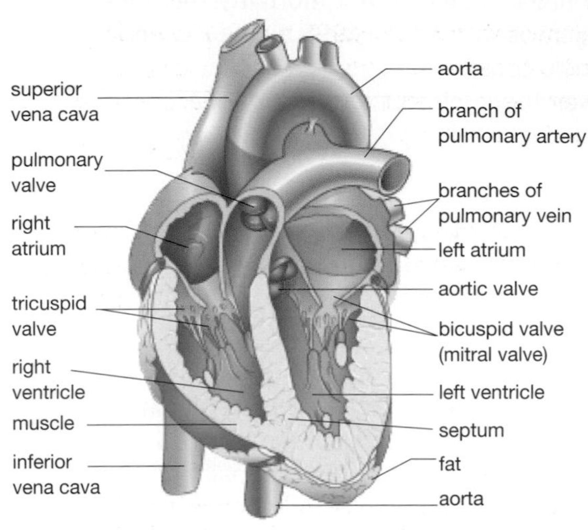

The heart.

heart

The **muscle** that pumps **blood** around the body (*see* **circulation**). The main parts are:

- the left **atrium**, which receives **oxygenated** blood from the **lungs**
- the right atrium, which receives de-oxygenated blood from the **venae cavae**
- the left **ventricle**, which receives blood from the left atrium and pumps it into the aorta
- the right ventricle, which receives blood from the right atrium and pumps it to the lungs.

There is a one-way flow of blood through the heart promoted by heart valves.

heart attack

A blockage in the **coronary artery** that can result in the **death** of part of the **heart muscle**. It is also known as **myocardial infarction**. A person having a heart attack will complain of pain in the centre of the **chest** and into the left arm, perhaps radiating across the jaw. This requires immediate **medical treatment**; an emergency ambulance should be called and the person kept calm until it arrives.

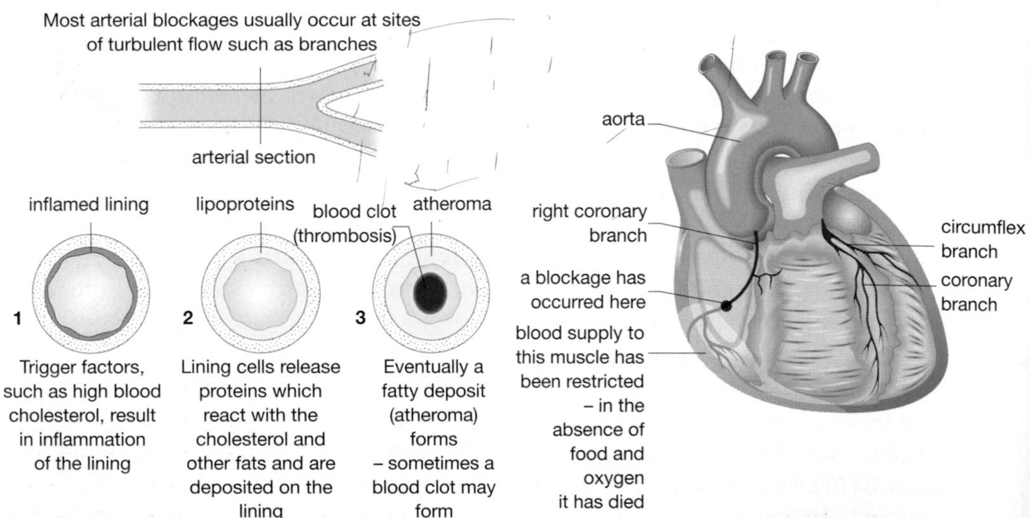

The events leading to a heart attack.

heart disease
Coronary heart disease (CHD), the commonest form, is caused by the **coronary arteries** becoming narrowed or blocked with fatty deposits of **cholesterol** and other substances (atherosclerosis). Other forms of heart disease are **infections** and cardiomyopathy, a **disease** affecting the functioning of the **heart muscle**.

heart rate
The number of times per minute that a heart beats. The average adult heart rate is around 70 beats per minute at rest; children's hearts beat faster. **Exercise** increases the heart rate, which is usually beneficial for healthy people, if done on a regular basis and built up gradually. The heart rate can be felt as a **pulse** at various points in the body where an artery crosses bone, but usually the wrist, neck and groin.

Heimlich manoeuvre
A first aid technique used if a person is choking. By standing behind the person and placing joined hands just below their diaphragm, then jerking sharply upwards, the object causing the choking is usually expelled. Potential risks mean that it should only be used following training.

hemiplegia
Paralysis affecting one side of the body usually as a result of a stroke or other brain damage or injury.

hepatic
Relating to the liver.

hepatitis
An **infection** causing **inflammation** of the **liver**. Currently five different types of **virus** (A, B, C, D and E) are identified as causing hepatitis. Each virus causes different **symptoms** with different levels of severity.

- Hepatitis A: This is the commonest form of hepatitis, has flu-like symptoms and **jaundice**, and usually clears up in a couple of weeks without any specific **treatment**. The virus is passed out of the body in **faeces** and is usually spread through contaminated **food** or water. It is most usually found in areas of the world where sanitation methods may not be efficient. **Personal hygiene**, particularly **hand washing**, is important in preventing further spread.
- Hepatitis B: This is a highly infectious virus that is carried in the bloodstream and bodily fluids of an infected person. It is 100 times more infectious than **HIV**. It is transmitted through unprotected **sexual intercourse**, sharing infected drug **needles**, **accidental injury** from infected needles, sharing razors, tattooing or body piercing with infected needles, and **blood transfusions** in countries where **blood** is not effectively screened for infection. Hepatitis B is an occupational **hazard** for people working in **health services** and **vaccination** is essential. Hepatitis B can be an acute infection that will clear up in a few months or can be a **chronic disease** that can cause long-term serious **liver** damage, including liver **cancer**.

- Hepatitis C: This is passed on through direct contact with infected blood from another person; it is more unusual for it to be passed on through other bodily fluids. People can remain symptom-free for many years and some remain well throughout their lives. About 20 per cent of infected people will go on to develop serious liver damage. No vaccination is available.
- Hepatitis D: This carries similar infection risks to hepatitis B, but the hepatitis D virus only occurs when the hepatitis B virus is also present; the two together make the symptoms and consequences more serious.
- Hepatitis E: This is similar to hepatitis A in that it is carried in the bowel and passed on through contaminated food and water. It is not passed on through contact with infected blood or bodily fluids. It is commonest in Africa, Asia, Central America and the Middle East, with low levels of infection in Western countries. It can, however, be serious for **pregnant** women and can cause **miscarriage** or a serious infection that can be fatal for about 20 per cent of infected women.

heredity
The passing on of **genetic** characteristics from one generation to the next.

heroin
An illegal drug derived from **morphine**, obtained from the opium poppy. It is a restricted Class A drug, used as an analgesic for people with severe **pain**. It is also used **illegally** as a drug to induce euphoria. Users of heroin can develop an **addiction** and the **symptoms** of **withdrawal** are unpleasant.

heterosexuality
Sexual attraction to people of the opposite sex.

hierarchy
A system that has a clearly set out order where each level is superior to the level below. This is most commonly seen in management of organisations where there is a hierarchy leading up to the Chief Executive or Director.

High Court
An **access** point for the **justice system**. The High Court deals with civil cases through three divisions:
- Chancery: wills, company **law**, taxation
- Family: **divorce**, custody and **adoption**
- Queen's Bench: claims involving money and awards of damages.

high density lipoprotein (HDL)
High density lipoprotein is in the bloodstream and carries **cholesterol** away from the cells and back to the liver where it is broken down or becomes a waste product. Is also known as 'good cholesterol'.

histogram
A chart similar to a **bar chart**, but with the columns touching each other. It is usually drawn with vertical columns and used to represent continuous **data** measured on the same scale. Unlike a bar chart, it would not usually be used to show comparisons between two distinct and different sets of data.

histology
The study of **human tissue. Microscopic examination** of **samples** of **tissue** can identify **disease** and disorders. Histology, for example, can determine whether a **cancerous tumour** is **malignant** or **benign** by looking at the tissue under a powerful **microscope** and examining the **cells**.

hoist
A piece of **equipment** designed to assist a person with restricted **mobility** to move from one place to another by lifting him or her. Hoists can be manual or electrically powered. They usually consist of a seat or sling into which someone can be secured and supporting metal frames that enable movement. Hoists should always be used rather than lifting a person manually, but instructions for use must be followed exactly or **serious injuries** to both the person being moved and the person operating the hoist could result. *See* **moving and handling**.

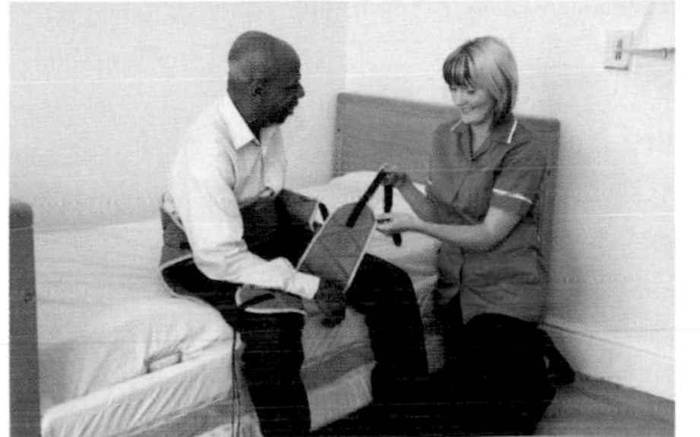

Place the sling around or under the service user.

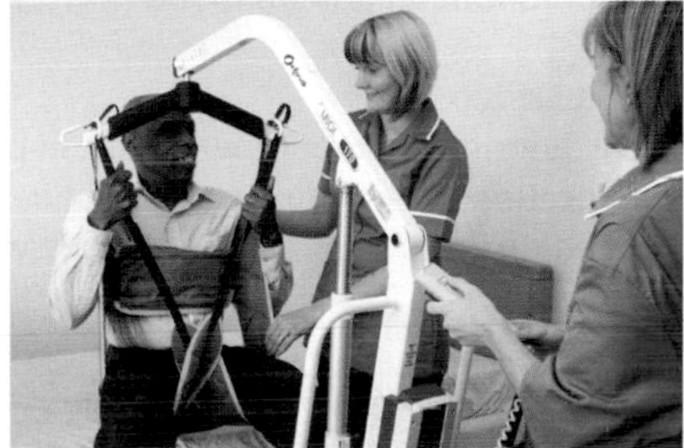

It is only necessary to have a small clearance from the bed or chair.

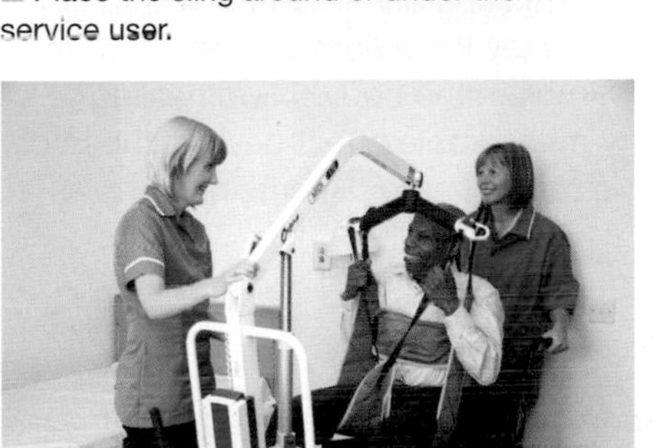

Place the wheelchair in position and make sure it is steady.

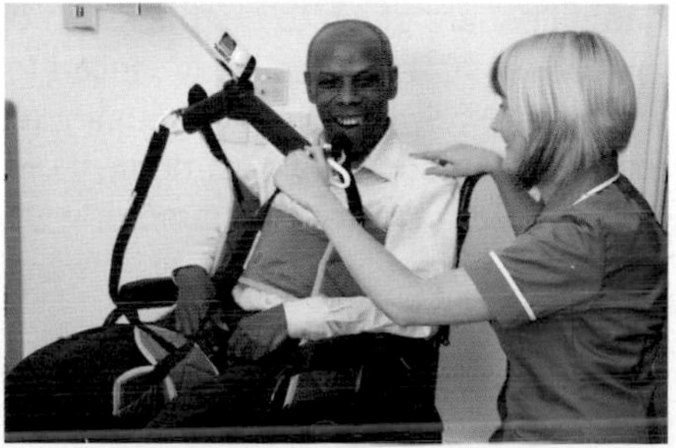

Make sure the service user feels safe and comfortable at the end of the move.

A B C D E F G H I J K L M N O P Q R S T U V W XYZ

holistic approach
A way of approaching the delivery of **health** or care that considers the whole person and not just the part that requires **treatment** or care. It takes into account a person's **culture**, **beliefs**, background, living situation, and social and emotional circumstances on the basis that all of these factors contribute to the current condition of the person and determine the best ways to meet their **needs**.

home care
The **provision** of **support** and assistance with daily living and **personal care** in a person's own home. This can often make the difference between someone needing residential support and being able to remain in the **community**. *See* **domiciliary care**.

home childcarer
Someone who is registered and approved to deliver childcare in the child's own home.

homeless
Without a permanent place to live. People become homeless for many reasons and may become **rough sleepers** or may move between temporary **hostels**. People who have **mental health problems** or those who have been in the looked-after **system** have a greater chance of becoming homeless.
More information can be found at www.crisis.org.uk

Home Office
The **government** department with **responsibility** for **law**, public order, public **safety**, **immigration**, passports and the **police**.
More information can be found at www.homeoffice.gov.uk

homeopathy
A **complementary** to traditional medicine. Based on treating the person and not the **disease**, it takes a **holistic approach** to **diagnosis** and **treatment**. The principle of the treatments is that minute quantities of natural substances, which would cause **symptoms** similar to those of the **patient** if they were administered in large quantities, are given to the patient in order to stimulate the body's own healing **processes**. Clinical trials have failed to find any measurable effect beyond those of a **placebo**; however, many thousands of people report improvements or cures as a result of homeopathic treatment.
More information can be found at www.trusthomeopathy.org/index.html

homeostasis
The **process** of maintaining the internal environment of the body in a constant and steady state despite varying **environmental** conditions. The body will adjust by sweating in order to counteract excessive **temperatures**, or similarly will shiver to counteract external cold. Blood sugar levels are kept constant by the supply

of **insulin** from the **pancreas**. The body's pH (measure of acidity or alkalinity) is homeostatically maintained at between 7.33 and 7.42.

Home-Start UK
A **voluntary organisation** providing parenting **support** to **families**. Support is provided by volunteers who are experienced **parents** and offer advice, reassurance and support to families who are struggling to cope.
More information can be found at www.home-start.org.uk

homophobia
A **fear** and hatred of **homosexuals**. This can result in **discrimination** and **hate crimes**.

homosexuality
Sexual attraction to people of the same sex.

hormonal
Brought about by hormones.

hormone replacement therapy (HRT)
A treatment providing additional **oestrogen** for women whose **ovaries** no longer supply sufficient amounts. This can be a result of the **menopause** or of **surgery** to remove the ovaries.

hormones
Chemical messengers present throughout the body. They travel in the bloodstream to **tissues** and **organs** and work slowly over time to affect, for example, growth and development, **metabolism**, sexual function, **reproduction** and mood. Endocrine **glands** – such as the **thymus**, **thyroid**, adrenal and **pituitary** – make hormones, as do males **testes** and female **ovaries**. Excess or insufficient hormone levels can have serious effects on the body. Levels can be checked in blood tests.

hospice
An **organisation** offering **palliative care** to people who are **terminally ill**, and **support** for their **families**. May also provide respite care for those with life limiting conditions.

hospital
Large institution providing **health care** for a local or regional **community**. There are over 350 **NHS** hospitals and over 180 in the **private sector** in the UK. Some hospitals provide specialist **services** to a region or even nationally, and others provide general medical services for a local community. Some hospitals are attached to universities and participate in the **teaching** and **learning** of **nurses**, **midwives** and **doctors**.

hospital acquired infections/healthcare associated infections (HCAI)
These are bacterial infections resulting from being in a hospital environment for other reasons and tend to affect vulnerable people such as older and younger patients with poor immunity that have had invasive procedures such as operations. Common hospital acquired infections are caused by *escherichia coli* (**E. coli**), *methicillin-resistant Staphylococcus aureus* (**MRSA**) and *Clostridium difficile* (**C. difficile**). These can be very serious life-threatening conditions and certain **antibiotics** are kept for their treatment. **Infections** resulting from other care environments may be termed healthcare associated infections.

hospital social workers
Social work teams based in a **hospital**. Social work **services** are provided for hospital **patients** and their **families**, and close liaison is maintained with local **community** services.

hostel
Temporary lodging for someone without a permanent home. Hostels are usually run for a specific **group** of potential users, such as people who are **homeless**, **young people** leaving care, people who have had **mental health problems**, people leaving prison, or women who are survivors of **domestic abuse**.

household
The people who share a living space.

Houses of Parliament
The place where **law** is made for the UK. It contains the House of Commons and the House of Lords. The House of Commons is for democratically elected members of **Parliament**. The **political party** with the majority of members forms the **government**. The House of Lords has members appointed by the government. Laws are made in the House of Commons; the House of Lords can question, amend or delay laws as they go through the **process**, but cannot override the decision of the democratically elected members of the Commons.

housing
General term to describe dwellings where people live. This includes private housing that is owned by the people who live in it, privately rented housing that is owned by a **landlord** where **rent** is paid by the people who live there, and social housing that is owned by a **local authority** or a **housing association**.

housing association
Independent, **not-for-profit organisation** for managing, building and renovating **housing**. Funded through central and **local government**, housing associations provide houses for **rent**, and some have schemes for purchase. They also provide

specialist housing such as **supported living** and **sheltered housing** developments. They are regulated through the Housing Corporation in England and Wales, and Scottish Homes in Scotland.

Housing Benefit
A means-tested benefit, paid through **local authorities**, to assist people with **housing** costs. Housing benefit can be paid directly to **landlords**.

human behaviour
The way that humans **interact** with each other. Behaviour results from each individual's **personality** and the factors that influenced his or her development. **Challenging behaviour** can be the result of illness or **disability** or factors in the background and development of individuals.

human development
The **process** of growth and progress through **life stages** for humans. Life stages are: **infancy** (0–2 years), childhood (3–11 years), **adolescence** (11–18 years), young **adulthood** (18–30 years), middle adulthood (30–60 years), older adulthood (60–80 years), old age (over 80 years). People pass through the stages at slightly different ages, but these are a general indicator. At each life stage people will have changing social, emotional, intellectual and physical **needs**.

Life stage	Age	Key features
Conception	9 months before birth	Egg and sperm fuse after sexual intercourse and create a new living being
Pregnancy (gestation)	9 months to birth	Physical development of embryo and foetus
Birth and infancy	0-3 years	Attachment to carers
Childhood	4-9 years	First experience of education
Adolescence	10-18 years	Identification with peer group – puberty takes place during this period
Adulthood	18-65 years	The right to vote, and manage one's own financial affairs happens at 18
Other adulthood	65 years onwards	65 is the current age when men (and women born after 6 April 1955 receive state pension
Final stages of life	variable	Physical 'decline'

Table 4.1 Life stages

A B C D E F G H I J K L M N O P Q R S T U V W X Y Z

human genome
The complete set of **deoxyribonucleic acid (DNA)** for an individual; all of the **genetic** material for one person that contains the 'pattern' or 'blueprint' of how they will develop. It seems likely that the complete human genome contains around 30–35,000 **genes**. *See* **genetics**.
More information can be found at http://genome.wellcome.ac.uk/

Human Immunodeficiency Virus (HIV)
The virus is most commonly transmitted between humans through:
- unprotected **sexual intercourse** with an infected person
- **transfusion** of contaminated **blood** or blood products
- artificial insemination with **semen** from an infected person
- a mother with HIV can infect her baby during **pregnancy**, during the **birth** process or through breastfeeding
- sharing unsterilised injection equipment with infected people.

The **virus** has a very small chance of:
- being transmitted to health care workers who are working with infected people provided that universal precautions are taken. Even when there is a needle stick injury, there is a very small chance of the virus being transmitted.
- being transmitted through kissing or other intimate physical contact that does not involve penetrative vaginal or anal sexual intercourse.

The virus cannot be transmitted through day-to-day activities such as sitting on a chair or using eating utensils that have been used by an infected person, nor can it be caught from lavatory seats, showers or baths that have been used by an infected person.

human resources
The **workforce** available to an **organisation** in order to carry out its work. Also the name given to some personnel departments in organisations.

human rights
The basic principles and entitlements of all human beings. The **Universal Declaration of Human Rights** of the United Nations, and the European Convention on Human Rights, identify the rights that every person should be entitled to. These are the basis of **legislation** to protect human rights in the UK.

human tissue
Material from a human body that consists of, or includes, **cells**. The uses and disposal of human tissue are regulated through **legislation** (the Human Tissue Act 2004) by the Human Tissue Authority. If human tissue is used for **research** or testing, there are clear procedures that must be followed and **consents** must be obtained.

Huntington's disease
A **genetic disease** that is presently incurable. It is caused by a faulty **gene** and results in slowly developing but major **changes** in movement and **personality**. The disease usually begins in **adulthood** and people's **motor control** decreases until they are making significant involuntary movements and have **mobility** problems. There are usually significant personality changes and people present quite **challenging behaviour**, with mood swings and frustration.

hydrocephalus
A condition where there is an excessive quantity of **cerebrospinal fluid** surrounding the **brain**. Normally about half a litre of this fluid is circulating around the brain at any time. If this is unable to drain away it will build up and create pressure on the **tissues** of the brain. In **babies** and **infants**, the head increases in size. In older children and adults, this is not possible as the **skull** has fused together. Valves or shunts can be inserted to drain away fluid. Babies born with **spina bifida** often also have hydrocephalus.

hydrolysis
The **process** of splitting a compound into separate fragments by adding water.

hygiene
The **processes** and methods of achieving and maintaining cleanliness. Hygiene procedures need to be followed for individuals and **environments** to ensure that any possibility of **contamination** is reduced. *See* **personal hygiene**.

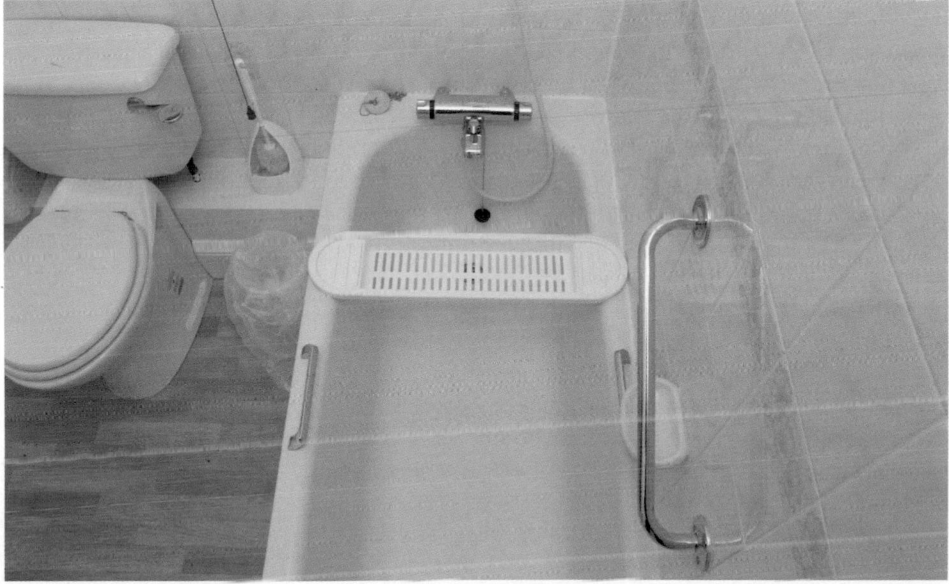

It is important to keep bathrooms clean.

A B C D E F G H I J K L M N O P Q R S T U V W XYZ

hypertension
Persistent resting raised **blood pressure** generally accepted to be over 140/90 mmHg. This causes the heart to work harder to pump blood around the body and may contribute to heart attacks and strokes. Antihypertensive drugs are prescribed to lower blood pressure and reduce such incidents.

hypoactivity
Under-activity where people may appear lethargic and to have no energy. This can be caused by various medical conditions, but most commonly through a thyroid gland disorder.

hypotension
Low blood pressure.

hypothalamus
A small and important **organ** in the centre of the base of the **brain** that interprets signals from the **environment** and controls **body temperature**, breathing, **heart rate** and **reproduction**. Also influences all autonomic functions.

hypothermia
The lowering of the human **body temperature** below the normal level. It occurs when the exterior environmental conditions are so cold that the body systems cannot maintain normal temperature. In these conditions people feel very tired and drift off to sleep. If the body temperature is not raised, death will result. When hypothermia requires medical treatment hospitals usually re-warm the patient from the inside by putting warm fluids into the body through a vein. In severe cases they may remove blood and warm it before returning it to the body. The key to providing first aid to someone who is hypothermic is to be gentle. Moving them to somewhere warm, removing wet clothes and wrapping them in blankets will all help. Warm drinks and foods high in carbohydrates can be given if the person is able to eat and drink. Do not give alcohol, rub the limbs or place a person in a hot bath as all of these can cause further problems.

hypothesis
A statement or question that forms the basis of a **research** project. The research will be designed either to answer the question or to test whether the statement is true. 'In our class more people have blue eyes than brown eyes' is a simple hypothesis that can be tested by research: **observing** and noting the colour of people's eyes. The results of the research will show clearly whether the statement is true. *See* **null hypothesis**.

I

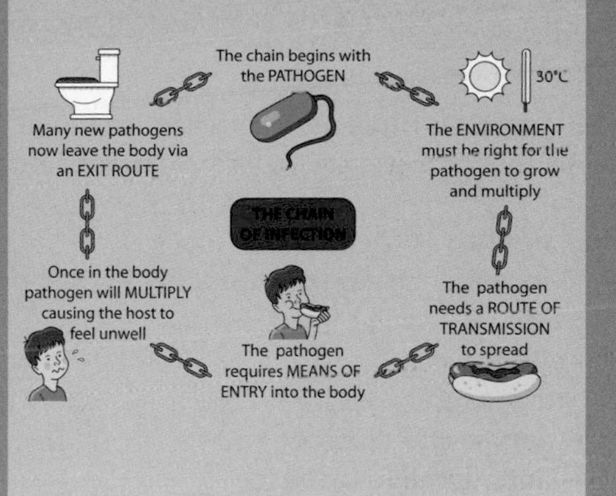
The chain begins with the PATHOGEN
30°C
The ENVIRONMENT must be right for the pathogen to grow and multiply
The pathogen needs a ROUTE OF TRANSMISSION to spread
The pathogen requires MEANS OF ENTRY into the body
Once in the body pathogen will MULTIPLY causing the host to feel unwell
Many new pathogens now leave the body via an EXIT ROUTE
THE CHAIN OF INFECTION

id
The **personality** component that works to satisfy basic urges, **needs**, and desires; according to **psychodynamic theory**, it is made up of **unconscious** psychic **energy**. The id operates on the pleasure principle, which demands immediate gratification of needs.

identity
How individuals see and **understand** themselves, and factors that they see as being important parts of who they are. These factors can include **culture**, music, **religion**, **family responsibilities** and **gender**.

ideology
A set of ideas and **beliefs** that influence and **motivate** behaviour and **decision making**.

ileum
The third and lowest section of the small intestine. It follows the duodenum and jejunum and is separated from the caecum (which connects the small and large intestines) by the ileocaecal valve ensuring a one-way flow.

illegal
Outside the **law**. Any act that deliberately, or accidentally, breaks or fails to comply with the law is illegal.

illegal/illicit drugs
Street **drugs** or **prescription medication** unlawfully used.

illegal immigrants
People who have entered a country and remained there without authority to do so. People in this position will be unable to claim any of the social and financial **benefits** offered by the country, and will be unable to work officially, thus leaving

themselves vulnerable to being exploited by employers who offer work **illegally** without proper wages, terms or conditions.

ill health
Disorder or **dysfunction** leading to the body not functioning as it should. This may be as the result of:

- **infection**
- **disease**
- **congenital disorder**
- **degenerative disease**
- **injury**.

Ill health may be short term (acute) and curable, or it may be long term (**chronic**) and treatable but have no cure.

illness
A subjective sensation of being unwell.

imagination
Creative thinking and the ability to see how things could be different using mental images. Children need to be able to **play** using imagination; it is an important part of **cognitive development**.

imitation
Copying the behaviour of others. This is important for children, who will imitate the behaviour they see around them as they develop.

immigrants
People who move to a new country with the intention of remaining permanently.

immigration
The movement of people into a new country. This can be through a formal **process** and be recognised by the host country, or people can arrive and live in countries without any formal, legal procedures and become **illegal immigrants**.

immune response
The **reaction** of the body to a **threat** from a foreign antigen. The body deals with foreign antigens by producing **antibodies** that surround them and make them harmless. The antibodies are produced by **white blood cells** called **lymphocytes** that are produced in lymphoid tissue (lymphocytes are not produced in bone marrow). This is adaptive immunity and is unique to **vertebrates**.

immune system
A complex **system** of **organs** and **cells** that defend the body against attack and

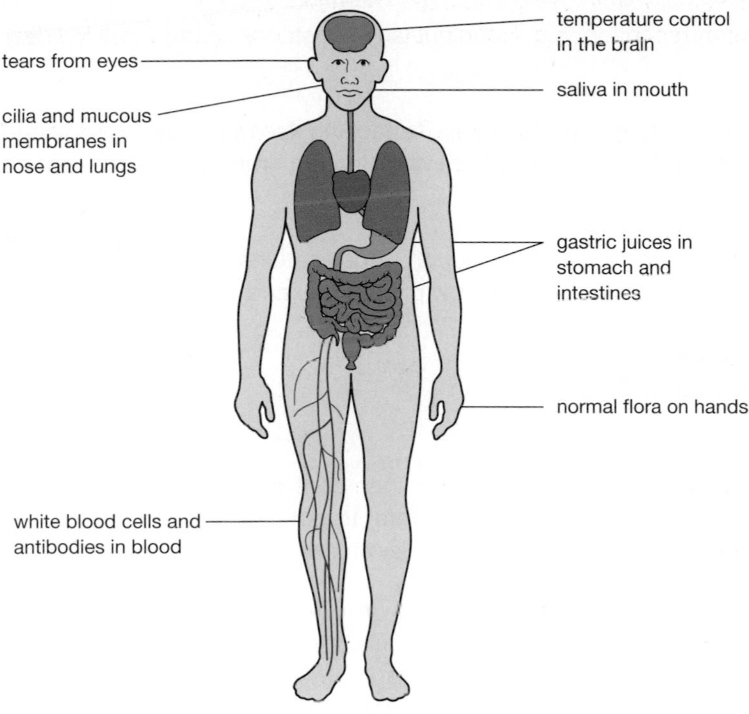

■ The body's defences against infection.

invasion from **bacteria**, **viruses**, **parasites** and other **pathogens**. There are some parts of the immune system that are present in all **vertebrates at birth**; they provide **innate immunity**. Humans also gain acquired immunity after exposure to pathogens through illness, **disease** or **immunisation**. *See* **lymphatic system**.

immunisation
The **process** of giving a **vaccine** to protect against **disease** through enabling a person to develop acquired immunity. Programmes provide **vaccinations** at the intervals necessary to maintain the immunity for diseases like **measles**, **mumps**, **rubella**, **tuberculosis** and **meningitis**.

immunity
Resistance to a particular disease caused by infection.

impairment
Loss of or reduction in a function of the body. This is usually used to refer to hearing, vision or speech.

implant
Method of contraception, e.g. Nonplant (any substance grafted into tissues).

implantation
The **process** of a **zygote** (fertilised egg) attaching itself to and embedding into the wall of the **uterus** and beginning to develop into an **embryo** and then a **foetus**.

implement
To carry out something, follow it through. Organisations may implement a government policy by introducing new procedures and practices.

implementation
Putting a decision or plan into action.

in house
Using an **organisation**'s own staff rather than **contracting** out. Often used to refer to **training and development**. Can also refer to **policies and procedures** that have been developed specifically for a particular organisation.

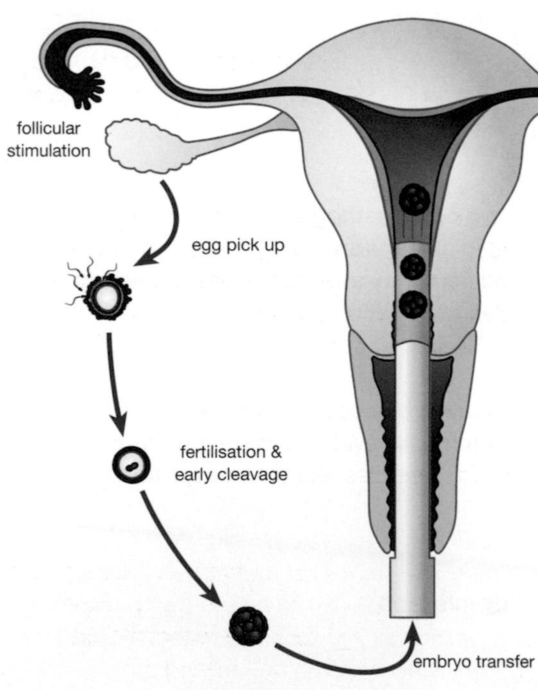

■ The process of in vitro fertilisation.

in vitro fertilisation (IVF)
The **process** of fertilising an egg and a **sperm** outside the body, then returning the fertilised egg into the woman's **uterus**. Women are given **hormones** to stimulate the production of eggs; at the right point in the **ovulation** cycle they are 'harvested' through a fine tube and placed in a **laboratory** dish; **semen** containing sperm is added, and fertilisation of several eggs takes place. Two or three of the fertilised eggs are then gently placed into the uterus through a fine tube. The sperm is usually that of the male partner in a **relationship**, but can be from an anonymous donor.

inappropriate behaviour
Ways of behaving that are not acceptable for the **social norms**, company, audience or setting. **Challenging** or disruptive behaviour is most usually an issue with children

and **young people**, and is usually most effectively dealt with by responding to behaviour that is appropriate and acceptable and not responding to the unacceptable behaviour. Some incidents cannot be dealt with in this way if they are the result of a **learning disability** or **mental health problems** and will require an approach to be agreed in a **support plan** for the particular individual.

incapacity
The inability to carry out some aspects of daily living because of illness or **disability**. This could include working, managing financial affairs, **personal care** and **decision making**.

Incapacity Benefit
Money paid to people who are unable to work for a period longer than 28 weeks because of illness or **disability**. The benefit is paid following a medical **examination** to confirm **incapacity**. Employment and Support Allowance was introduced in October 2008 to replace some incapacity benefits.

incidence
The number of times something happens in a given time period. The term can be used to refer to **diseases, accidents, challenging behaviour**, crime or any events that need to be **recorded** and **reported**.

incidents
Occurrences that require immediate attention to avoid possible danger and harm to people, goods and/or the environment. An example could be, a disclosure of abuse would be described as an 'incident' of abuse.

inclusivity
An approach that ensures that all the views and **needs** of minority and **under-represented groups** are taken into account in the planning of **services** and **facilities** so that no one is left out. The approach means that the potential **barriers** that people may face have been considered and steps taken to overcome them.

income
Money obtained by an individual or **family** from **work**, investments or other means. In an organisation's budget income refers to the monies coming in to the organisation through grants, fees, donations, charging policies.

incontinence
The inability to retain **urine** in the **bladder** or **faeces** in the **rectum** until a suitable place is found for release. This can be caused by **disease**, or **injury** to the **nerves** and **muscles** that control the bladder or rectum. It can also be caused by injury or disease affecting the **brain** or **nervous system**. Urinary incontinence is more common than faecal incontinence. Both conditions can often be improved by **exercises** or **medication**. There are **aids** that can improve the **quality of life** of people with either condition.

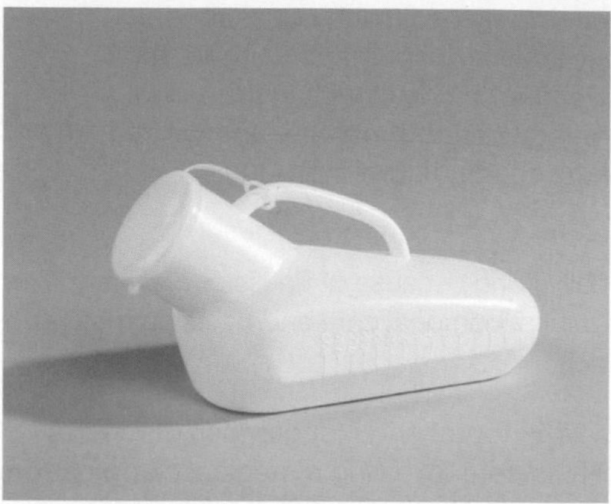

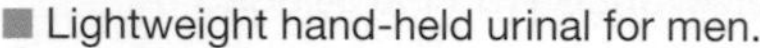

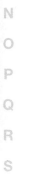

■ Lightweight hand-held urinal for men.

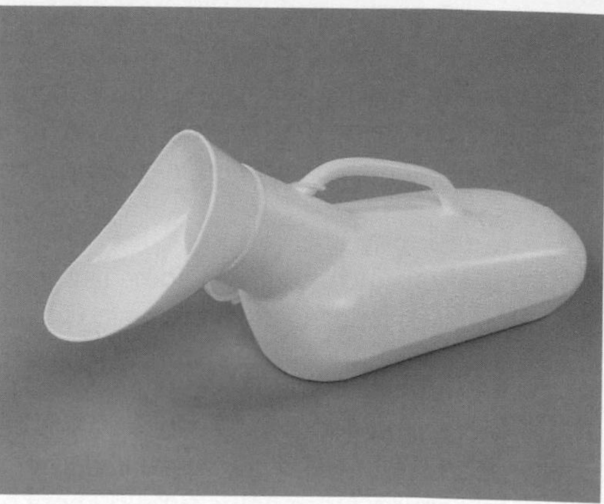

■ Lightweight hand-held urinal for women.

In control

The projects that have led the implementation of **direct payments** for disabled people across the country.

incubation period

The length of time between initial contact with an **infectious disease** and the development of the first **symptoms**. Chickenpox, for example, takes on average 14–16 days (but can be 10–21 days) following contact with an infected person before the first symptoms appear.

independence

Freedom from being **dependent** on others; a right to choose and be in control of one's own life.

Independent Living Fund (ILF)

Money to enable **disabled** people to live **independently** in the **community**. A means-tested **benefit** is paid to people between 16 and 65 who meet the **eligibility criteria**.

independent sector

The non-**statutory organisations** providing **health** and care **services** for adults or children and **young people**. This can include **not-for-profit organisations** such as **charities** and **social enterprise companies**, and private businesses that make a profit from providing services.

index

A list showing contents and where they are located. This could be in a book, a computer disk, a library or any reference facility.

individual budget
The amount of **resources** assessed for the **provision** of **services** for an individual. The system of individual budgets places the people who receive the **support** in control of how they want the money to be spent. They can continue with existing services if they are happy with them, or can develop a plan for doing things in a different way that suits them better.

individual rights
Service users have a range of rights that are established in codes and legislations, as shown in the diagram.

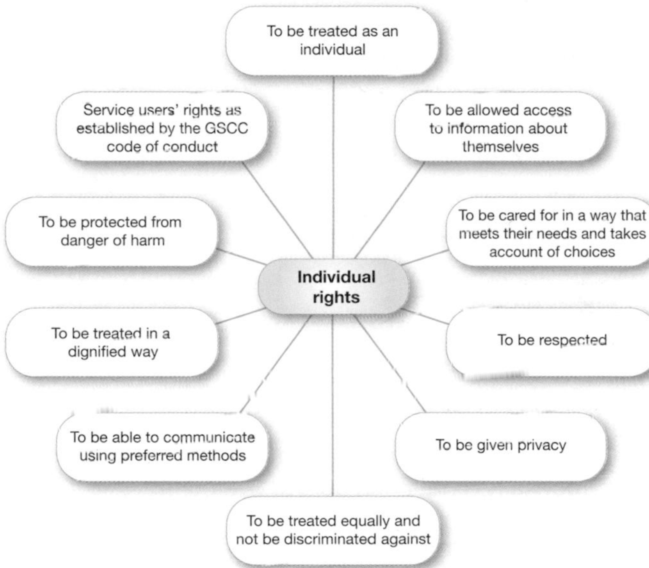
Individual rights
To be treated as an individual
To be allowed access to information about themselves
To be cared for in a way that meets their needs and takes account of choices
To be respected
To be given privacy
To be treated equally and not be discriminated against
To be able to communicate using preferred methods
To be treated in a dignified way
To be protected from danger of harm
Service users' rights as established by the GSCC code of conduct

■ Service users' individual rights.

Individual Support Order (ISO)
A court order for a 10- to 17-year-old which can be attached to an **Anti-Social Behaviour Order** (ASBO) and impose positive conditions on the **young person** to address the underlying causes of the behaviour that led to the ASBO.
An ISO may last up to six months and can require a young person to attend up to two sessions a week under the **supervision** of the **youth offending team**. Breach of an ISO is a criminal **offence** which may be punished by a financial penalty.

individuality
The unique nature and **personality** of every person that grows and develops from life experience and other factors such as **culture**, background, **social class**, age, **ethnicity** and **gender**.

induction
An introductory programme when starting **work** or a **learning** programme.

induction standards
A set of **standards** identifying the levels of knowledge and **performance** to be achieved within a specified time from starting **work** in **health** and **social care** and childcare. More information can be found at www.skillsforcare.org.uk

industrialisation
The change that took place in Britain between the middle of the 18th century (around 1750) and the end of the 19th century (around 1900) when **society** moved from being based in rural areas, with agriculture and small-scale crafts, to a factory-based manufacturing economy centred on towns and cities.

inequality
Differences in **treatment** or opportunities experienced by whole **groups** of people based on **gender**, ability, age, **ethnicity**, **religion** or **sexual orientation**. *See* **Black Report**.

infancy
The **life stage** from **birth** to 2 years.

infant
A child under the age of 2 years.

infant mortality rate
The number of **deaths** during the first year of life expressed as the number per 1,000 live **births** in any given **population**.

infection
The result of the invasion of the body by **pathogens** that the body's **immune response** has not been able to overcome.

infection control

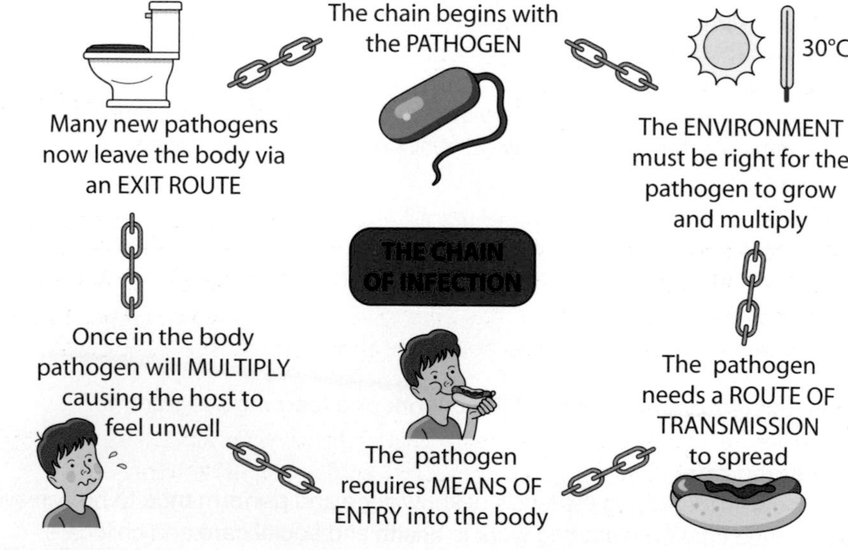
The chain begins with the PATHOGEN
30°C
The ENVIRONMENT must be right for the pathogen to grow and multiply
The pathogen needs a ROUTE OF TRANSMISSION to spread
The pathogen requires MEANS OF ENTRY into the body
Once in the body pathogen will MULTIPLY causing the host to feel unwell
Many new pathogens now leave the body via an EXIT ROUTE
THE CHAIN OF INFECTION

■ Chain of infection.

The measures put in place to try to stop the spread of **health care**-associated **infections** (HCAIs) within an **organisation**, usually a **hospital** or **residential care** setting. These can include **hand washing**, **protective clothing**, barrier protection, reduction in antibiotic use, isolation and segregation of **patients** and improvements in **hygiene** and cleaning.

In order to control infection effectively, it is necessary to break the 'chain of infection' (*See* diagram opposite). Any break in the chain will stop or reduce the infection. The purpose of infection control is to break one of the links in the chain of infection.

infertility

The inability to achieve a **pregnancy** after one year of unprotected **sexual intercourse**, or the inability to carry a pregnancy to a live **birth**.

infestation

The presence of a large number of insects, vermin or **parasites**. These can be in, or on, a person or in a house, **hospital** or other building. Infestations usually require expert assistance to deal with them effectively.

inflammation

A localised response to an **injury** or **allergic reaction** that causes damage to **tissues**. Inflammation can result in heat, redness, pain and swelling of the affected area.

information

Messages containing facts and knowledge. Information may be **communicated** by word of mouth, electronically or in written form.

information and communication technology (ICT)

The **equipment** and **skills** needed to process and **access information** electronically using computers and electronic devices.

informed consent

Agreement given by a person who has the ability to make a decision after being given all the facts and **information**. Any action, **treatment** or procedure undertaken in **health** and **social care** should be fully discussed with the relevant individuals and only carried out when agreement has been given. Those involved need to be made fully aware of all the information needed to make an informed decision.

infringement of rights

The situation where a person's entitlements have been disregarded and **access** to entitlements has been blocked through deliberate or **accidental** actions.

ingestion

The taking of **food**, liquid or **medications** into the body by mouth.

A B C D E F G H I J K L M N O P Q R S T U V W XYZ

Inhalers are used by people with asthma.

in good faith
Used to describe professional acts that are carried out with the best of intentions and in the light of the knowledge available at the time. Sometimes actions can later turn out to have been wrong, but having carried out something 'in good faith' and with no intent to do harm is usually acceptable in terms of professional accountability.

inhale
To breathe air into the body. This occurs when the diaphragm contracts, moving downward and expanding the chest cavity, allowing air to flow into the lungs.

inhaler
A device to deliver **medication** into the body through being breathed into the **lungs**.

inheritance
The passing on of **genetic** characteristics from one **generation** to the next.

inherited disorder
A condition resulting from the passing on of a defective **gene** from one generation to the next.

initiative
A new approach and plan, usually one developed by **government** and **promoted** throughout the **health**, **social care** and children and **young people**'s sectors.

injection
A medical procedure that forces liquid into the subcutaneous tissues, the blood system or an organ.

injunction
A court order forbidding a particular activity or course of action. Injunctions are frequently sought to forbid harmful **access** to a person or place or to stop **harassment**.

injury
Damage to **tissues** or **organs**. This could be as the result of an **accident** or a physical attack.

innate immunity
The body's natural defences, which everyone is born with, and which form the first line of defence against foreign **pathogens** entering the body.

- The **skin** provides a waterproof (also micro-organism roof) protective layer covering the entire body.
- Ciliated mucous membranes lining the gut and **airways** trap invading **bacteria**.
- **Stomach** acid kills bacteria that have been taken in with **food**.
- Helpful bacteria in the bowel keep out **harmful** bacteria.
- **Urine** flow washes out bacteria from the **bladder** and **urethra**.
- **White blood cells** called neutrophils seek out and overwhelm invading bacteria.

inoculation
The introduction of a substance, usually a **vaccine**, into the body in order to protect against **infectious disease**.

in-patient
Someone receiving medical treatment in hospital rather than at home.

inquest
An investigation carried out by a Coroner to establish a cause of death.

inquiry
An investigation held because of concerns about a specific incident, or about an area of **health**, **social care** or children and young people's practice.

insomnia
A condition where people have difficulty **sleeping**.

inspections
Examinations and audits of **organisations** providing **services**, such as **hospitals**, **schools** and **residential provision**. The examinations and audits are carried out using a set of **standards** and the **performance** of the organisation is measured against the standards. The results are **recorded** and **reported** publicly.
More information can be found at www.ofsted.gov.uk, www.csci.gov.uk, www.cqc.org.uk

inspectors
Suitably qualified and experienced **professionals** who carry out **inspections**.

institutional abuse
Abuse or harm that occurs because an **organisation** providing a **service** is run for the benefit and convenience of the organisation or staff, rather than for the benefit of those receiving the **support**. People can be abused by having **choices** removed, **privacy** violated, **dignity** not **respected** and **rights** infringed.

institutionalisation
The possible negative effects of being in **hospital** or **residential care** for a prolonged period. Individuals may only feel safe and comfortable with the **routine** they have become used to and may have become **passive**, finding it hard to make any decisions, make enquiries or take control of their lives. Putting people in control of their lives and **decision making** is essential, whatever the length of stay.

instrumental delivery
Medical assistance to deliver a **baby** by using forceps or **ventouse** suction cup. This **intervention** is used if **labour** is not progressing as it should and either the baby or the **mother** is becoming stressed.

insulin
A **hormone** naturally produced by the **pancreas** and can also be medically produced. Its function is to control the **glucose** levels in the body. If the pancreas produces insufficient insulin this results in **diabetes**.
There are four main types of insulin:

- Rapid-acting insulin (Lispro) reaches the blood within 15 minutes after injection. It peaks 30 to 90 minutes later and may last as long as 5 hours.
- Short-acting (regular) insulin usually reaches the blood within 30 minutes after injection. It peaks 2 to 4 hours later and stays in the blood for about 4 to 8 hours.
- Intermediate-acting (NPH and lente) insulins reach the blood 2 to 6 hours after injection. They peak 4 to 14 hours later and stay in the blood for about 14 to 20 hours.
- Long-acting (ultralente) insulin takes 6 to 14 hours to start working. It has no peak or a very small peak 10 to 16 hours after injection. It stays in the blood between 20 and 24 hours.

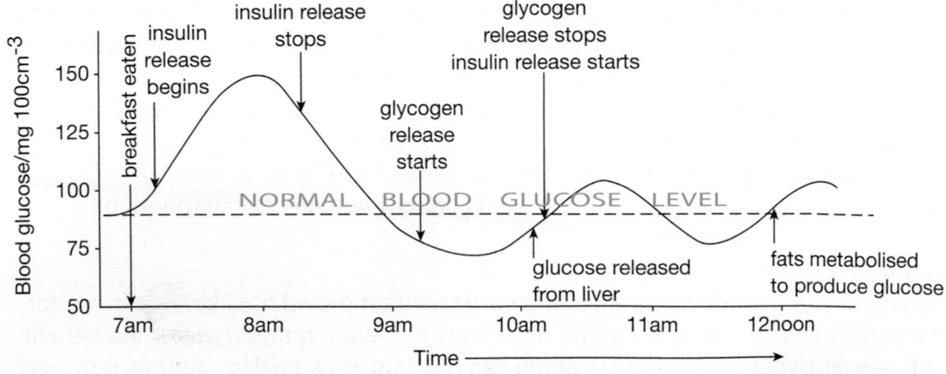

■ Insulin and glycogen together regulate blood sugar levels.

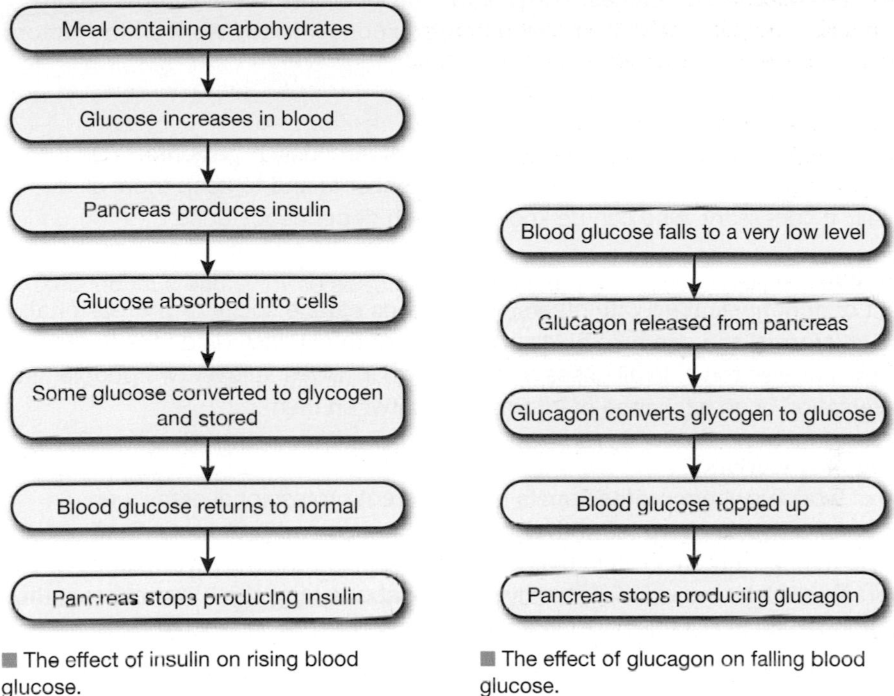

■ The effect of insulin on rising blood glucose.

■ The effect of glucagon on falling blood glucose.

integrated community equipment services
Services provided by **local authorities** to supply the **aids** and **equipment** people need to live **independently** and undertake daily living tasks.

integrated working
A way of working where **professionals** from different specialities work together in the same **team**. Team **management** may be provided by someone from any discipline, but professional management is available for each of the special areas. This way of working recognises the importance of a **holistic approach** and the sharing of **skills** and knowledge to provide benefit and **support**.

intellectual development (cognitive development)
The growth of the **brain** and the development of **thought processes, reasoning, problem solving, memory**, comprehension and **understanding**.

intelligence
The ability to comprehend, **understand** and benefit from experience.

intensive supervision and surveillance programme (ISSP)
Rigorous, **community**-based programme for repeat young offenders and those who

commit the most serious crimes. The programme involves intensive **supervision** (25 hours per week for the first three months) and concentrated work on the factors causing the **offending behaviour**.

intensive therapy unit (ITU)
Hospital unit providing specialist care for the most seriously ill **patients**. ITUs use highly sophisticated technology to **monitor** patients and to keep them alive artificially if necessary. Also can be known as high dependency units.

interaction
The act of **communicating** with others. Interactions can be social or **professional**, formal or informal and can take place in a variety of forms, including face to face, telephone, or electronic. In all cases an interaction involves at least two people and a conversation or an exchange of **information** between them.

inter-agency working
A way of working where **professionals** from different professional areas work together for a specific purpose with agreed procedures and **protocols**. Staff remain in their own **teams** within their own **organisation**, but may work together to **support** a particular individual or **family**. **Organisations** may agree to work together to support a particular project or **initiative**.

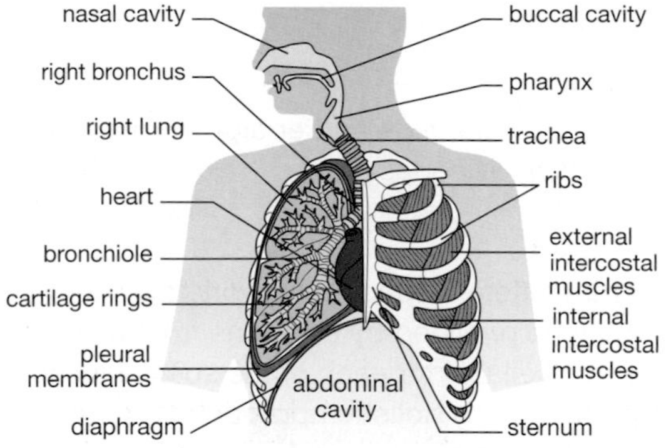

■ The intercostal muscles and the process of breathing.

intercostal muscles
Respiratory muscles that are attached from the bottom of one **rib** to the top of the next rib and contract and expand during **breathing**.

interests
Those things that draw your attention, that you want to get involved with and spend time on. *See* **well-being**.

interim care order
A court order placing a child or **young person** in the care of the **local authority** on a temporary basis. This is usually for 8 weeks initially, while further investigations or planning takes place.

intermediate or interim care
Services to provide any immediate **support** necessary to enable a person to return home from **hospital**. Services may include **personal care**, nursing care and **equipment**, and will be provided for the short term to **promote independence** and recovery.

internal audit
A **review** and check of **performance** and financial **management** by auditors from within an **organisation**.

internalisation
The **process** of deeply understanding and embedding **learning** so that it will not be forgotten. Once learning has been internalised, people are able to apply it to solve problems in a range of situations.

internal verifier
The person from within an **organisation** providing **vocational qualifications** who has the **responsibility** for checking that evidence is sufficient to meet the requirements of the qualification and that the assessment **process** is being correctly undertaken.

International Classification Of Diseases (ICD)
A catalogue of **diseases** published every decade by the **World Health Organization**.

International Classification Of Disorders
Information published by the **World Health Organization** on various disorders, whether physical or psychological.

Internet
The World Wide Web, a shared global **information resource**.

interpersonal skills
The abilities necessary in order to **communicate** and **interact** successfully with other people. **Skills** include the ability to listen effectively, to communicate and to **empathise** with others.

interpreter
Someone who is able to listen to what a person is saying in one language and to **translate** it and communicate the meaning in another language. **Professional** interpreting is highly **skilled** and should always be used in **health** and **social care** situations where there are language differences. **Family** members should not be used to translate in personal or sensitive discussions.

intervention
Action by a **professional** to change the path that an individual is following or the course of a **disease** or disorder.

intervertebral disc
A tough pad of fibro-cartilage that separates the **vertebrae (bones)** of the spine. Collectively they act as shock absorbers and protect the vertebrae from **injury**.

interview
A face-to-face meeting. Interviews are often used in **research** to find out **data**. The term is also used to describe a **therapeutic** session when working in **social care** with adults, children or **young people** and in the employee selection process.

intestines
The part of the **digestive system** that extends from the lower opening of the **stomach** to the **anus**. It is divided into the large and small intestine. The small intestine is where all the absorption of nutrients from food takes place. It is about 5 metres long, much longer than the large intestine, but its diameter is smaller. It starts at the duodenum and food is moved along through the jejunum and the ileum by peristalsis. Digestive juices containing enzymes and bile is added to the food during this process in order to aid the absorption of nutrients. By the time food reaches the end of the ileum, only indigestible food remains and this is passed into the large intestine. The large intestine is the wide lower section of the intestine that extends from the end of the small intestine to the anus. The large intestine acts mainly to absorb water from digested materials and solidify faeces. It includes the cecum, colon and rectum.

intimidation
Threatening or **bullying** behaviour intended to force someone to do something.

intravenous
Directly into a **vein**. A substance can be delivered directly into a vein by inserting a cannula into a vein and then connecting it to a tube containing the substance. **Medications**, **anaesthetic**, fluids or **nutrition** can be administered in this way.

introversion
A **personality trait** that means people are likely to be reserved and not outward-going or sociable. They may find it difficult to relate to others or not take much interest in other people.

involuntary muscle
Smooth muscle that is not under the conscious control of the individual, for example the muscles of the **oesophagus** that move a **food** bolus into the **stomach** are involuntary. If they are examined under a **microscope**, smooth muscles have a different structure from **voluntary muscles**.

iodine
A **mineral** that is used as an antiseptic in liquid form. Iodine is essential to the **thyroid** gland for its production of the thyroid **hormones** that control the body's metabolism, growth rate and other functions. If there is insufficient iodine in the diet, the thyroid gland will not produce enough thyroid hormones.

iron
A mineral essential in a **healthy balanced diet**, it is found in leafy green vegetables, meat, beans and peas. It is needed for the production of **haemoglobin**.

irregular heart rhythm
A change in the usual steady heartbeat. **Changes** in **heart** rhythms may be a sign of **disease** and should always be medically investigated. Some causes of irregular heart rhythms can be treated. *See* **electrocardiogram**.

Islets of Langerhans
The hormone-producing cells of the **pancreas** that produce **insulin**, glucagon and somatostatin directly into the blood flow.

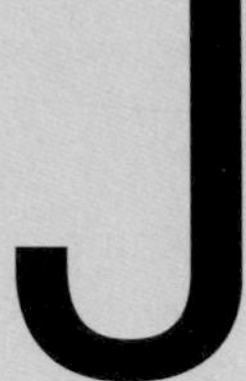

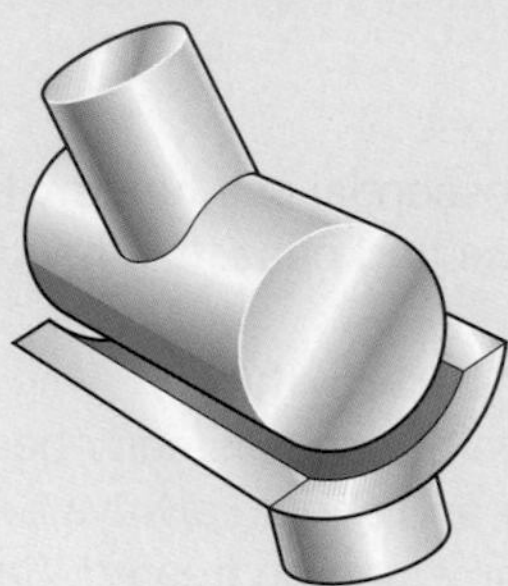

jargon

Words used by a particular profession or **group** as a '**professional** shorthand' that are hard for others to **understand**.
More information can be found at www.plainenglish.co.uk

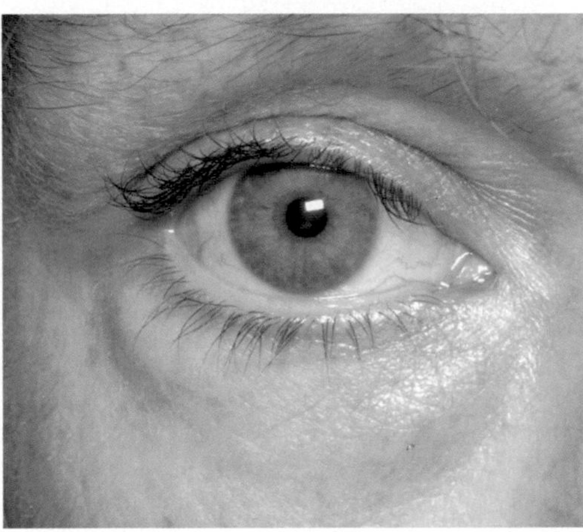

Jaundice.

jaundice

A yellowing of the **skin** and the whites of the eyes as the result of an excess of a pigment called bilirubin. This is a normal by-product of the breakdown of **red blood cells** that is usually **excreted** in the bile after being broken down by actions of the **liver**. Jaundice normally indicates a liver problem, but it can also result from **blood** or **spleen** disorders. **Neonatal jaundice** is common in **newborns** as the liver can take a few days to start functioning properly; it is not usually an indication of a **health** problem.

job description

Information about what is entailed in a particular job role. It is likely to include:

- information about the employing **organisation**
- the location of the job
- the tasks to be undertaken
- the hours of **work**
- the person to whom the job holder is **accountable**
- details of any staff who are accountable to the job holder
- the terms and conditions of the job
- the salary offered.

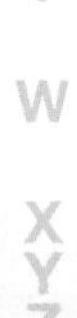

Job descriptions are also useful to refer to during **performance reviews** and **appraisals**, and when planning **professional development**.

SUNNYSIDE

ANYTOWN

JOB DESCRIPTION

JOB TITLE: Care Assistant

PAY: £5.60 per hour

HOURS: 21

REPORTING TO: The manager

ABOUT SUNNYSIDE

Sunnyside is a purpose-built residential home for up to 48 older people who are infirm and most of whom need some assistance with their personal care. There is a shared dining and recreational area which offers a programme of activities for residents each week.

The post holder will work as part of the care assistant team as directed by the home manager and the care assistant team leader.

PERSON SPECIFICATION:

Essential

- aged 18 years or over
- education qualifications at Level 2 e.g. GCSE, NVQ, BTEC
- ability to communicate appropriately with others
- patience, understanding and ability to be flexible in approach to meeting residents' care needs

Desirable

- NVQ Level 2 in Care/Health and Social Care or willingness to work towards this within an agreed timescale
- experience of work in health or social care
- knowledge of the National Minimum Standards for Social Care

MAIN DUTIES:

The post holder will:

1. assist residents with personal care in accordance with their individual care plan
2. promote the well-being of residents at all times, including assisting residents to participate in recreational activities
3. maintain residents' dignity and privacy at all times
4. work in accordance with Sunnyside's policies and procedures.

RESPONSIBILITIES:

The post holder will be expected to:

- assist residents with washing, toileting, bathing, dressing, feeding and drinking in accordance with each individual's care plan
- respect the confidentiality of residents and their relatives at all times both on and off duty
- assist in maintaining the comfort of residents
- contribute to the planning and delivery of the recreational activities programme and support individual residents to participate as appropriate
- assist residents who have limited mobility to use walking and moving aids as specified in the individual's care plan
- support residents to maintain contact with their family, friends and community
- under the supervision of a senior care assistant, assist with the safe administration of medication in accordance with the administration of medication policy and procedures
- maintain records of all care provided on individual care plans
- when directed by the manager, escort residents on outings to attend, for example, GP or hospital appointments
- inform and discuss matters relating to the care of residents with the care team leader and/or the manager
- undertake certain cleaning, laundering and ironing duties as they relate to the delivery of personal care
- promote the health, safety and security of residents and staff at all times
- contribute to creating a friendly and homely atmosphere for residents through all actions and communications with residents and staff
- receive and report verbal and written communication including answering the telephone and maintaining written records in accordance with policies and procedures
- attend and participate in staff meetings
- attend training in accordance with legal requirements and personal development plan
- after six months in post, and thereafter at an annual performance review, agree and implement

Part of a job description for a care assistant.

job opportunities

The **employment** that is available. Some people have less **access** to job opportunities than others, either because they have not had the chance to gain the necessary **qualifications**, or because they are unable to move from an area of high **unemployment** to an area where **work** is available, or are unable to overcome **barriers** such as childcare **provision** or travel costs.

Jobseekers Allowance
A **benefit** paid to people over 16 years and under **retirement** age who are available and looking for work. The allowance can be non-means tested if sufficient **National Insurance** contributions have been paid, or means tested if not. People receiving the benefit usually have to report every two weeks on the progress they are making in looking for work.

Joint Area Review (JAR)
An **inspection** of all children's **services** within a local area undertaken by a **team** of **inspectors** from **Ofsted**, the Commission for Social Care Inspection, the **Healthcare Commission**, the Adult Learning Inspectorate and the **Audit Commission**.

joint planning and commissioning
Where two or more **organisations** work together to plan and **commission services**. Organisations may pool budgets or may contribute to shared costs.

joints
Where two, or more, **bones** meet. Various types of joint allow different amounts and different types of movement. The types are:

- fixed joints, such as the joints in the **skull**, which cannot move
- slightly moveable joints, such as those between the **vertebrae** in the **spine**, which have a very small amount of movement
- **synovial joints** – the majority of joints are synovial, and these are the most moveable joints in the body, filled with synovial fluid which lubricates the joint.

The most mobile of all the synovial joints are ball-and-socket joints such as hips and shoulders. These can move in many different directions. Hinge joints such as elbows

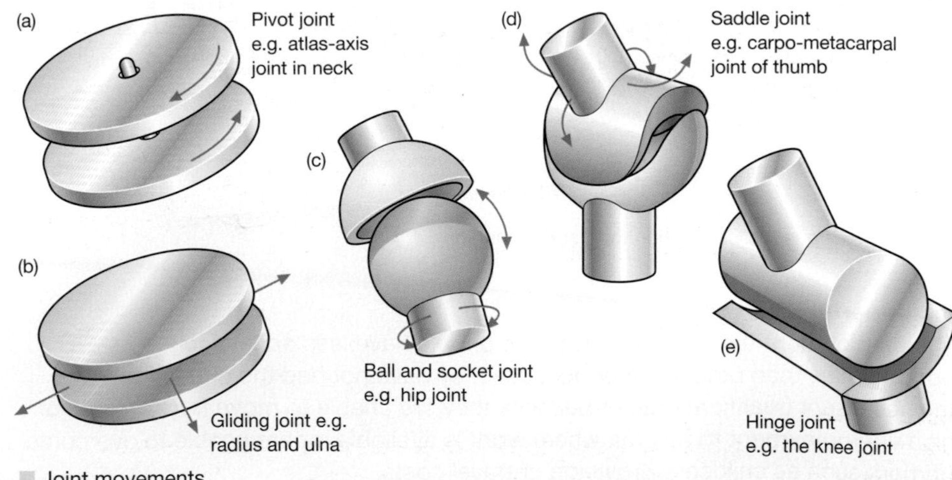

Joint movements.

and knees can move in two directions only, like a hinged door. Pivot joints, such as the neck, allow limited rotational movements, and ellipsoidal joints such as the wrist allow bending, rocking and extending but very limited rotational movement.

joint working
Where two or more **organisations** work to a shared and agreed plan. Staff remain working for their own organisations and do not become part of an integrated **team**.

journal
A **professional** publication providing information so that people can remain up to date on current developments and issues in their own particular area of **work**.

judge
The person responsible for delivering decisions, making judgements and overseeing justice in the **courts**.

judgemental
Taking a position that approves or disapproves of the actions of others, often based on **prejudice** rather than evidence

judicial review
A legal challenge to the **process** of **decision making** by a public body such as a **local authority** or a **hospital** trust. A **judge** will **review** the process followed by the public body and make a judgement as to whether the process was lawful. The **court** does not take a view on the correctness or otherwise of the decision, just the way it was arrived at.

junk food
Processed food containing large amounts of fat, salt or **sugar**. Junk food is not a healthy choice for eating, and children should be strongly encouraged to eat healthy alternatives.

jury
A group of citizens who are sworn to give a true **verdict** after listening to all the evidence in a **court of law**. Juries usually have 12 members, and anyone over the age of 18 years can be asked to sit on a jury.

Justice of the Peace (JP)
See **magistrate**.

justice system
The **organisations**, **processes** and people that administer and deliver justice through the investigation, **prosecution** and **court services**.

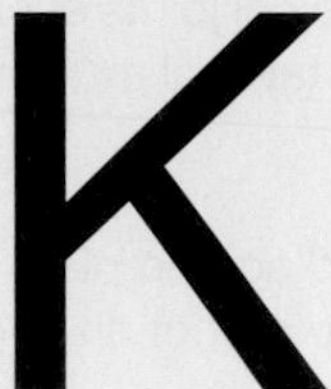

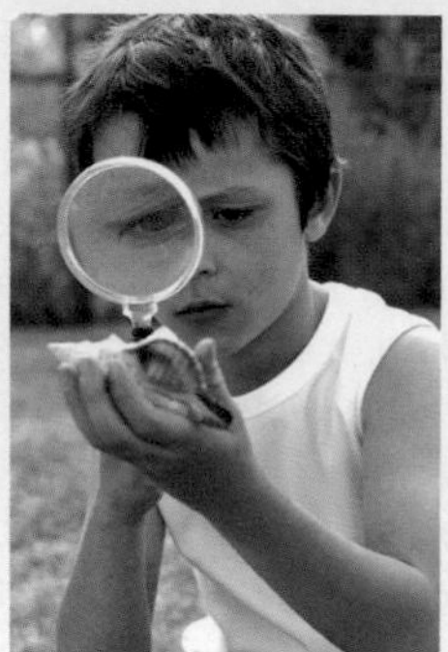

K, vitamin
See vitamins.

keratin
A protein produced by keratinocytes and found in hair, the outer layer of skin and nails.

key people
Those people who are important to an adult, child or young person's health and **well-being**.

keyhole surgery
Laparoscopic surgical procedures carried out using special instruments that require only very small incisions, thus giving a shorter recovery time and reducing the risks of surgery and **infection**.

key worker
Someone who does an essential job in the **public services** and is eligible for special **support** for **housing** under a **government** scheme. The government defines key workers as **nurses** and other **NHS** staff, **police** officers and probation staff, **social workers**, **educational psychologists** and **local authority occupational therapists**. The term is also used to describe a named member of staff who takes **responsibility** for the care of a particular individual in a **residential** or **day care** setting. For children and **young people**, this role is taken by a lead **professional**.

kidneys
Organs situated on either side of the back. They are the main organs of the urinary system and their function is to filter waste products. **Blood** containing metabolic waste, **toxins** and water enter through the renal **artery**. The **kidneys** then filter out waste, toxins and excess water to form urine which pass into the **bladder**, from where they are **excreted** as **urine**. Cleansed, filtered blood is returned to the circulation through the renal **vein**.

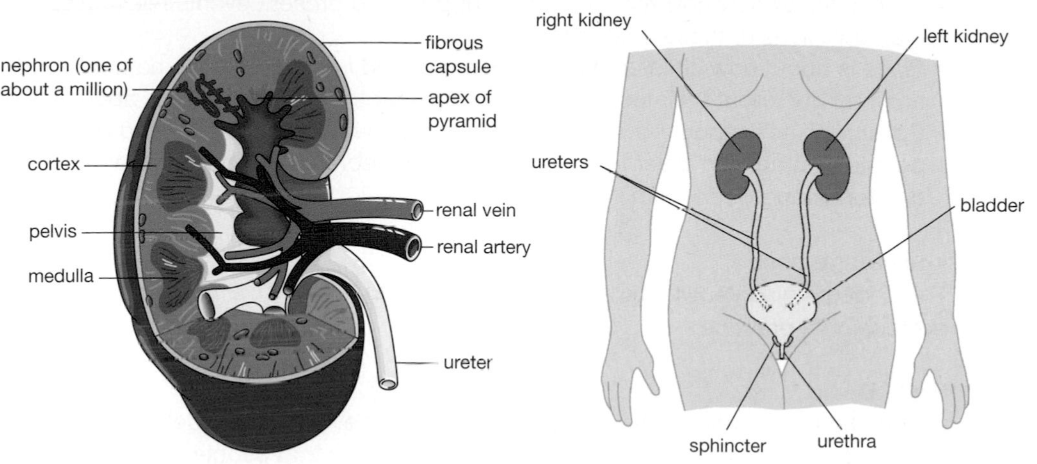

Section through a kidney.

The gross anatomy of the renal system.

kinaesthetic learning
A style of learning that involves physical experience; touching, feeling and doing.

King's Fund
An independent **charitable** foundation that funds **research** and undertakes **analysis** to help inform **health** policy. The King's Fund has a particular focus on health in London. More information can be found at www.**kingsfund**.org.uk

knowledge and understanding of the world
One of the six areas of **learning** in the **early years foundation stage** made up of the following aspects.

- *Exploration and Investigation* is about how children investigate objects and materials and their **properties**, learn about **change** and patterns, similarities and differences, and question how and why things work.
- *Designing and Making* is about the ways in which children learn about the construction **process** and the tools and techniques that can be used to assemble materials creatively and safely.
- *ICT* is about how children find out how to use appropriate information technology such as computers and programmable toys that **support** their learning.

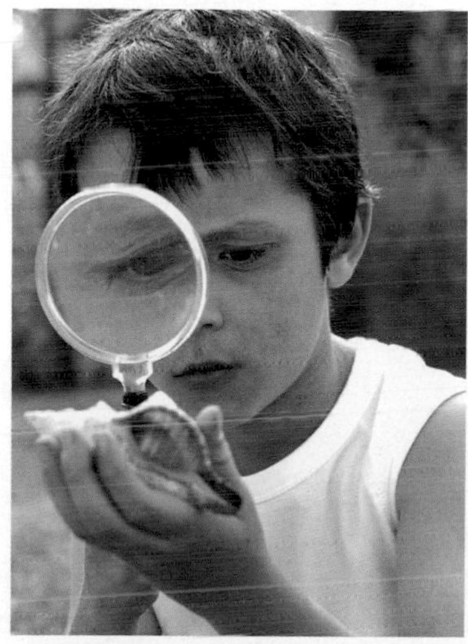

Exploration and investigation.

- *Time* is about how children find out about past and present events relevant to their own lives or those of their **families**.
- *Place* is about how children become aware of and interested in the natural world, and find out about their local area, knowing what they like and dislike about it.
- ***Communities*** is about how children begin to know about their own and other people's **cultures** in order to **understand** and celebrate the similarities and differences between them in a diverse **society**.

knowledge base
The underpinning knowledge and **understanding** that forms the basis for all **professional practice**.

Kolb, David
An American educational theorist (born 1939) who developed a widely used theory about how people learn from experience. The theory is that people:
- have an experience
- think about it (reflect)
- reach a conclusion about what the experience tells them
- plan how to use what they have learned.

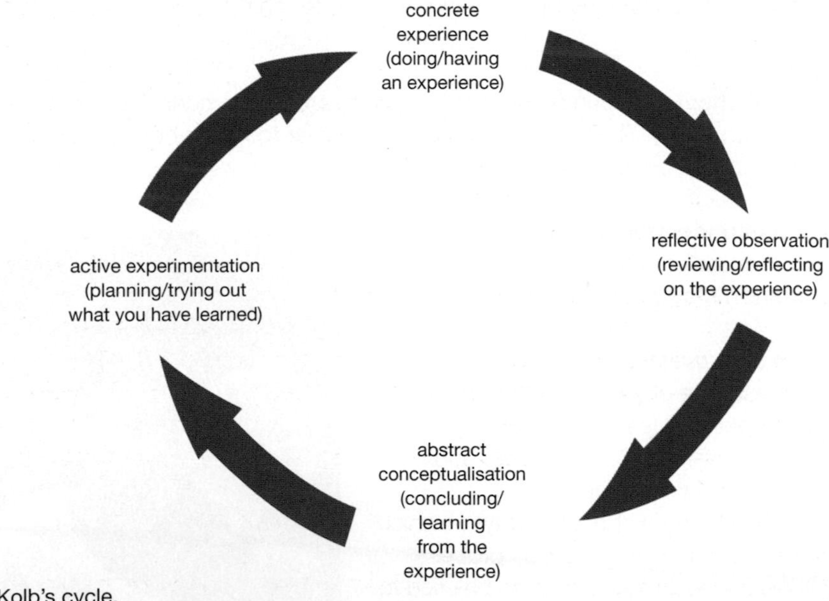

Kolb's cycle.

kosher food
Food prepared in accordance with the **dietary laws** of the Jewish **religion**. Requirements include: pig meat must not be eaten; animals must be butchered in a particular way; meat and dairy foods may not be cooked or eaten together.

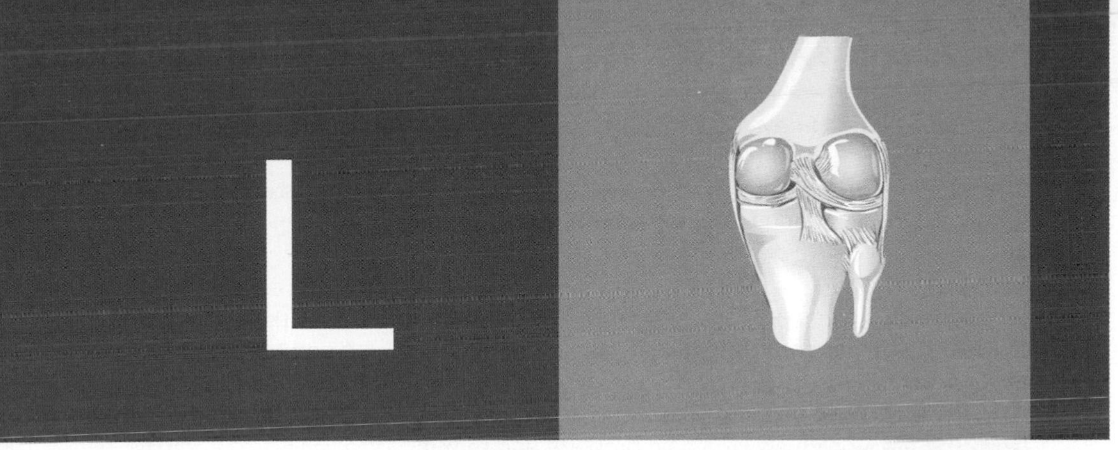

L

labelling
A negative process which identifies people as members of a particular **group** and assuming that they conform to **stereotypes** of the group.

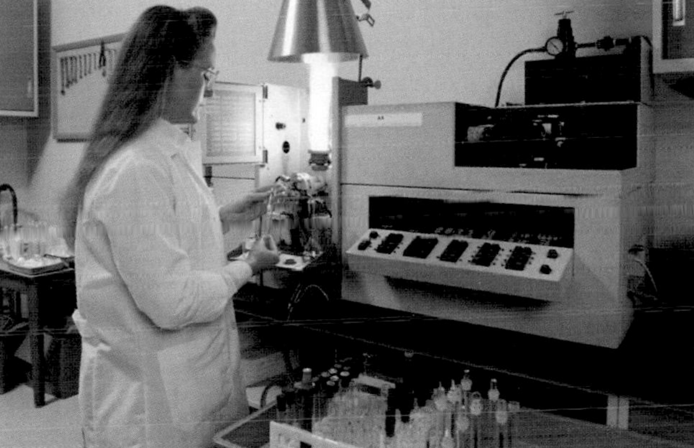
■ A laboratory.

laboratory
A place equipped for scientific **research** or **experimentation**.

labour
The **process** of giving **birth**, during which the **uterus** contracts and pushes the **baby** out through the **vagina** (birth canal) over a period of several hours. There are three stages.

- Stage 1: the uterus contracts and the **cervix** gradually dilates (opens) until the baby's head is able to pass through
- Stage 2: contractions push the baby out of the uterus and through the vagina (birth canal)
- Stage 3: after the baby has been born, the uterus contracts again to expel the **placenta**.

laissez faire
Literally 'leave things alone'. In **child development**, a theory based on the work of the French philosopher Jean-Jacques Rousseau (1712–1778). He taught that children learned naturally and were programmed to learn certain things at certain times; their development would proceed anyway whether or not there was a significant influence from adults or the **environment**. Developmental scales were first developed as a result of the laissez faire approach, as they assume that there

is a 'normal' rate of development and most children will be at an approximate point at a given age.
The term is also used to describe a **leadership** style that is 'hands off' and takes a non-directive approach to **management**.

landlord
Someone who owns property and **rents** it to **tenants** to live or work in. The owner of rented property has **responsibilities** in respect of repairing and maintaining the property and the right to have rent paid and to be able to **re-possess** the property under certain circumstances. There are different types of landlords. *Private landlords* are individuals who own property and rent it. *Social landlords* such as **housing associations** will rent property to people who are at risk of exclusion and offer ongoing support to their tenants. **Local authorities** can also be landlords, and in the past used to build and rent large estates of 'council houses', but there are very few new local authority **housing** schemes.

language
The means of spoken or signed communication between humans. There are 6,809 recorded languages in the world, although many thousands of these are only spoken by a few people, and many cannot be written. Languages are unique to specific racial or national groups and are an important means of maintaining cultural identify if people are in another country and they still wish to maintain using their own language to communicate with friends and family. **British Sign Language** uses signs not speech and is an important part of the culture of the Deaf Community.

language development
The **process** of children **learning** how to **communicate** using words. Each child varies, but generally children develop language in the following stages:

Birth to 1 year	The baby babbles, coos, and approaching 12 months has simple words such as 'dada' or 'mama'. The baby will also follow simple instructions such as 'put it down'.
1 to 2 years	The child's words are more recognisable, and have intonation like conversation. The child begins to put two words together, and by 18 months knows 50 words. A 2-year-old knows about 200 words.
2 to 3 years	The child uses question words such as 'why?' puts 3- or 4-word sentences together, uses 'and' to join ideas together, and knows about 1,000 words.
3 to 4 years	Sentences are longer. The child uses 'the' and 'it', and **understands** the linking of ideas – for example, by using 'because'. Language is used to communicate and to tell stories, repeat rhymes and join in imaginative **play**. The vocabulary is around 5,000 words.

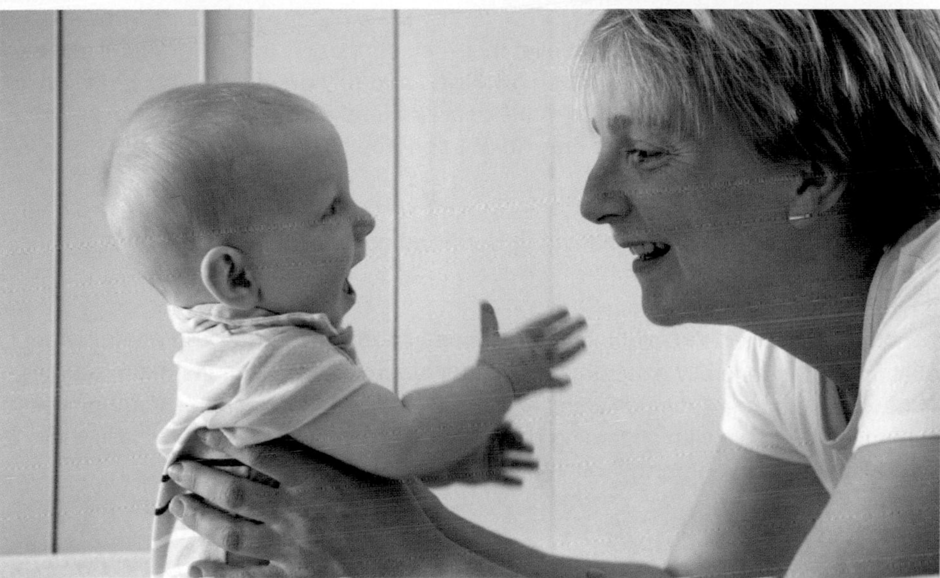

Infants develop language as part of the process of maturation

laparoscopy
A surgical endoscope is passed through a small incision in the abdominal wall to view the organs inside.

laparotomy
Laparotomy is exploratory surgery carried out using a larger incision. Both are usually performed when the diagnosis is not clear.

laser treatment
Procedure where energy is concentrated in a very fine, highly concentrated beam of light and used to perform **surgery**, to unblock **arteries**, correct short or long sight, remove disfiguring marks from the **skin** or remove unwanted hair.

laws
Regulations that set out the **rights and responsibilities** of individual citizens and **organisations**. They are made by **Parliament**, interpreted by **judges** and upheld through the **courts**. Sanctions and punishments are decided by the courts.

leadership
The skills and duties of inspiring, **motivating**, instilling **confidence** and taking **responsibility** for the **outcomes** of a **group** or **organisation**.

lead professional
The person who takes responsibility for co-ordinating the work of a team who are supporting an individual and their family.

learned helplessness
Where people have developed a belief that they cannot do things for themselves and should give up control over their own lives and rely on others. Everyone should be encouraged and **supported** to make decisions, take control and do as much as possible for themselves so that they do not become **dependent** on others.

learning
The development of knowledge and **understanding** or acquisition of a skill.

learning disabilities
Conditions that result in learning taking place at a different pace and at a different level from that generally expected or from environmental conditions that create a delay in development. The causes can be **genetic** or as the result of **trauma**, illness or **accident**. People with a learning disability can function very effectively in the right enabling **environment**.

learning style
The way in which a person learns best. There are different theories that describe ways of learning, but one of the most widely used identifies three different types of learning styles.

- *Visual* learning involves the use of seen or **observed** things, including written instructions, pictures, diagrams, demonstrations, displays, **handouts**, films, flip-chart, and watching others (also known as '**sitting next to Nellie**').
- *Auditory* learning involves the transfer of **information** through listening to the spoken word, of oneself or others, and to sounds and noises.
- *Kinesthetic* learning involves physical experiences, such as **touching**, feeling, holding, doing, and practical hands-on experiences.

Everyone learns using a combination of styles, but most people are likely to find that one type of learning is dominant.

learning theory
A theory resulting from the **transmission model**. There are broadly two schools of thought. Learning theory sees children as reacting to what goes on around them and absorbing **information** from their experiences. It also recognises that **human behaviour** can be modified by consequences (called 'reinforcement' in the **models**), for example if a child puts a hand on a hot iron, he or she will get burned and will not be likely to repeat the act. **Social learning theory** accepts the basics of learning theory but also emphasises that children learn behaviours by **observing** and **imitating** adults, especially those adults who are important to them.

learning, training and development opportunities
Programmes to enable individuals to learn, develop and maximise their own potential and independence.

lecture
Information given to learners by a single teacher/lecturer/expert. Usually, verbal information is accompanied by visual information and delivered by standing in front of the audience, often in quite a formal way and to a fairly large audience.

legal aid
Financial **support** to enable people on **low incomes** to **access** the legal **system**.

legislation
Laws that have been passed by **Parliament**.

leisure
Free time when people are not working and are able to spend time on other activities and interests.

lesbian
A woman who is romantically or sexually attracted to other women or has **sexual relationships** with other women.

leucocytes
One type of **white blood cell** made in the bone marrow hat helps to fight **infections** and attacks **pathogens** by engulfing them (known as phagocytosis).

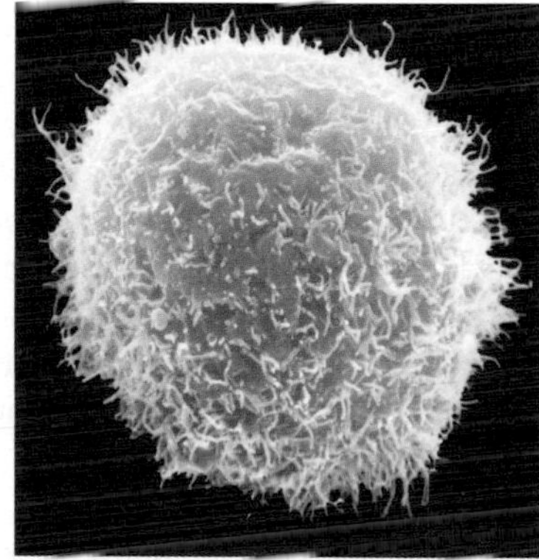
Leucocytes under a microscope.

level of development and understanding
Covers the **cognitive**, **physical**, **social**, **emotional** and **intellectual** level of children and young people. It can be related to chronological age but where children and young people have disabilities this form of development may be delayed.

libido
Sex drive, in the commonly understood use of the term. It comes from psychoanalytic theory and describes the **energy** that comes from sexual and survival drives.

life chances
Aspects of children and young people's life that can inhibit or promote the chance they have to maximise and realise their full potential, educationally and socially.

life event
Any particularly important thing which takes place or happens during the life span.

life expectancy
The average number of years a person can expect to live from **birth**. This is calculated **statistically** for a given **population**; however, it can be calculated from any age and the results will differ depending on the age at which the calculation is done.

life stage
The phase of life of a person at a given point in time. People move through **infancy**, childhood, **adolescence**, early **adulthood**, late adulthood and **old age**. *See* **human development**.

lifestyle
The **choices** people make about how they live, spend money, use **leisure** time, eat and **exercise**.

lifting and handling
See **moving and handling**.

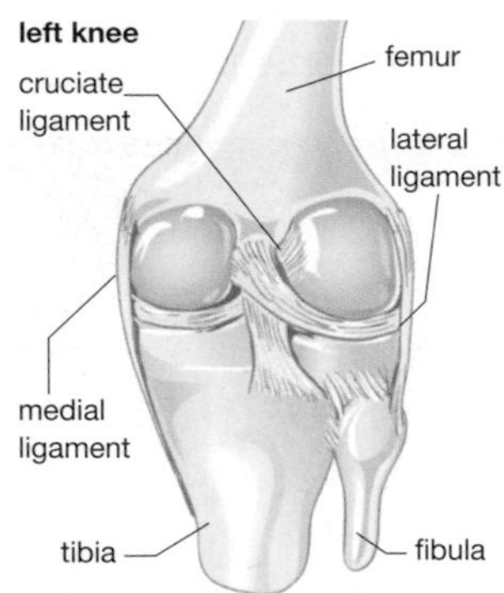

■ Knee joint ligaments.

ligament
A tough band or sheet of fibrous **tissue** that connects **bone** to bone or cartilage at a **joint**, or supports an **organ**.

lipids
Substances such as **fats**, oil or wax that dissolve in alcohol but not in water. They are found in all plant and animal **cells** and are easily stored in the human body as a source of **energy**. They include fatty acids, **cholesterol**, triglycerides, neutral fats and steroids.

lip reading
A means of communication for deaf people who participate in verbal communication through recognising the shapes made by people's lips as they speak.

lip speaking
A means of communication for deaf people who prefer to **communicate** through lip reading and speech rather than through signing. People can train as lip speakers and then will provide communication support for deaf people in education, meetings, conferences and day-to-day situations.

listening skills
The ability to build an **understanding** of another person's position through using **questioning skills**, **reflective listening**, reading **non-verbal communication** and giving positive encouragement to others to **communicate**.

literacy
The ability to read, write and **understand** the written and spoken word. The United Nations Educational, Scientific and Cultural Organization (UNESCO) defines it as: 'the ability to identify, understand, interpret, create, **communicate** and compute, using printed and written materials associated with varying contexts. Literacy involves a continuum of **learning** to enable an individual to achieve his or her **goals**, to develop his or her knowledge and **potential**, and to participate fully in the wider **society**.'

literature review
A search of current writings and background **information** about an area that is being **researched**. This is normally done at the outset of a research project.

liver
The second largest **organ** in the body. The adult human liver normally weighs between 1.4 and 1.6 kg (3.1 to 3.5 pounds). It is located on the right side of the upper **abdomen**, to the right of the **stomach**. It has many functions, including:

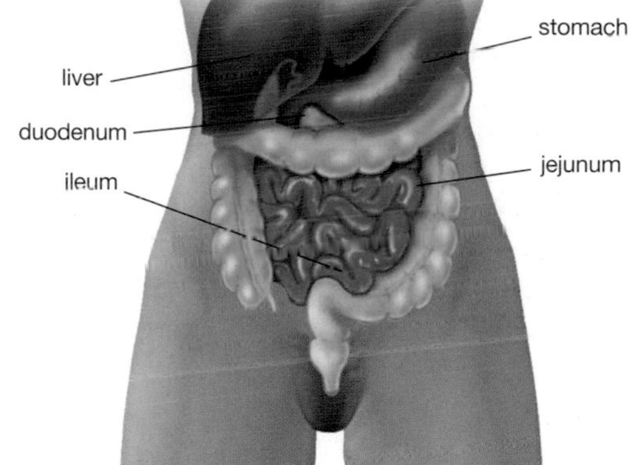

■ Position of the liver.

- processing **digested food** from the **intestine**
- controlling levels of **fats**, amino acids and **glucose** in the **blood**
- combating **infections** in the body
- clearing the blood of particles and infections, including **bacteria**
- neutralising and destroying drugs and **toxins**
- manufacturing bile
- storing iron, **vitamins** and other essential chemicals
- manufacturing, breaking down and regulating numerous **hormones** including sex hormones
- making **enzymes** and **proteins** which are responsible for most chemical **reactions** in the body, for example, those involved in blood clotting and repair of damaged **tissues**.

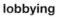

lobbying
The act of arguing a case to decision makers for a particular cause or point of view.

local area agreements
Agreements between national and **local government** and their partners that include up to 35 **targets** that reflect national and local **priorities** around children and **young people**, safer and stronger **communities**, healthier communities, **older people**, and economic development and enterprise. These are measured against a set of indicators during the annual comprehensive area assessment.

A B C D E F G H I J K L M N O P Q R S T U V W X Y Z

local authorities
Elected bodies with **responsibility** for the **local government** of a particular area. Responsibility lies with elected members (**councillors**) who have to make policy and budget decisions, but the day-to-day **administration** of local **services** is undertaken by employed officers.

local government
The body of elected local **councillors** who have the **responsibility** to provide a safe and secure local **environment** and **services** to meet the **needs** of a local **population**.

lone parent
A person bringing up children without a partner, through **choice**, **divorce**, **separation** or **bereavement**.

longitudinal studies
Research projects carried out over a period of time, where the same set of **data** is **recorded** at specified intervals.

long-term memory
Recall of events in the distant past. A feature of **dementia** is that some people may have excellent long-term memories but be unable to recall recent events.

loss
The experience of being bereaved or of losing a key part or aspect of life. People experience **feelings** of **bereavement** and loss not only at the **death** of someone close, but following amputation of a limb, breast removal, or hysterectomy. For some people losing a job or a house can result in similar feelings.

low density lipoprotein (LDL)
Also known as 'bad cholesterol'. Transports cholesterol to cells. A surplus can build up causing damage to the lining of blood vessels.

low income
An income of less than 60 per cent of the **median** disposable **income** in the UK. More information can be found at www.lowpay.gov.uk

lumbar puncture
Also called a 'spinal tap', a **process** to take a **sample** of **cerebrospinal fluid** in order to **diagnose** conditions such as **meningitis**, **brain tumour** or **inflammation**. It can also be used to diagnose some **diseases** of the **immune system** such as **multiple sclerosis**. The sample is obtained by inserting a hollow **needle** into the space around the spinal nerves inside the **vertebrae** in the lower spine.

lung capacity
The volume of air that can be breathed out of the lungs after breathing in as deeply as possible. This can also be called 'forced vital capacity'. Trained athletes are likely to have the largest lung capacities. Men generally have larger lung capacities than women and tall people have a larger capacity than short people. **Asthmatics** and people with lung **disease** generally have small lung capacities.

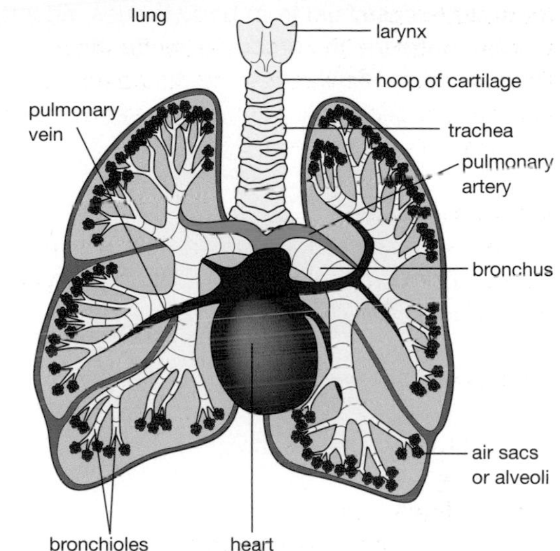

■ The lungs.

lungs
The main **organs** of the **respiratory system**. They are large, sponge-like structures that lie on either side of the **heart** in the air-tight **thoracic cavity**. Each lung expands rhythmically with the ribs to accommodate inhaled air and recoils due to elastic fibres surrounding the **alveoli** to expel air. Lungs consist of berry-like, thin-walled alveoli lined with a film of moisture and connected to the outside by tubes – bronchioles, bronchi and the **trachea**. Their function is to carry out gaseous exchange.

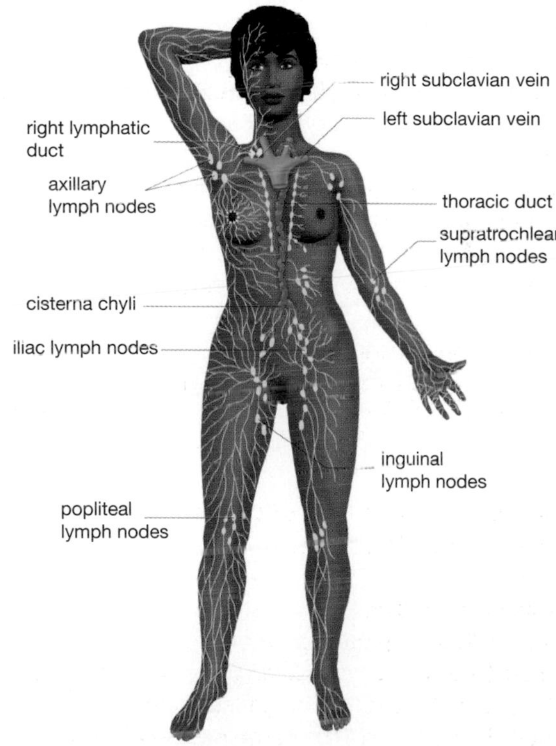

■ The body's lymphatic system.

lymphatic system
The **tissues** and **organs**, including the **bone** marrow, **spleen**, **thymus**, and **lymph nodes**, that produce and store **cells** that fight **infection** and **disease**. The **system**

removes excess fluid from body tissues, absorbs fatty acids, transports fat into the bloodstream and produces **white blood cells** such as **lymphocytes** which produce antibodies.

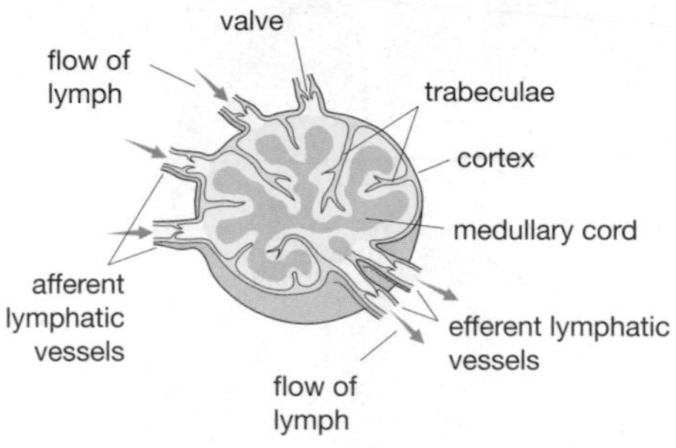

■ A lymph node.

lymph nodes
Bean-shaped structures found throughout the body that are honeycombed with **connective tissue.** They filter and trap **pathogens** that are then destroyed by **lymphocytes.** During an **infection,** lymph nodes may be swollen as large numbers of lymphocytes fight the invading pathogens.

lymphocytes
White blood cells that fight **infection**, produced in lymphoid tissue. There are two main types, B **cells** and T cells. B cells produce the **antibodies** to neutralise antigens on the surface of micro-organisms, and T cells have wide-ranging functions in the **immune system**.

lysergic acid diethylamide (LSD)
A **hallucinogenic** drug that causes visual and aural **hallucinations**, and changes in levels of awareness and **understanding**. Effects can be unpredictable and can result in a 'bad trip' with frightening and disturbing hallucinations. Use of the drug can also result in **paranoia**, **anxiety** and long-term **mental health problems**.

M

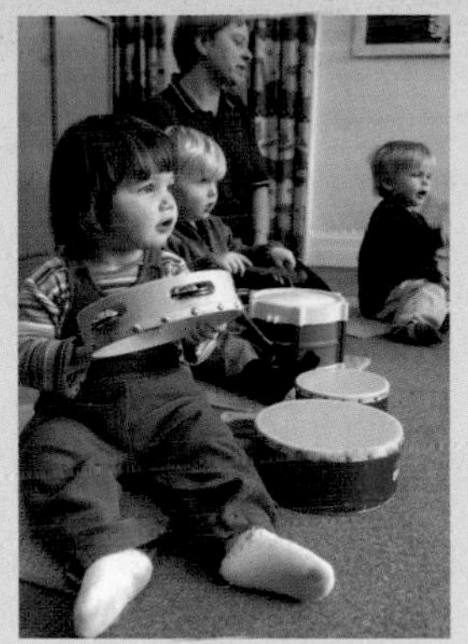

macronutrients
The largest **food** groups that humans need, and which make up the bulk of the necessary daily food intake: **proteins**, **carbohydrates** and **fats**. They are large complex molecules which need to be broken down by enzymes before they can be used in the body. Macronutrients supply the calories for energy.

magistrate
Also known as a Justice of the Peace, the person responsible for dealing with most criminal cases in local **courts** involving the less serious crimes, such as minor theft, criminal damage, public disorder and motoring **offences**. A magistrate considers the evidence, reaches a **verdict** and sets a **sentence**. When sitting in the Family Proceedings Court, magistrates deal with a range of issues affecting **families** and children.

Magistrate's Court
The first tier of the **criminal justice system**. All criminal cases start there, and only 3 per cent go on to be heard in the Crown Court. These courts are administered by Her Majesty's Courts Service and **accountable** to the Department for Constitutional Affairs.

magnetic resonance imaging (MRI)
A way of producing images of soft body **tissue** using magnetic and radio waves to produce an image. This has the advantage of not exposing people to radioactive **X-rays** and also allows images to be taken from all angles.

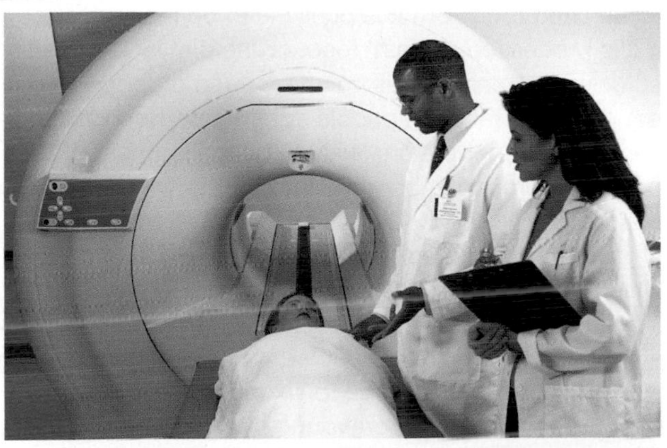

Magnetic resonance imaging is a way of producing images of soft body tissue using magnetic and radio waves to produce an image.

main carer
The person with the primary role in caring for a child or **vulnerable adult**. The **relationship** between a **baby** and its main carer (usually the **mother**) is important for future **emotional development**.

mainstream schools
Establishments that provide **education** for all children. They must take all reasonable steps to ensure that **disabled** children are able to **access** education and that the **teaching** and/or building does not present **barriers** for children with **special education needs**.

Makaton
A form of simple signing, used to support speech. It was developed in the 1970s in the UK for **deaf** adults who also had a **learning disability**, and it is used in many other countries.
More information can be found at www.makaton.org

male reproductive system
See **reproductive systems**.

malignant
Term used to describe a **tumour** which has the potential for progressive and uncontrolled growth and spread into surrounding **tissue**, which is dangerous to **health** and can be life-threatening.

malnutrition
The condition that results from an inadequate or insufficient **diet**. People in countries where there is famine become malnourished because of **starvation** and insufficient **food**. But it is possible to be malnourished while eating plenty of food if it is processed or 'fast' food, or the diet is very limited and does not contain sufficient **nutrients**. This can happen to **older people** who either cannot or do not eat properly. Tests on people admitted to **hospital** show that as many as 10 per cent of older people are likely to be malnourished. Disorders that result in food not being properly absorbed into the body are another cause of malnutrition.
Malnutrition in the UK is defined as:

- having a **body mass index (BMI)** of less than 18.5
- unintentional weight loss greater than 10 per cent in the last three to six months
- a BMI of less than 20 coupled with unintentional weight loss greater than 5 per cent within the last three to six months.

Malnutrition causes poor **wound** healing, **muscle** wasting and fatigue, and can result in more serious and irreversible deterioration of major **organs** and body **systems**.

mammography
Specialist **X-rays** used to check the breasts for **tumours** and cysts. The UK has a national **screening programme** where all women over 50 years are offered a mammogram every three years.

management
The **process** of planning, organising and maintaining **resources** in order to deliver **objectives** and **outcomes** for an individual or organisation.

manicure
Treatment caring for the hands and nails.

manipulation
Usually carried out by an **osteopath**, a **chiropractor** or a **physiotherapist**, it is a means of moving parts of the body in order to aid recovery from **illness or injury**. If used in connection with **behaviour**, it means someone using people or situations in a deliberately deceitful way in order to achieve what they want.

marginalisation
The **process** where certain **groups** or individuals are pushed to the edge (or margins) of **society**, where they have little say in **decision making** and are denied the means to improve their position. This can be based on **race**, **gender**, **sexual orientation**, level of ability or age.

market analysis
Research undertaken by **commissioners** and **providers** of **services** in order to **understand** and forecast the levels of demand and supply for services, and to identify **needs** and the extent to which they are met.

Maslow, Abraham
An American **psychologist** (1908–1970) best known for developing the 'hierarchy of **needs**', a theory that suggests basic physiological needs such as **food** and shelter and **safety** must be met before people can move on to meet other needs such as love, social **relationships** and intellectual stimulation.

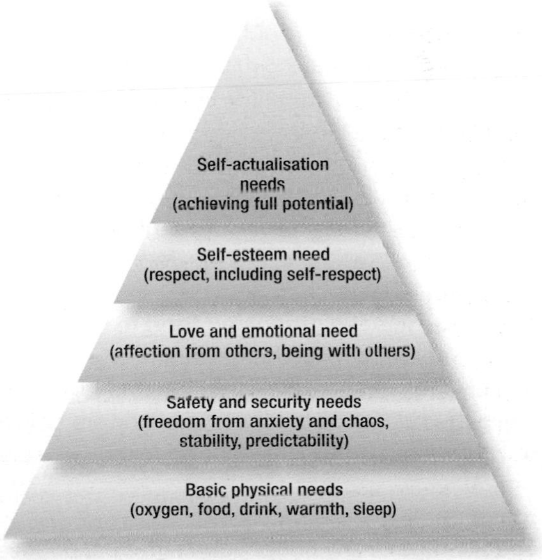

Maslow's hierarchy of needs.

A B C D E F G H I J K L M N O P Q R S T U V W XYZ

massage
Manual manipulation (movement) of the skin and muscles for a therapeutic purpose using different techniques. Massage should be smooth and rhythmical with an even depth and pressure, which may be adapted for the size and condition of the client.

massage therapy
Manipulation of **soft tissues** of the body by kneading, pushing, squeezing and stroking to provide **relaxation**. **Aromatherapy** massage, a form of **complementary therapy** uses essential oils combined with massage to enhance relaxation and a feeling of **well-being**.

maternal deprivation
The condition a young child experiences if separated from the **mother** or main carer for long periods of time. Children become **anxious** and fretful, and ultimately withdrawn. The impact can last throughout life, making it difficult to make and sustain loving **relationships** and resulting in low **self-esteem** and **confidence**. The first **psychologist** to identify this was **John Bowlby** (1907–1990) in his theories about the importance of **attachment**.

matriarchal
A term used to describe a **society**, **community**, **group** or **family** where **power**, control, **decision making** and **responsibility** are undertaken by women.

matrix
Elements arranged in such a way as to show how they are interconnected. Also a background material in which different cells and fibres can be embedded that is characteristic of connective tissue. The matrix can be a liquid such as blood, or hard such as bone.

maturation
The **process** of progressing through expected stages of development.

meals on wheels
A **service** delivering prepared **food** to people in their own homes. This can be important for people who have difficulty in shopping for or preparing food, but it can also reinforce **social isolation** and loneliness as there is no need for people to leave the house. Traditionally, meals were delivered fresh each day, but many are now prepared for the freezer and microwave and can be delivered in bulk.

mean
The average of any set of figures (terms) of collected **data**. It is arrived at by adding up all the terms and dividing by the number of terms included.

means testing
The **process** of working out people's entitlement to **benefits** and free or reduced-price **services** based on an **assessment** of how much **income** and savings they have. Most benefits and services require a **contribution** or the payment of full cost from people who have financial **resources** above certain levels.

measles
An acute, highly contagious viral **disease** that begins after a 10- to 12-day **incubation period** and appears mainly in children. It usually begins with a mild to moderate **fever**, persistent cough, runny nose, sore eyes and sore throat. Two or three days later, small bright red spots, called Koplik's spots, appear on the insides of the cheeks followed by a red blotchy **rash** on the skin, usually on the face, along the hairline and behind the ears. The rash rapidly spreads to the **chest** and back, then to the thighs and feet. The rash fades over about a week in the same sequence that it appeared. Measles is so contagious that 90 per cent of contacts of an infected person will develop it. **Immunity** develops after being infected or being **vaccinated**, and measles cannot be caught twice.
See **MMR vaccine**.

measurements
Recorded checks on key body functions and risks, such as **heart rate** (by checking the **pulse**), risk of **heart disease** or **stroke** (by checking **blood pressure**), the production of **insulin** (by checking **blood glucose**) or **lung** function (by checking the **peak flow**).

media
Public channels of **communication** such as television, radio, newspapers, magazines and electronic **networking** websites.

median
The middle figure (term) in a set of collected **data**, where there is an odd number of terms. Where there is an even number of terms, it is the average of the two terms in the middle.

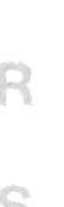

mediation
A **process** for resolving disagreements in which an impartial third party (the mediator) helps the people in dispute to find a mutually acceptable resolution. Mediation is based on the principles that:

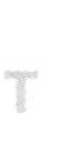

- all parties in a dispute need to work to find a solution that is acceptable to all – there should always be a win/win
- it is necessary to look forward and not to re-live (or apportion blame for) situations in the past
- **feelings** need to be acknowledged as well as the facts of a situation, as only then can people let go and move forward.

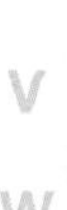

medical history
A complete description of a patient's physical and mental condition, past and present.

medical model
An approach to a range of social issues that looks for what is 'wrong' with the individual or **family** involved. **Assessment** is about '**diagnosing**' a problem, and the action plan is about how to 'cure' the problem. This is less likely to be seen in current **practice**, although this terminology can still be heard from some practitioners.

medical practitioners
Registered, qualified **doctors** who are on the General Medical Council's list of Registered Medical Practitioners. There are specialist lists for different aspects of medicine and for general **practice**.

medical records
Information relating to the **health** of an individual. Key records are held by a person's **general practitioner**, but additional records will be held at any **hospital** where investigations or **treatment** have been provided. All medical records are **confidential** and can only be shared using **Caldicott principles**.

medical treatment
Assistance given by a **doctor** or other **health professional** to alleviate, cure or improve a medical condition, illness or **disease**.

medication
Drugs given as part of **medical treatment**. Drugs for people to use at home are given with clear instructions as to how they are to be used, and must include the name of the drug, the **patient**'s name and the date on the label. Drugs given as part of **treatment** in **hospital** are administered by qualified **health professionals**.

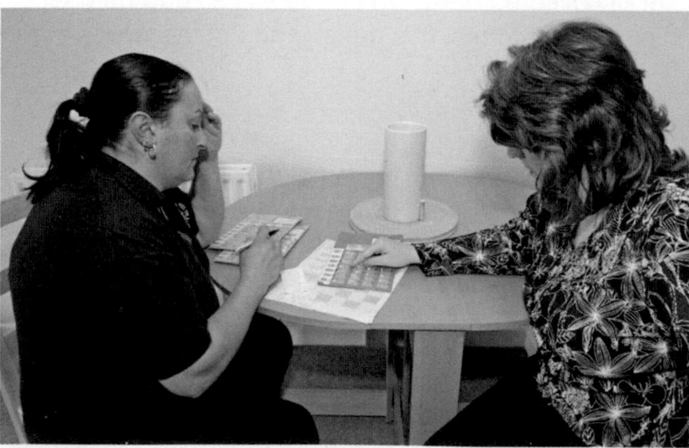

Medication.

All medication should be regularly **reviewed** by a **doctor** to see if it is still required or if any **changes** need to be made. It is very important that people only take drugs that have been **prescribed** for them; serious effects can result from taking medicine prescribed for someone else.

medication administration record
The documentation on which the medication has been ordered/prescribed – this will vary across care settings and environments, such as hospital and community settings, including medications prescribed by GPs and dispensed by community pharmacists where the instructions will be found on the medication packaging.

medicine
Medicine falls into three categories: 1. The whole of the diagnosis and treatment of disease and the maintenance of health; 2. Diagnosis and treatment that does not involve surgical procedures; 3. Any drug or remedy used to treat diseases and disorders.

melanin
A pigment in the **skin**. Dark-skinned people have more melanin than light-skinned people. Melanin protects the skin from ultraviolet radiation (sunlight). It is produced by **cells** called melanocytes that increase their production of melanin in response to sun exposure. Freckles are small, concentrated areas of increased melanin production.

Member of Parliament
A person who is elected to represent one of the parliamentary constituencies in Parliament.

memory
The ability to store and later **recall** events and **information**. The ease of recall varies between individuals, but generally it becomes more difficult to recall recent events and information with age. **Dementia** involves a gradual loss of memory function; there is often excellent recall of details from many years previously, but no memory of recent events.

menarche
A woman's first **menstrual** period. The average age when this occurs is 13 years, but it can be as young as 8 years or as late as 18 years. Anywhere between 10 and 16 years is considered normal.

Mencap
A national charity, with local branches, that represents the interests of people with a learning disability. The organisation lobbies on behalf of people with learning disabilities and provides information, advice and support.
More information can be found at www.mencap.org.uk

meninges
Three layers of membranes surrounding the **brain** and **spinal cord**, which provide a barrier from the rest of the body and act as a protection from **infection**.

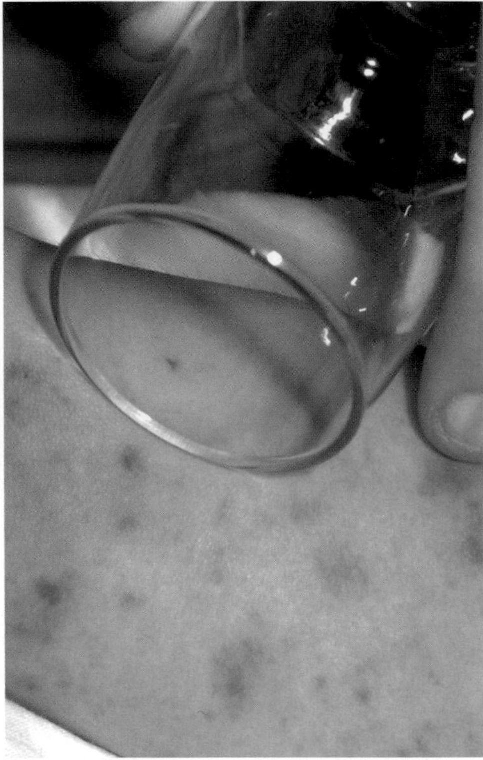

Bacterial meningitis is very serious and can progress rapidly.

meningitis
Inflammation of the **meninges**, caused by **bacteria** or a **virus**. The disease is spread through prolonged contact with an infected person, through sneezing, coughing or kissing. Bacterial meningitis is very serious and can progress rapidly. **Babies** and young children are most vulnerable, but the **disease** can be fatal, or cause permanent damage, at any age. Viral meningitis is usually less severe and less likely to have long-term effects, but it is still serious and requires urgent medical attention. **Symptoms** in babies and **infants** may include:

- a high **temperature**, **fever** (possibly with cold hands and feet)
- **vomiting** and refusing feeds
- high-pitched moaning or whimpering cry
- blank, staring expression
- pale, itchy complexion
- floppiness
- dislike of being handled
- becoming fretful
- neck retraction, with arching of the back
- convulsions
- being lethargic and difficult to wake
- a tense or bulging fontanelle (soft spot on the head).

Symptoms in adults and older children may include:

- a constant, generalised headache
- confusion
- a high temperature, although hands and feet may be cold
- drowsiness
- vomiting, **stomach** pain, sometimes with **diarrhoea**
- rapid breathing
- neck stiffness
- a **rash** of red or purple spots or **bruises** that does not fade when you press a glass tumbler or finger against it – this may not be present in the early stages
- **joint** or **muscle** pain
- sensitivity to bright lights, daylight or even the television.

Medical attention must be sought at once for any combination of these symptoms.

COMMON SYMPTOMS OF MENINGITIS

IN BABIES & TODDLERS

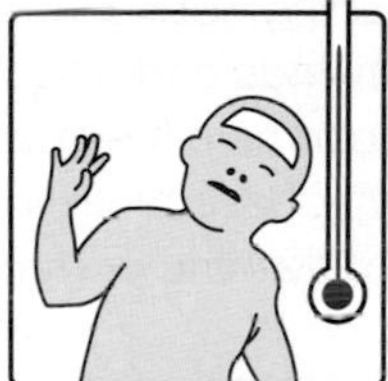

Fever – hands & feet may also feel cold

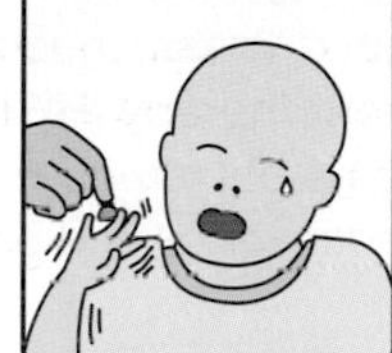

Refusing feeds or vomiting

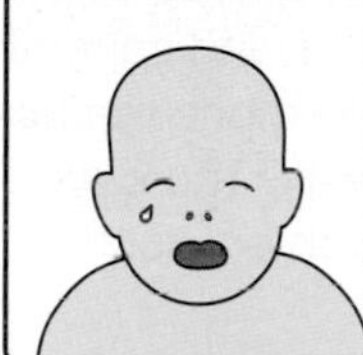

High pitched moaning cry or whimpering

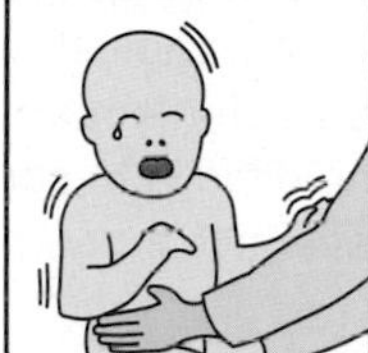

Dislike of being handled, fretful

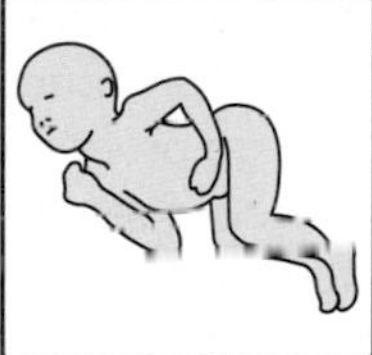

Neck retraction with arching of back

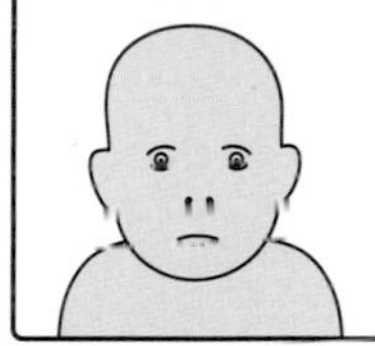

Blank & staring expression

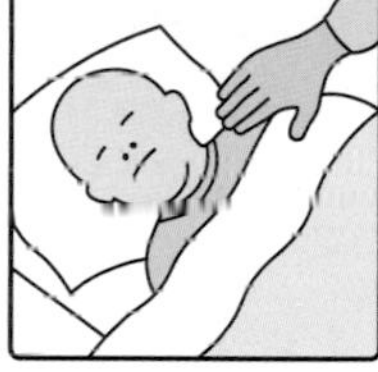

Difficult to wake, lethargic

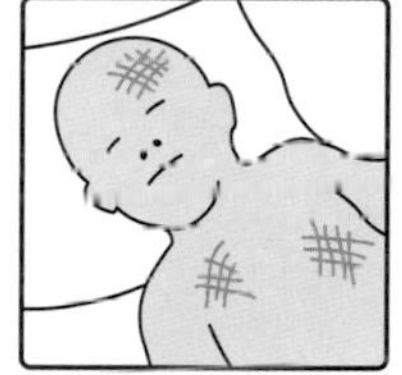

Pale blotchy complexion

IN ADULTS & CHILDREN

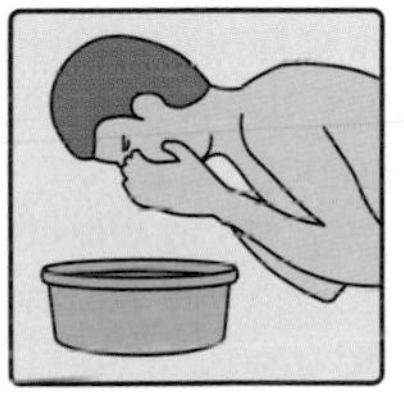

Vomiting

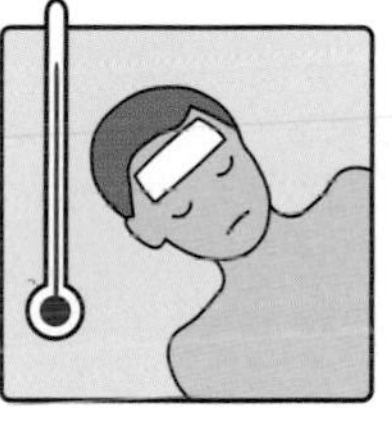

Fever

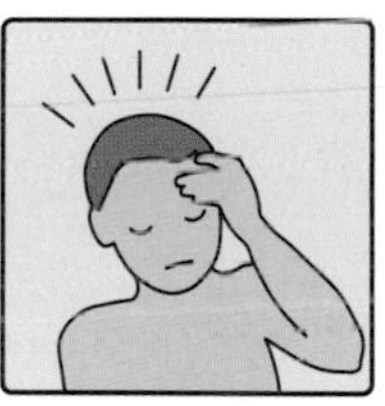

Headache

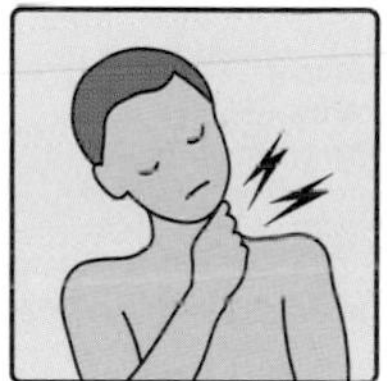

Stiff neck

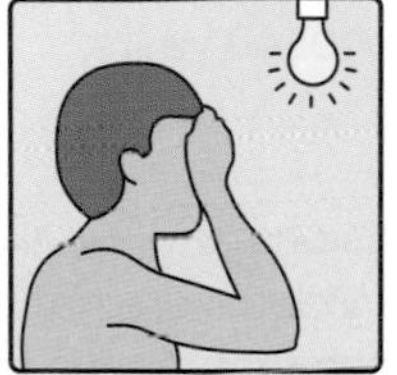

Light aversion

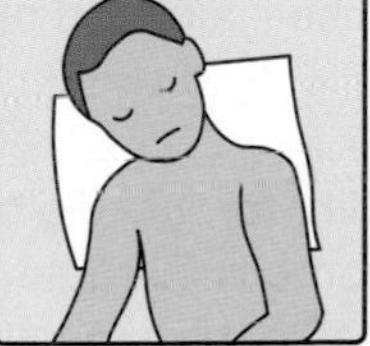

Drowsiness

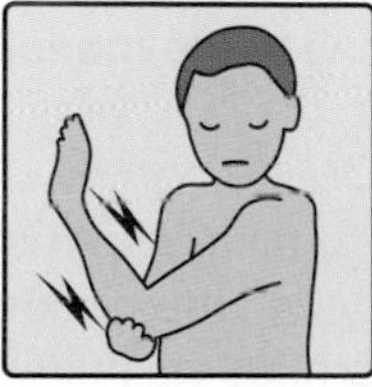

Joint pain

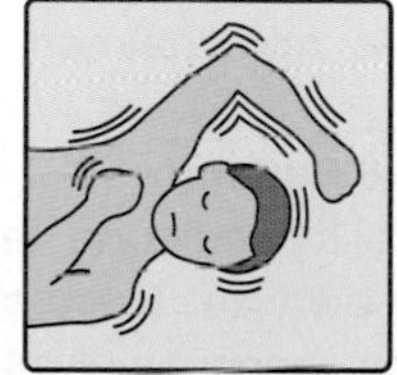

Fitting

The symptoms of meningitis.

menopause
The end of a woman's fertility. **Menstrual** periods become less frequent and then stop, and the **ovaries** no longer produce eggs. This is brought about by the falling production of **oestrogen**, the female **hormone**. The menopause is considered to have been reached when a woman has not had a menstrual period for a year. In the UK, the average age for the menopause is 52 years. When going through the menopause, 80 per cent of women experience **symptoms** including hot flushes and sweats, **vaginal** dryness and general **skin** dryness, mood swings and frequent **urinary** tract **infections. Hormone replacement therapy** (HRT) can help if symptoms become difficult to cope with. There are also herbal remedies that have been found to be effective for some women, such as starflower oil and oil of evening primrose.

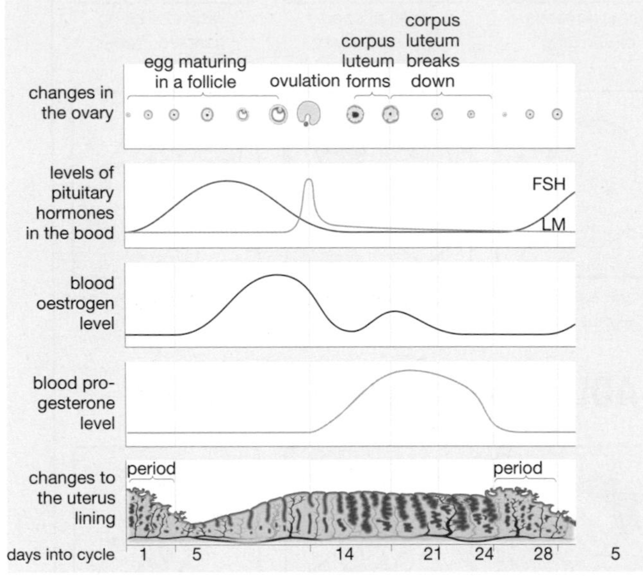

Changes during the menstrual cycle.

menstruation
The bleeding that follows the breakdown of the lining of the **uterus** every four weeks if the egg produced by the **ovaries** remains unfertilised. As the egg is produced by the ovaries, the lining of the uterus thickens in preparation for an **implanted zygote**. If the egg is not fertilised, the lining breaks down and, over about five days, it is discarded from the body, along with **blood**, through the **vagina**. The uterus lining then begins to thicken again in preparation for the next egg. This is the 'menstrual cycle'. Each cycle lasts about 28 days and will be continuous during the years that a woman is fertile, from the **menarche** to the **menopause** – a period of about 40 years.

mental capacity
The ability someone has to take **responsibility** for making decisions and running his or her own life. There may be times when some vulnerable individuals are not able to cope, because of a **learning disability**, **dementia**, or an illness that means they are not conscious. The **law** in this area is underpinned by a set of five principles:

- a presumption of capacity – every adult has the right to make his or her own decisions and must be assumed to have capacity to do so unless it is proved otherwise

- the right for individuals to be **supported** to make their own decisions – people must be given all appropriate help before anyone concludes that they cannot make their own decisions
- individuals must retain the right to make what might be seen by others as eccentric or unwise decisions
- anything done for or on behalf of people without capacity must be in their best interests
- there must be the least restrictive **intervention** – anything done for or on behalf of people without capacity should be the least restrictive of their basic rights and freedoms.

mental disorder

The general term now used in **legislation** to describe a whole range of conditions and illnesses that were previously defined separately. The term now includes conditions previously referred to as:

- mental illness
- mental **impairment**
- severe mental impairment
- psychopathic disorder.

mental health

A person's mental state and **well-being**. Many factors can have an impact on a person's mental health, such as **stress**, **relationships**, **lifestyle**, **substance misuse**, **social isolation** or exclusion, and economic deprivation. Additionally, failure to take prescribed **medication** will have an impact on someone with a history of **mental health problems**.

Mental Health Act Commission

A public body whose role is to **safeguard** the interests of people detained under the Mental Health Act 1983 (as amended by the Mental Health Act 2007). The Mental Health Act Commission is a **monitoring** body rather than an inspectorate or **regulator**. Its concern is primarily the legality of detention and the protection of individuals' **human rights**. In addition to a visiting programme, where **patients** can be **interviewed** in private, the Commission provides important safeguards to patients who lack capacity or refuse to **consent** to **treatment**, through the Second Opinion Appointed Doctor Service. The Commission can hear complaints from detained patients and can **review** decisions likely to involve human rights issues, such as the withholding of mail. The responsibilities of the Commission are being brought together with those of the Healthcare Commission and the Commission for Social Care Inspection with the Care Quality Commission in October 2008.
More information can be found at www.mhac.org.uk

mental health problems
Mental illness, or mental distress, that changes how people think, feel or behave. About one in four people in the UK will suffer from a mental illness at some point in their lives, but there is still considerable **prejudice** and **fear** around a **diagnosis** of mental illness. Mental illness/distress covers a range of conditions, including **depression** (as opposed to unhappiness), **anxiety** (as opposed to being worried), **obsessive compulsive disorder**, **phobias**, bipolar disorder and **schizophrenia**.

mentoring
The act of providing one-to-one **support**, guidance and an example to someone to help him or her grow, learn and develop and to reach **goals**.

meritocracy
An **organisation** or **community** where reward and recognition is based on achievement and ability.

metabolism
The biochemical **processes** that break down (catabolism) and build up substances from one formto another (anabolism) in the human body, and the **energy** and exchanges involved. The sum of all chemical reactions in the body.

metacognition
The **process** of a learner **understanding** that **learning** is taking place. Commonly referred to as 'thinking about thinking' or 'knowing about knowing', metacognition enables learners to plan and organise learning and to develop **strategies** to learn more effectively.

methadone
A chemically produced synthetic **opiate**. It is prescribed as a substitute for people who are coming off **heroin**, as it has longer-lasting effects.

methicillin-resistant staphylococcus aureus (MRSA)
A **health care**-acquired **infection** that is prevalent in **hospitals** and also in **nursing homes**, although people living at home can also have it. Also referred to as a '**superbug**', this particular bacterial **infection** is resistant to almost all antibiotics and people may need to take high doses of powerful antibiotic over long periods of time to overcome it. The **bacterium** is very common and large numbers of people have it in their throats without it causing a problem; it is noticed in hospitals because when it is transmitted to someone who is already ill, it can cause serious illness.

methods
Ways of doing something, or an approach to a task or issue, for example someone may use a particular method of changing a dressing, or may find a particular method of reflection to be useful when thinking about practice.

microbiology
A biological science that studies **micro-organisms** and their effects on humans.

micronutrients
The **trace elements** of a balanced **diet**. These are **vitamins** and **minerals** taken in small amounts that are essential to maintaining **health**. A diet which is low in one or more of the trace elements can result in illness or **disability**. Micronutrients are only needed in small quantities and do not produce calories.

micro-organisms
Minute **organisms** including **viruses**, fungi, **bacteria**, algae and single-**cell** organisms such as **protozoa**.

microscope
Laboratory equipment to magnify the image of objects too small to be seen with the naked eye. There are electron, laser and **X-ray** microscopes, but the optical microscope is the one most commonly seen.

microscopic
Too small to see without using a **microscope**; this includes **cells**, **bacteria** and **viruses**.

midwife
A **health professional** who is an **autonomous** practitioner with **responsibility** for the care and **well-being** of pregnant women and their **babies** throughout **pregnancy**, **labour** and delivery, and following the **birth**. Midwives are responsible for normal pregnancies and deliveries and for recognising complications that require the **intervention** of a **doctor**. Advanced Midwifery Practitioners are also able to perform **instrumental deliveries**, prescribe some drugs and assist at **caesarean sections**.

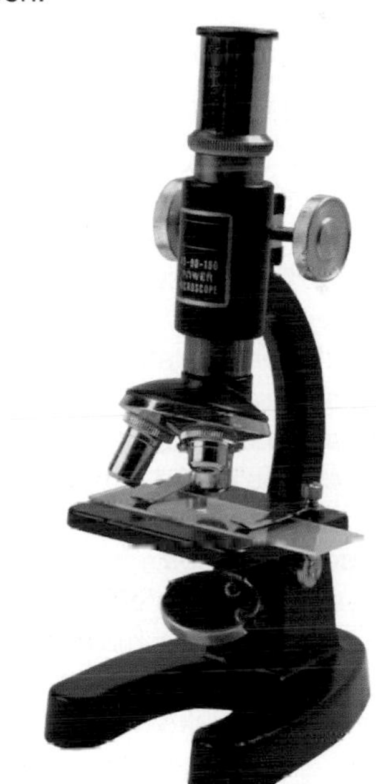

A microscope shows objects too small to be seen with the naked eye.

milestones
Measurable points in **development**. The term is usually used to describe stages in children's development where progress can be measured. It can also be used to

identify stages of recovery from illness, and is used in **contracts** to identify what a **provider** has to deliver at a certain point.

minerals

Micronutrients that are essential for a healthy, balanced **diet**.

- Major minerals: a healthy diet needs more than 100 mg a day
- **Trace elements**: a healthy diet needs less than 100 mg a day, but they are just as essential.

Major minerals	Trace elements
Calcium	Chromium
Magnesium	Copper
Phosphorus	**Iodine**
Potassium	Iron
Sodium	Manganese
	Selenium
	Zinc

minimum standards

The basic requirements of acceptable **practice** or **service** delivery. Services in **health** and **social care** are inspected in all the UK countries and compared against minimum standards. These set out the least that can be done to make a service adequate. Some **service providers** will work to achieve higher quality standards in order to ensure the best possible levels of service, while others will be content to meet the standards required for **inspection**. National minimum standards documents can be found at the link below.

More information can be found at www.dh.gov.uk

minority ethnic communities

Cultural or **racial communities** of people who are living in a country where another cultural or racial **group** is in the majority. Minority cultures are an important part of the **diversity** of any **society**, but sometimes such communities are **marginalised** and excluded rather than **valued**.

minutes

The written **record** of what has happened in a meeting or conference. These can be very detailed and record all the individual comments (these are called 'verbatim' minutes). Minutes usually record the main decisions that were made and any actions that were agreed. Copies are usually circulated to everyone present at the meeting, and they have the opportunity to comment and suggest any corrections before the minutes are finalised.

miscarriage
The failure of a **pregnancy** before 24 weeks. After this time it is called a **stillbirth**. About 15 per cent of confirmed pregnancies result in miscarriage. It can happen for a range of reasons: a **chromosomal** abnormality in the **foetus**, **hormonal** imbalance, a structurally weak **cervix** that dilates too early, **blood** clotting disorders, and **infection**.

mission statement
An **organisation**'s public statement about its purpose and **goals**.

mitochondria
Structures in human **cells** that turn **nutrients** into **energy** for the cells. They are sometimes called the 'powerhouse' of the cells.

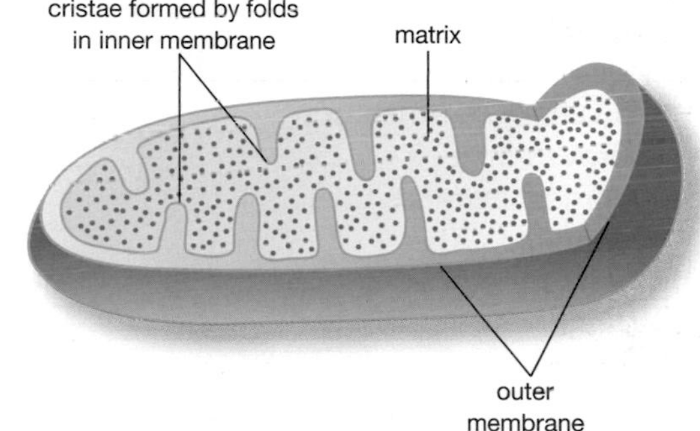

Structure of a single mitochondrion.

mitral valve
A valve in the **heart** that divides the left **atrium** and left **ventricle** (also known as the left atrio-ventricular valve and the bicuspid valve). As the left atrium contracts, the mitral valve opens so that **blood** can flow into the left ventricle. When the valve closes it stops blood flowing back into the left atrium. Closing of the valve is responsible for the first heart sound heard with a **stethoscope**.

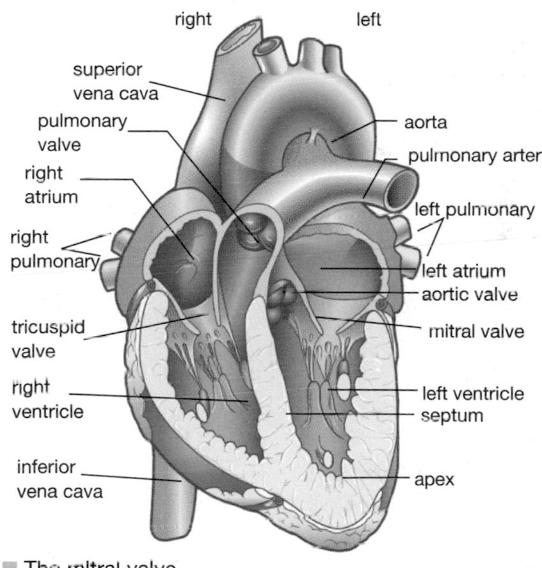

The mitral valve.

MMR vaccine
A combined **vaccine** to protect children against **measles**, **mumps** and **rubella** (German measles). There has been controversy following a well-publicised study that seemed to suggest a link between the vaccine and autism. Other studies did not support this, but large numbers of **parents** stopped having their children **vaccinated**. This has resulted in significant increases in the **incidence** of the **diseases**.

mnemonics
A technique for assisting **memory** by using aids such as rhymes, phrases, acronyms and diagrams. Examples include: 'I before E except after C' is a rhyme to help people remember the spelling rule; 'spring forward, fall back' is a way to remember which way the clocks move at which season.

mobility
The ability to move around. People's mobility can sometimes be improved through development activities or **walking aids**. The **environment** is also a key aid to mobility, and considerable improvements can be made by adapting someone's living environment.

Date	No.	PATIENT'S NURSING NEEDS/PROBLEMS AND CAUSES OF PROBLEMS (NB Physiological, Psychological, Social and Family Problems)	Objectives	Nursing Instructions	Review On/By	Date Resolved
1.5.07	8	Mobility:			8.5.07	
		Due to suffering from a	To prevent complications	a) Encourage Mr K to be as	15.5.07	
		congenital foot deformity,	of immobility and	independent as possible.	22.5.07	
		Mr K is unable to bear	maintain Mr. K's safety	b) Always give clear, consise	29.5.07	
		weight and needs the hoist	as far as is reasonably	instructions when moving and	5.6.07	
		to be used when moving	practicable	handling to gain full	12.6.07	
		and handling		co-operation.	19.6.07	
				c)The hoist must be used at all	26.6.07	
				times with either the Quickfit	3.7.07	
				deluxe sling or the toiletting	10.7.07	
				sling - depending on	17.7.07	
				circumstances.	24.7.07	
				d) Ensure safe practice maintained	31.7.07	
				when moving and handling.	7.8.07	
				e) Observe for any problems and		
				reassess appropriately.		
				f) Review problem weekly		

An example of notes on an individual's mobility in his plan of care.

model
An example of how to do something, for example when working with children and young people it is important to model the behaviour that is expected of them, so that they can see what it is that they need to do.

modelling
Showing the behaviour that is expected from others. This technique is commonly used when working with children and **young people**. Continual exposure to a way of behaving will have an impact on the behaviour of others, and changes will be seen.

molecules
The smallest particle of a substance that still has the **properties** of the substance.

Mongolian blue spot
A blue/black discolouration usually on the base of the spine or buttocks of a **newborn** child. This is most common among Asian and Afro-Caribbean **babies**, but can also be seen in Caucasian **infants**. The marks are harmless and will fade over the first few years of life, but they are regularly mistaken for **bruises** and can lead to **child protection** concerns.

monitoring
Checking at regular intervals, measuring against known criteria and **recording** the results. A **patient**'s **pulse** and **temperature** may be monitored every 4 hours;

they will be recorded and the criteria that would cause concern and require action are known.

monoplegia
Paralysis affecting only one limb.

morals
Views, **beliefs** and principles about what is right. They are an individual matter, but people's morals are influenced by many factors, such as **family** background, personal experience, **religious** beliefs and **cultural** beliefs.

morbidity
A state of illness or **disease**. Morbidity rates show the **incidence** of illness and disease within a particular **group** over a specified period of time. Morbidity **data** can show related **information** such as **hospital** admissions or **GP** consultations.

morphine
A powerful **opiate** drug which is used as an analgesic. Because it is a strong **painkiller**, and can be given in quick acting or slow-release forms, morphine is commonly used to treat severe pain in conditions such as **cancer**.

mortality
Mortality rates are the numbers of **deaths** per thousand in a given **population**.

mother
The woman who gave **birth** to a child is the 'birth mother', but the 'mother figure' in a child's life is the main carer, regardless of whether this is the father, an **adoptive** mother, grandparent, **foster carer** or **nanny**. **Babies** need to be able to form **attachments** and to **bond** with a constant carer.

motivating
Inspiring and encouraging. In order to be an effective **leader** of a **team** or **organisation**, it is necessary to be able to motivate people. People can also be motivated by a **goal** they want to achieve, a reward, or a cause that they **support**.

motor control/motor development
The ability to control body movements. This is divided into gross motor control, the ability to make large movements such as waving or lifting a leg, and fine motor control, the ability to make more complex movements such as holding a pencil or building a tower of bricks. Both are **milestones** in a child's development, with gross motor control being achieved earlier.

A
B
C
D
E
F
G
H
I
J
K
L
M
N
O
P
Q
R
S
T
U
V
W
X
Y
Z

motor neurone disease

A progressive **degenerative disease** for which there is no cure. The cause is unknown. Motor **neurones** are the **nerve cells** through which the **brain** sends instructions, in the form of electrical impulses, to the **muscles** or **glands**. Degeneration of these cells leads to weakness and wasting of muscles. Ultimately, people with the condition become almost completely immobile, but the disease does not affect the brain or the intellect. More information can be found at www.mndassociation.org

mouth care

The cleaning of someone's mouth when he or she is unable to do so because of illness or **disability**. It is important for the prevention of **infections** and for making people feel more comfortable.

moving and handling

The **process** of assisting people to move from one place to another. **Risk assessments** are essential before moving anyone and the correct **equipment** must be used. It is not safe for the person being moved, or those doing the moving, to lift anyone manually. Aids and equipment for lifting are widely available in all places where health and care services are delivered.

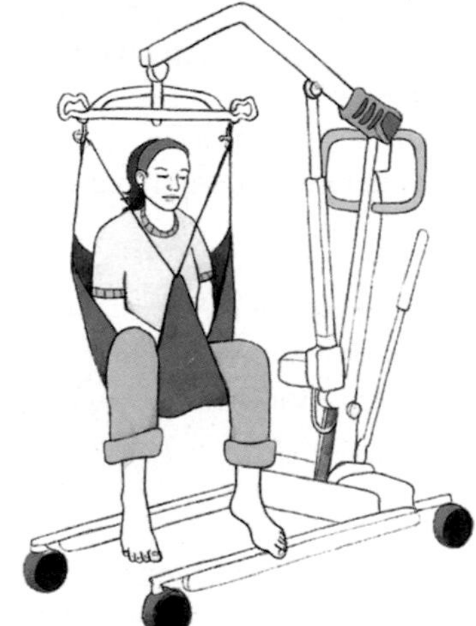

Using a hoist.

mucous membranes

The lubricated pink inner lining of the mouth, nasal passages, eyelids, **vagina** and urethra.

multi-agency working

Where **agencies** work together, following agreed **protocols** and procedures. This way of working can be effective for people who need **services** from more than one agency. If agencies work together following an agreed plan, there is less chance of duplication of effort.

multi-disciplinary teams

Health and care **professionals** working together as a **team** in order to combine their **skills** in response to the **needs** of individuals and **families**. **Management** of multi-disciplinary teams can be from any discipline, and people will normally have a professional lead from their own discipline for **supervision**.

multiple sclerosis (MS)

A **chronic degenerative disease** of the **central nervous system** where the fatty sheath (myelin) that coats the **nerves** is gradually destroyed. This can cause a range of **symptoms** including **muscle** weakness, muscle spasms, changes in sensation, balance problems, visual problems and speech difficulties. The progress of MS is very individual and is likely to be varied in different people.
More information can be found at www.mssociety.org.uk

mumps

A **disease** usually occurring in children. The salivary **glands** swell up and become painful, causing a swollen face, particularly just below and in front of the ear. The swelling of the glands increases over two to three days and gradually decreases as the high **temperature** falls. The **incubation period** for mumps is 14–21 days.

Munchausen's syndrome

A **mental disorder** where a person will fake the **symptoms** of an illness that does not exist, or will **harm** himself or herself in order to create symptoms, then present at a **hospital** for investigations and **treatment**. Many people have had unnecessary investigative **surgery** on several occasions. Such people will often visit different hospitals and **doctors** to avoid detection. When people invent symptoms of illness in others or cause harm to others for this purpose (usually their children or someone they are caring for) it is called 'fabricated' or 'induced illness'; it was previously known as 'Munchausen's syndrome by proxy'.

muscles

Body **tissues** that are attached to the **bones** by **tendons** and can contract and relax in order to create movement.

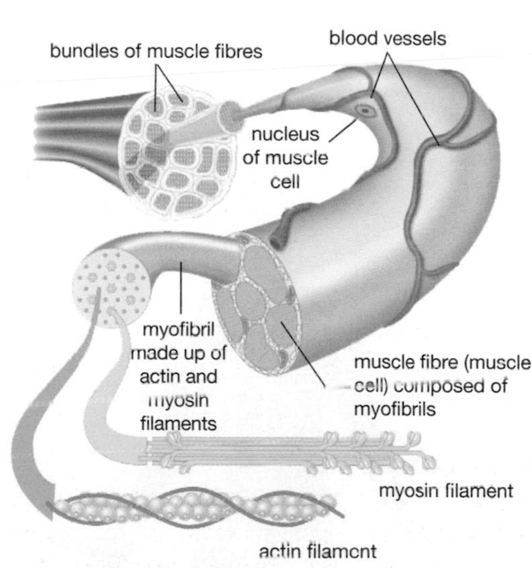

Muscle structure.

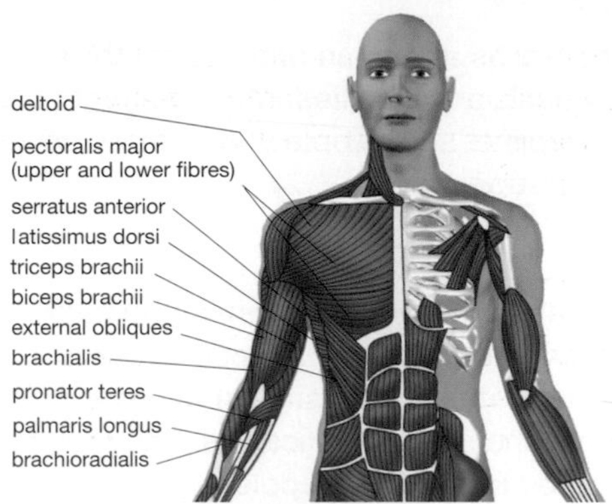
deltoid
pectoralis major
(upper and lower fibres)
serratus anterior
latissimus dorsi
triceps brachii
biceps brachii
external obliques
brachialis
pronator teres
palmaris longus
brachioradialis

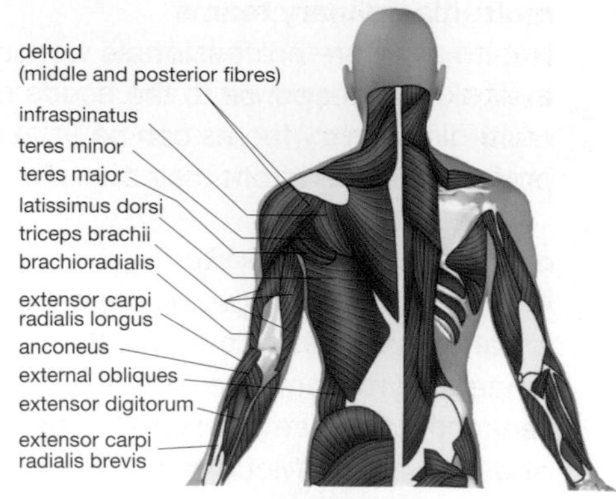
deltoid
(middle and posterior fibres)
infraspinatus
teres minor
teres major
latissimus dorsi
triceps brachii
brachioradialis
extensor carpi
radialis longus
anconeus
external obliques
extensor digitorum
extensor carpi
radialis brevis

Arm and shoulder muscles.

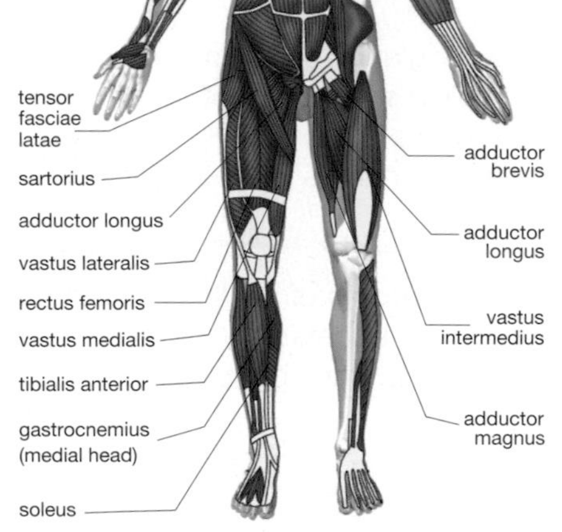
tensor
fasciae
latae
sartorius
adductor longus
vastus lateralis
rectus femoris
vastus medialis
tibialis anterior
gastrocnemius
(medial head)
soleus
adductor
brevis
adductor
longus
vastus
intermedius
adductor
magnus

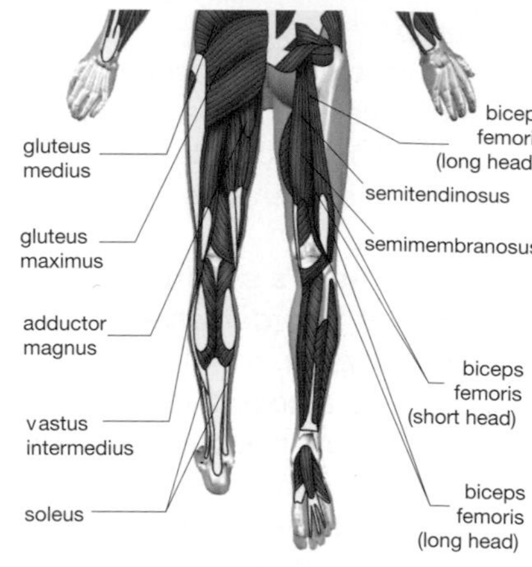
gluteus
medius
gluteus
maximus
adductor
magnus
vastus
intermedius
soleus
biceps
femoris
(long head)
semitendinosus
semimembranosus
biceps
femoris
(short head)
biceps
femoris
(long head)

Leg and hip muscles.

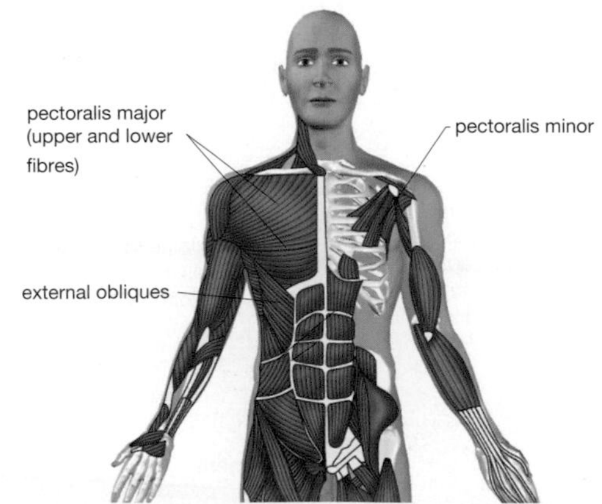
pectoralis major
(upper and lower
fibres)
external obliques
pectoralis minor

Chest and abdomen muscles.

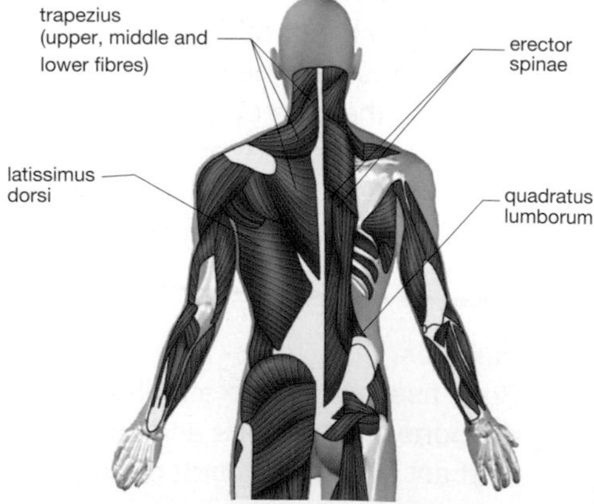
trapezius
(upper, middle and
lower fibres)
latissimus
dorsi
erector
spinae
quadratus
lumborum

Back muscles.

muscular dystrophy

A group of **genetic** conditions that cause the **muscles** to lose their ability to contract, thus creating serious **disability**. There are several different types of muscular dystrophy, and some have more serious effects than others. The **disease** is most common in boys, although it occurs in girls occasionally.

musculo-skeletal system

The **skeleton** and its associated **muscles, ligaments**, cartilage and **tendons**. The skeleton provides the form of the human body and protects the body cavities. **Bones** are joined together by ligaments, and muscles are joined to bones by tendons. Movement occurs by muscles shortening and lengthening (contracting and relaxing) and thus causing the skeleton to move.

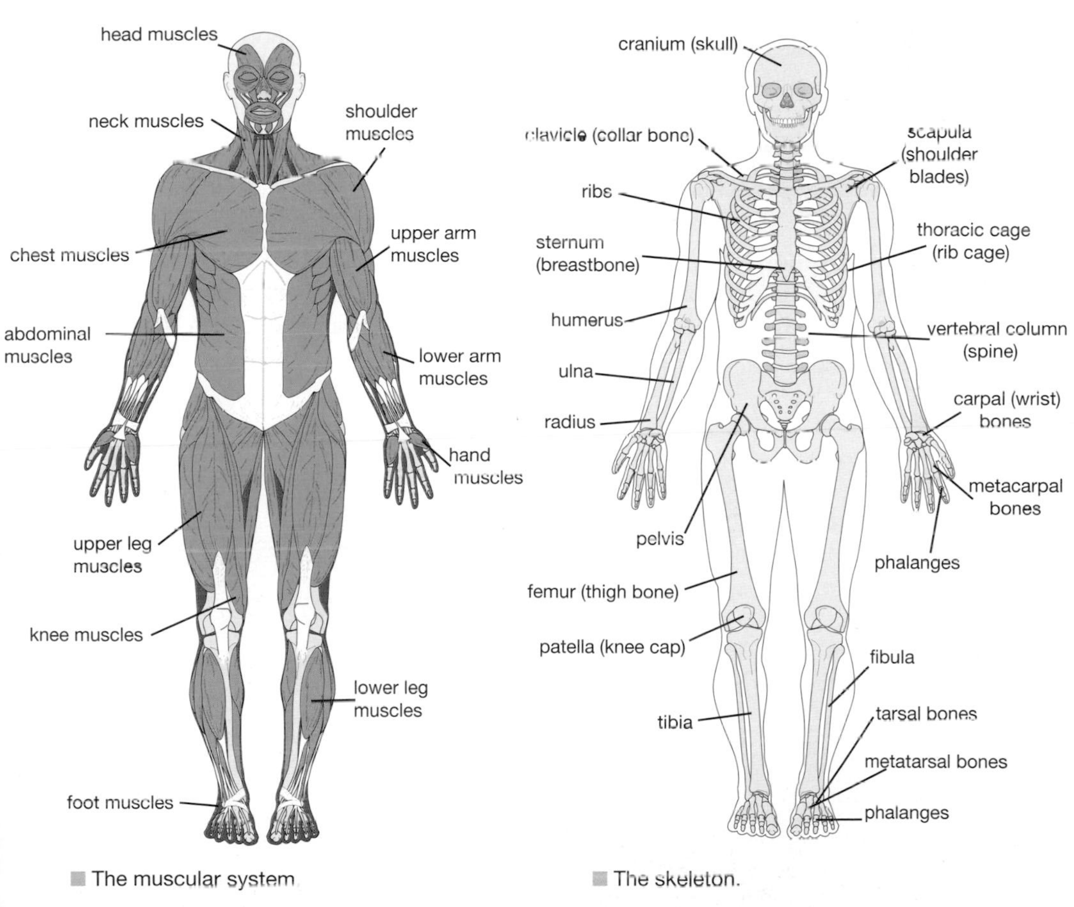

The muscular system

The skeleton.

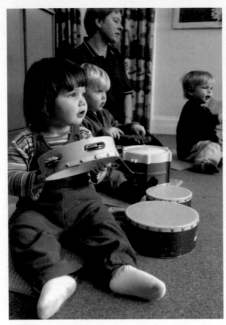

Music therapy.

music therapy
A therapy involving listening to or creating music, often used with children and **young people** with **challenging behaviour**, or with people with **mental health problems.** Music can be helpful for relaxing, but can also help people to change moods and **feelings** when they listen to or create different types of music.

myalgic encephalomyelitis (ME)
A condition causing extreme fatigue, **joint** and **muscle** pain and dizziness. It often occurs following a **viral infection**, can last for a long period of time and can be very disabling, sometimes confining people to bed. Causes are unknown and there is little **treatment** except rest.
More information can be found at www.afme.org.uk

myocardial infarction
A **heart attack**. It is usually caused by a **blood** clot in the **coronary artery**. Immediate medical help is necessary as irreversible damage will occur to the **heart muscle**.

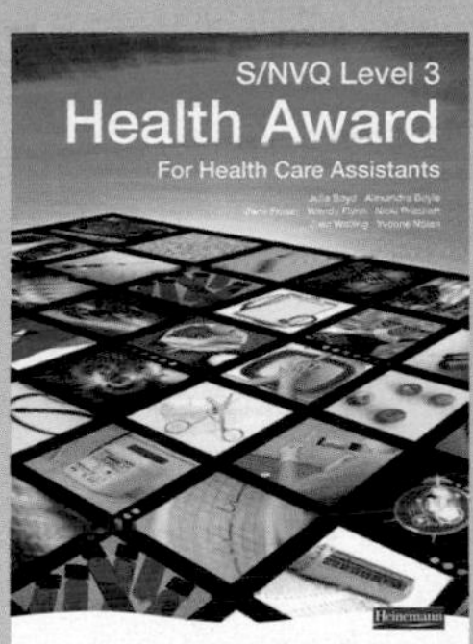

nanny
Someone who looks after a child or children in the child's home. Nannies usually live in, but can also care for children on a daily basis. There is no requirement for nannies to be qualified, although many are; they are not **regulated**. Nannies in England can choose to place themselves on the voluntary section of the Childcare Register; this will enable **parents** to know that they have had a **Criminal Records Bureau** check and hold a recognised **qualification.** Because nannies are not regulated, parents choosing a nanny do not qualify for the childcare element of Working Tax Credit, unlike parents choosing a home childcarer.

National Autistic Society
A national charity, with local branches, that represents the interests of people who have communication disorders that are on the autistic spectrum. The organisation lobbies on behalf of people with **autistic spectrum disorders** and provides information, advice and support.
More information can be found at www.nas.org.uk

National Children's Bureau
An **umbrella body** for **organisations** working with children and **young people**. It **promotes** the interests of children and young people and is a **network** for **professionals** working in any aspect of this. It works closely with the **agencies** Children in Wales and Children in Scotland, which perform similar roles.
More information can be found at www.ncb.org.uk

National Council for Voluntary Organisations (NCVO)
An **umbrella body** for **voluntary organisations**. It **promotes** the views and interests of civil **society** and lobbies and campaigns on issues of importance. It provides **networks** for those working and volunteering in the sector.
More information can be found at www.ncvo-vol.org.uk

National Curriculum
The legally required framework of education that must be delivered in all **schools**.

The National Curriculum sets out:

- the subjects taught
- the knowledge, **skills** and **understanding** required in each subject
- **standards** or attainment **targets** in each subject – **teachers** can use these to measure a child's progress and plan the next steps in their **learning**
- how a child's progress should be assessed and **reported**.

The subjects that must be taught are:

- art and design
- citizenship
- design and technology
- English
- geography
- history
- **information and communication technology** (ICT)
- mathematics
- modern foreign languages (MFL)
- music
- PE
- science.

The National Curriculum also includes **religious education**, careers education, work-related studies and personal, social and **health** education (PSHE).

National Health Service (NHS)

The **organisation** that provides **health care** throughout the UK. The **NHS** began in 1948 and was the result of the **Beveridge** Report, where the need to alleviate the serious **public health** problems of the time was identified. The underpinning principles of the NHS are that it is a universal **service**, available to all and free at the point of use. The NHS is the largest employer in the UK and spends around £92 billion annually. Services are arranged in three **groups**.

- Primary: all health care in the **community**, including **GPs**, community nursing, **midwifery** and dental care. The **provision** is the **responsibility** of 152 primary care trusts in England, and there are similar arrangements in Scotland, Wales and Northern Ireland.
- Secondary: general **hospital** care including maternity services, **accident** and emergency, and paediatric services. These are provided through hospital trusts, of which there are 394. **Mental health** services are provided through mental health trusts.
- Tertiary: specialist health services such as **spinal injury** units, eye hospitals and **oncology** units.

More information can be found at www.nhs.uk

National Institute for Health and Clinical Excellence (NICE)

An independent body responsible for providing guidance on health-related matters, particularly in three areas of **health**:

- **public health** – guidance on the **promotion** of good health and the prevention of **ill health** for those working in the **NHS**, **local authorities** and the wider public and **voluntary sector**
- health technologies – guidance on the use of new and existing medicines, **treatments** and procedures within the NHS
- clinical **practice** – guidance on the appropriate treatment and care of people with specific **diseases** and conditions within the NHS.

NICE **guidelines** must be followed by **health professionals** in prescribing medicines and providing treatment.
More information can be found at www.nice.org.uk

National Insurance
A system of contributions, made by people who are working, towards the cost of **benefits**. They are deducted from the wages of all people earning above a certain level, and also have to be made by employers for each employee. Every person in the UK has a National Insurance number, which is used as identification for the purposes of tax, insurance and benefits.
More information can be found at www.hmrc.gov.uk/nic

national minimum wage
The lowest hourly rate that an employee can legally be paid in the UK. There are separate rates for young workers aged 16 or 17 and from 18–21 years. Many jobs in **health** and **social care** are paid at minimum wage rates. Current minimum wage rates are set by the Low Pay Commission.
More information can be found at www.lowpay.gov.uk

National Occupational Standards (NOS)
A series of statements about what needs to be done in order to carry out **work** in an occupational area, e.g. **health** and **social care** or childcare. These are accompanied by a series of **performance criteria** that identify how the work should be done. The **standards** also include statements about the knowledge that needs to underpin the work. National Occupational Standards are used for a range of purposes, including training, **appraisals**, benchmarking, **job descriptions**, **person specifications**, **qualifications**, continuing **professional development**, and **funding** proposals. NOS are usually developed by **Sector Skills Councils** and are **reviewed** on a regular basis to reflect **changes** in ways of working.
More information can be found at www.ukstandards.org

National Service Frameworks (NSF)
Long-term **strategies** developed by the **NHS** through expert **reference groups**. They set out measurable **goals** within timeframes, and **standards** to improve **performance** and consistency. There are NSFs for the following areas:

- **coronary heart disease**
- **cancer**

- paediatric intensive care
- **mental health**
- **older people**
- **diabetes**
- long-term conditions
- renal **services**
- children, **young people** and maternity services
- chronic obstructive pulmonary disease (COPD).

National Society for the Prevention of Cruelty to Children (NSPCC)
A voluntary **organisation** that campaigns to end cruelty to children. It raises money, publicises issues around child cruelty and runs various **family support** projects and helplines for children who are being **abused**. It passes on **referrals** from the helplines to **professional social workers** in **local authority** children's services departments. More information can be found at www.nspcc.org.uk

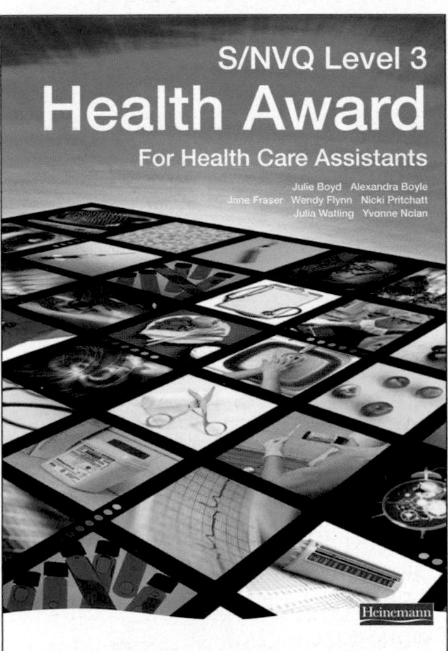

National Vocational Qualifications (NVQs)
Work-based learning and **assessment**; **qualifications** that assess **performance** as well as knowledge. They are available for all occupational areas and are especially appropriate for people who prefer not to take tests or exams, and who like to learn in a **workplace** rather than a classroom. All NVQs are based on **National Occupational Standards** and are available at a range of levels depending on the nature of the work in a particular sector.

natural childbirth
Giving birth without any medical intervention, **drugs** or assistance. Women giving birth in this way will still have the support of a **midwife** who will deliver the **baby**. The National Childbirth Trust is a support organisation that promotes natural childbirth. More information can be found at www.nct.org.uk

nature–nurture debate
The different theoretical viewpoints about the most significant influences on children's development. The 'nature' side of the argument maintains that children develop as they do because of **genetic** factors, and that physical, social and **emotional development** will happen at more or less the same rate for all children regardless of the **environment** in which they live. The 'nurture' argument is that very little development is due to

inherited factors and that the way children develop is a result of the environment in which they are brought up. It is likely that development is a combination of both influences, but there is still no final agreement on which is the stronger.

nausea
Sensation or feeling of going to vomit or be sick.

need to know basis
Giving information about a person only to those who need to know.

needle
An instrument used for delivering drugs or **vaccines** into the body, either under the **skin** (**subcutaneously**), into muscle (intramuscularly) or into a **vein** (**intravenously**). Needles are a hollow bore, of various sizes, and attached to a syringe containing the substance to be delivered. All used needles should be discarded properly in a '**sharps box**' and then disposed of safely as they pose a serious **infection** risk. People who are abusing substances will sometimes share needles, or reuse dirty needles, which is a major cause of infection.

needle-stick injury (NSI)
An **accidental** or deliberate **injury** involving a 'used' **needle** puncturing the **skin** of a **health professional** or member of the public who was not the person for whom the needle was intended. Such injuries have the potential for serious consequences if the needle is contaminated with a **blood-borne infection** such as **hepatitis** or **HIV**.

needs
Requirements for achieving a state of **health** and **well-being**. These include basic needs such as **food** and shelter, but also higher-level emotional needs such as being loved and **valued**, and feeling fulfilled. See **Maslow's** hierarchy of needs.

negative behaviour
Aggressive, **bullying**, anti-social or unacceptable ways of responding to others. This can include **violence** or outbursts of **temper**; it can also include silent, sulking or **uncommunicative behaviour**. **Guidelines** are available for dealing with negative behaviour regardless of the age of the person or setting where it occurs. All behaviour is a means of **communication**, so it is also important to **understand** what the person is trying to communicate through the behaviour.

neglect
Failure to care for a child or **vulnerable adult**. This can include failure to provide warmth, shelter, **food**, **medical treatment**, **exercise** and social contact. Neglect can be deliberate, which can result in a **prosecution**; or it can be due to a **carer**'s inability to cope or to **understand** the care that is needed, in which case help is available for the carer.

negligence
Failure to carry out a task or a **responsibility** as a result of carelessness, incompetence, laziness or lack of attention. Making a mistake is not necessarily negligence if the person was acting in good faith.

neighbourhood watch
Locally run schemes where people take note of any unusual or suspicious activity in their local neighbourhood in order to help reduce crime and anti-social behaviour. A local committee will take **responsibility** for the schemes and they will attempt to reduce crime in an area by vigilance, taking responsibility for making local checks, and providing **information** to local people.
More information can be found at www.neighbourhoodwatch.net

neonatal jaundice
A very common, and usually harmless, condition occurring in 50 per cent of full-term **babies** and 80 per cent of **premature** babies. When babies are born, their **livers** do not always begin to function immediately, and so are not able to process the orange/red **blood** pigment, bilirubin. This can mean that babies develop the yellow eye and **skin** typical of **jaundice**. This will gradually reduce over the first 10 days of life. The condition responds well to ultraviolet light, and special lights are used in **hospital** to provide **phototherapy**. Occasionally jaundice can be an indication of a more serious condition, so it is always carefully **monitored**.

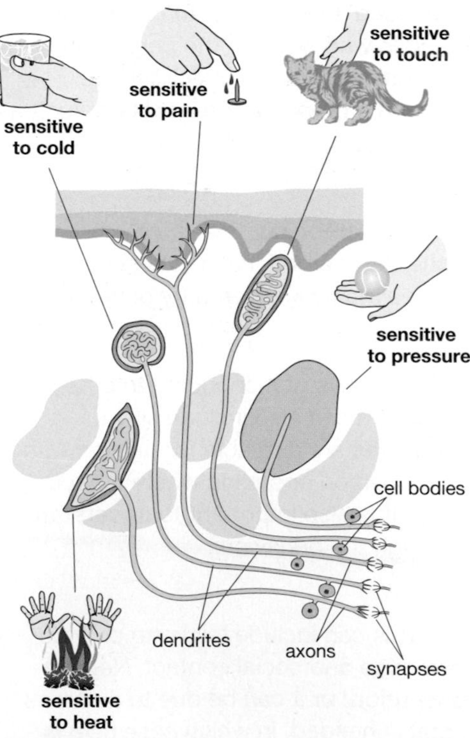

■ Nerve receptors in the skin.

neonatal nurse
A specialist **nurse** or **midwife** who has undertaken additional training to work with **newborn babies** who require special care. This can be in the **special care baby unit** (SCBU) of a general **hospital**, or in a neonatal intensive care unit (NICU) likely to be in a larger, regional centre. Babies may require care because they are **premature** or because they have been born with **health** problems.

nerves
Bundles of fibres that vary in thickness, which carry messages to and from the **brain** through the

spinal cord and **nervous system**. There are sensory (receptors) nerves that carry messages about the senses (hearing, sight, smell, taste, **touch**) and motor nerves (effectors) that carry messages about movement. Autonomic nerves supply internal organs. There are a total of 43 pairs of nerves to carry messages to and from the brain and various parts of the body.

nerve tissues
Tissues composed of **nerve cells** called **neurones**.

nervous conduction (heart)
Specialised **muscle** fibres that generate the impulses to make the heart beat without the requirement for a signal from the nervous system mean that the heart can continue beating without any input from the nervous system. The conduction system will cause the heart to beat between 70–80 times per minute, but the rate at which the **heart** beats will be altered by the **autonomic nervous system**.

nervous system
The body's **communication system**. There are two parts; the **central nervous system**, which includes the **brain** and the **spinal cord**, and the **peripheral nervous system**, which includes the sensory, motor and autonomic nerve fibres that send messages all round the body.

network
An interconnected **system** that enables people to share ideas and **information**. Connections can be made in person or electronically. There are several social networking websites where people can keep in touch with each other, and there are **professional** networks that meet on a regular basis. Information networks are the routes that enable information to circulate around an **organisation**, which can often be informal and not involve the expected **communication** channels.

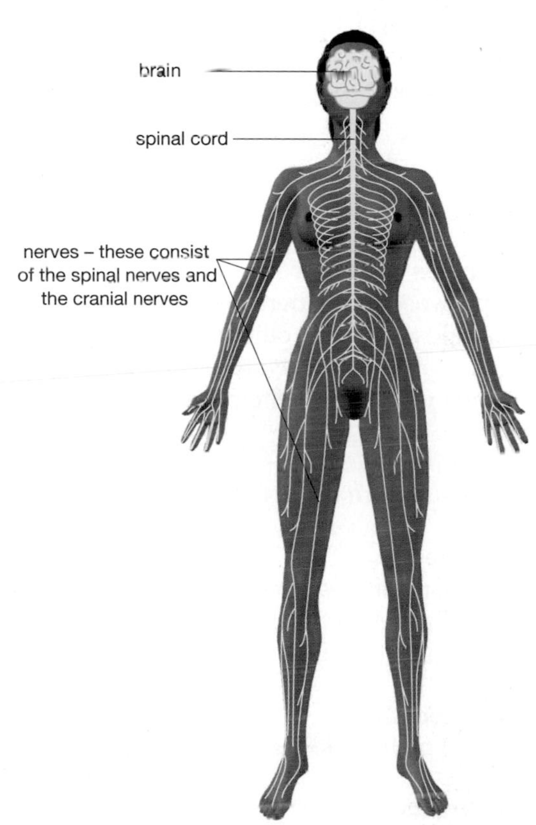

■ The nervous system.

neurology
The study, **diagnosis** and **treatment** of disorders of the **nervous system**.

neurones
The **cells** and their associated fibres (axons and dendrons) that make up **nerve tissues**.

neuropathy
A disorder involving the **peripheral nervous system**.

neurosis
A form of mental or emotional disorder that may involve **anxiety**, **depression**, obsession or **phobia**, but does not involve an altered view of reality. The term is no longer generally used as a **diagnosis** of mental illness, but may be used when describing a particular type of **personality**.

neurotransmitter
A chemical that allows nervous impulses to, or from, the **brain** to move across the minute gap (synapse) between **neurones**.

■ Structure of a neurone.

new types of worker
People working in a **person-centred**, **holistic** way that involves some different **skills** and knowledge other than those traditionally associated with work in **health** and **social care**. New types of workers may deliver **services** in different ways, or in different places or at different times, than has been the case in the past.

newborn
A **baby** just born or neonate; the term usually refers to the first 4 weeks of life.

NHS Direct
A 24-hour, **nurse**-led helpline providing **health** advice and **information** via the Internet, telephone lines and digital television.
More information can be found at www.NHSdirect.NHS.uk

NHS Executive
The part of the **NHS** that provides central **management** and strategic leadership.

NHS Trusts
NHS hospitals and Primary Care Trusts (PCTs) which are independent bodies and employ staff to deliver health care.

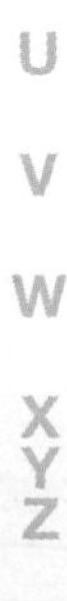

A B C D E F G H I J K L M N O P Q R S T U V W X Y Z

nicotine
A highly **addictive** alkaloid obtained from the dried leaves of the tobacco plant. It is the substance in cigarettes that makes them addictive. Nicotine can also be obtained through chewing tobacco, but it passes into the bloodstream very quickly when **smoked**.

nits
The eggs or young of head lice. They are found in the hair, and spread very easily among children when their heads touch each other. They can be removed through the use of specialist shampoos, but children regularly become re-infected.

Nolan Committee on Standards in Public Life
A committee set up in 1994 and chaired by Lord Nolan to **report** on **standards** of behaviour for those holding public positions. It later became the Commons Committee on Standards in Public Life. The committee makes sure that MPs and other people holding public office follow the necessary standards of behaviour, such as declaring if they have a vested interest in a matter being discussed, or disclosing all sources of **income**, including any gifts received.

nominal data
Data or statistics that can be counted, but not ranked or placed in order, for example, the number of males and the number of females in a data set, or the **ethnicity** of people taking part in a study.

non-judgemental
Not viewing a person's actions, behaviour or **lifestyle** in a negative way or taking a view that is based on personal **prejudice**. Being non-judgemental is an essential part of working as a **health** or **social care professional**.

non-starch polysaccharide (NSP)
Roughage or fibre, an important part of a balanced **diet**. Fibre is mainly found in cereals, beans, lentils, fruit and vegetables. It cannot be broken down by the **digestive system** and so provides bulk that helps to reduce constipation and lower **cholesterol**. In the UK, most people do not eat enough fibre. The recommended intake is 18 g per day, but most people eat around 12 g per day.

non-verbal communication (NVC)
Body language, the most important way in which people **communicate**. Only 7 per cent of communication is through words; everything else is communicated through body language. NVC is about **posture** and how bodies are placed, for example, if you sit in a relaxed way, face the person who is talking to you and lean slightly forwards, this shows that you are interested and ready to listen. Sitting slightly turned away from someone with arms and legs folded indicates

not listening, or being uninterested in what is being said. **Facial expression** is also a vital part of NVC; people read faces and can judge interest, concern, honesty and trustworthiness as well as moods such as joy, anger, resentment and deceitfulness.

normal development

The expected **process** of development for most children. Developmental charts identify the ages at which children are expected to have reached certain **milestones**. Although not every child develops at the same rate, it is possible to identify concerns if there is significant delay in children reaching expected milestones. The term 'normal', or preferably 'expected', must always be applied to the development stages and not to the individual child. Every child has his or her own level of development that is 'normal' for the child and his or her circumstances.

normal distribution curve

A bell-shaped curve shown on a **graph** of scores from any test. This visually demonstrates a normal distribution, which means most scores will be in the middle and there will be smaller numbers of scores at either extreme.

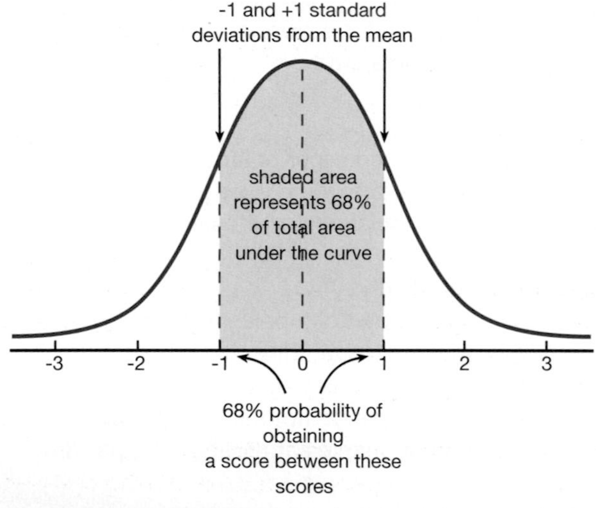

A normal distribution curve.

norms

Accepted or typical behaviours within any social **group** or **community**. Norms vary between different groups depending on age, **culture** and background. Behaviour that is outside the norms of a particular group is usually not tolerated by the members of that group.

A B C D E F G H I J K L M N O P Q R S T U V W X Y Z

The term can also be used **statistically** to identify the scores of a well-defined group, used as a standard against which to measure others' **performance**.

Northern Ireland Social Care Council
Established in 2001 by the Health and Personal Social Services Act (Northern Ireland), it is the regulatory body for the social care workforce. The council is response for ensuring that the workforce meets standards of conduct and it is also responsible for training the social care workforce.

Norton Scale
A scale that measures the risk of the development of **pressure sores**.

note taking
The **process** of a trained **communication support worker** working alongside a **deaf** learner, usually in further or higher **education**. The note taker will take notes in **lectures** and seminars for the learner to read later, because a person using **British Sign Language** cannot do so and take notes at the same time. Note takers can also take notes sitting beside a learner so that he or she can read them at the same time. Note takers can take notes manually or electronically. They undertake specialist training and **qualifications**.

not-for-profit organisation
A trading **organisation** that re-invests any profits back into the organisation and does not distribute them to shareholders, as most businesses do. Many **private hospitals** are run in this way. Such organisations can be **charities**, companies limited by guarantee, trusts, or foundations. They, along with **voluntary sector** organisations, are considered to be the **third sector**.

notifiable diseases
A range of **infectious diseases** that are required by **law** to be notified to the 'proper officers' (usually **environmental health** officers) of the **local authority**. The long list is maintained by the Health Protection Agency; it includes **AIDS**, ***Clostridium difficile*** and dysentery, for example.
More information can be found at www.hpa.org.uk

not in employment, education or training (NEET)
A term used to categorise **young people** aged 16–19 who have left **education**, do not have a job, and are not undertaking a college course or a **work**-based **learning** programme. This **group** of young people are a major focus for Connexions advisers, and assistance is offered to help them become engaged with training and learning or finding work. There are about 150,000 such young people in the UK and the figures show that they are 20 times more likely to commit a crime and 22 times more likely to become a teenage **parent**.
More information can be found at www.connexions-direct.com

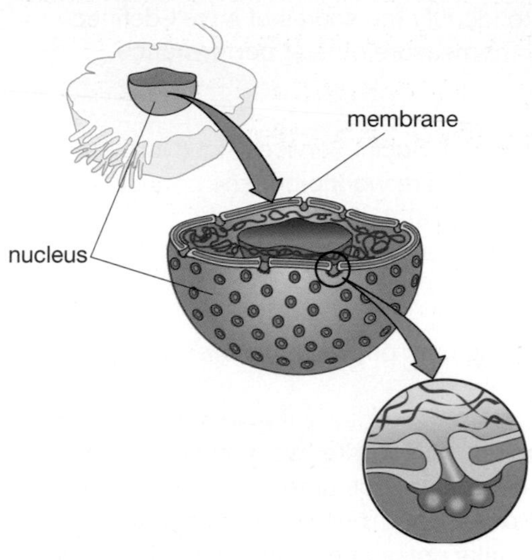

■ Structure of nucleus showing nuclear envelope and nucleolus.

nuclear family
A small **family** unit consisting of two **parents** and a child or children.

nucleus
The part of a **cell** that contains most of the **chromosomes**, and is separated from the rest of the cell by a nuclear membrane. It carries the blueprints for the processes occurring in a particular cell.

null hypothesis
In **research**, the statement of no effect; a statement that the research is expected to find that whatever is being researched will make no difference. One such null hypothesis is that there may be a **hypothesis** that a drug to treat **cancer** will have no effect. The research would then prove or disprove the hypothesis.

numeracy
Knowing about and **understanding** how numbers work and relate to each other, how they can be used and how **information** about numbers can be collected.

nurse
A qualified **health professional** who has clinical **skills** to provide care and **support** for people to improve, maintain or recover **health**. May work in a hospital, another health care seating or in the community.

nursery
A setting that provides early years care and **education** for children under **school** age. Nurseries are regulated and inspected, and there are requirements for **professional qualifications** for the staff who work in them.

nursery nurse
A **professional** qualified in early years care and development, likely to be working in a **nursery**, but may also work in a **hospital** or **school**. A nursery nurse is qualified to Level 3 and sometimes they are referred to as Early Years or Child/Care workers/practitioners.

Nursing and Midwifery Council
The **regulatory** body for **nurses** and **midwives.** It holds the registers, and ensures that all nurses and midwives keep their **practice** up to date. People can be removed from the register for misconduct or **professional negligence**. More information can be found at www.nmc-uk.org

The NMC Code of professional conduct: standards for conduct, performance and ethics

As a registered nurse, midwife or specialist community public health nurse, you are personally accountable for your practice. In caring for your patients and clients, you must:

- respect the patient or client as an individual
- obtain consent before you give any teatment or care
- protect confidential information
- co-operate with others in the team
- maintain your professional knowledge and competence
- be trustworthy
- act to identify and minimise risk to patients and clients.

These are the shared values of all the United Kingdom health care regulatory bodies.

The Nursing and Midwifery Council Code of professional conduct.

nursing home
An organisation providing residential nursing care for **older** or **disabled** people with long-term, **chronic conditions** that cannot be provided for in the **community**.

nutrients
The components of **food** that provide for a balanced **diet**. These include **carbohydrates, proteins, fats, sugars, minerals** and **vitamins**. Also a general term used for the digested products of the major food groups such as glucose, amino acids, glycerol and fatty acids.

nutrition
The way that **food** is used by the body for healthy growth and development; also the study of different **diets** and their impact on **health** and **well-being.**

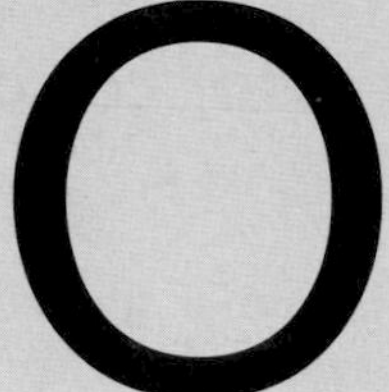

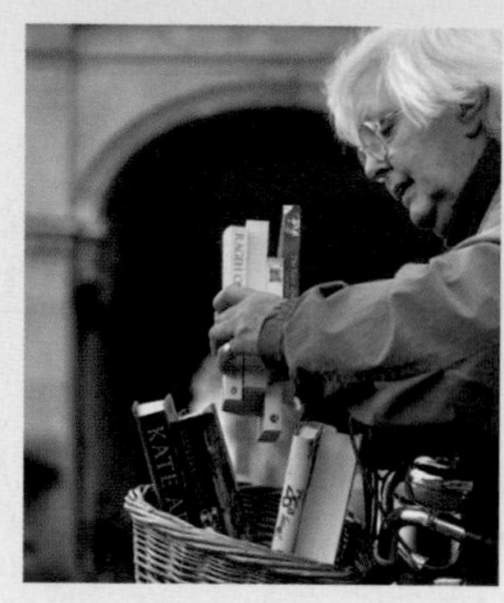

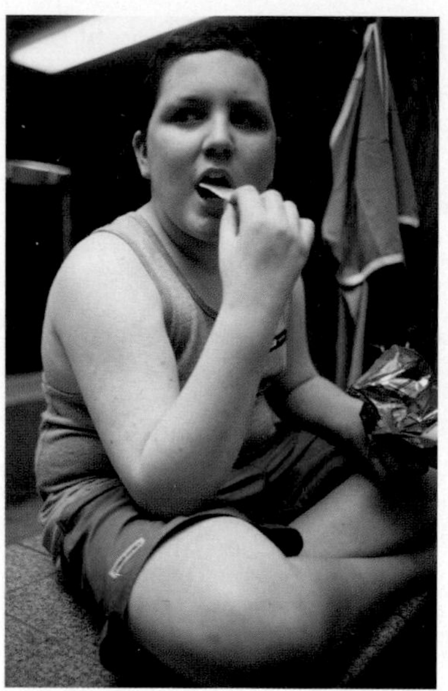

Obesity in children is becoming an increasing problem.

obesity

The condition of having excess body fat. Obesity is defined as having a **body mass index** of more than 30. Obesity causes **health** problems such as **diabetes**, **stroke**, **heart disease** and **arthritis**. It results from not using all the calories that are being consumed, thus leaving the excess to be stored as fat.

objectives

The practical **goals** to be reached as part of achieving an overall aim. Best practice uses SMART objectives that are **S**pecific, **M**easurable, **A**chievable, **R**ealistic and **T**ime-based.

object permanence

The fact that an object is still there, even when it cannot be seen. **Babies** usually **understand** this at around 8 months of age, according to work done by **Piaget**, although there is some recent work that suggests it may be as early as 3 months for some babies. Once this understanding is there, children will reach for an object hidden behind a cushion, whereas earlier they will assume it has gone and lose interest.

observation

In child development work, the **process** of carefully watching a child and taking note of all aspects including **non-verbal communication** and signals, physical condition, behaviour, **relationship** to others and how children **play**.

The term is also used to describe the nursing procedure of checking physical **measurements** such as **temperature**, **pulse** and **blood pressure** and maintaining a watch on a **patient**'s general condition. The process of observing the **practice** of an **S/NVQ** candidate is an essential part of the **assessment** process.

obsessive compulsive disorder
A mental or emotional disorder that involves states of high **anxiety** around particular actions. The affected person may feel that some actions have to be repeated continually, such as **hand washing**, cleaning rooms or locking doors. The condition only requires **treatment** if it interferes with daily life, for example, if the person has problems leaving the house because he or she has to keep going back to check that the door is locked. Many people will return once or twice to check the door, but if this escalates to 20 or 30 times, help is needed.

occupational disease
An illness directly related to or caused by the job that a person does such as a person who may have worked with asbestos may develop mesothelioma; people working in **health** and **social care** have a high **incidence** of back **injuries**; and people who work using a keyboard may develop repetitive strain injuries.

occupational health
The study, **diagnosis** and **treatment** of **work**-related **health** problems. Many large employers will have an occupational health **team** on site with specially trained staff Both **doctors** and **nurses** can specialise in this area.

occupational therapist
A **health professional** with a role in **rehabilitation** and **re-ablement** following illness or **injury**. They work with people to **promote** purposeful activity in order to help overcome **disability** resulting from **ageing**, mental or **physical illness** or **accident**. In the **community**, one of the key roles is to assess for **aids and adaptations** that people may need in order to return, or to remain at, home.

oesophagus
The muscular tube that leads from the mouth to the **stomach**. **Food** is chewed, mixed with saliva and rolled into a bolus in the mouth and it is then **swallowed** and pushed along the oesophagus and into the stomach by means of **peristalsis**. There are no enzymes secreted by the oesophagus. The **digestive process** continues in the stomach.

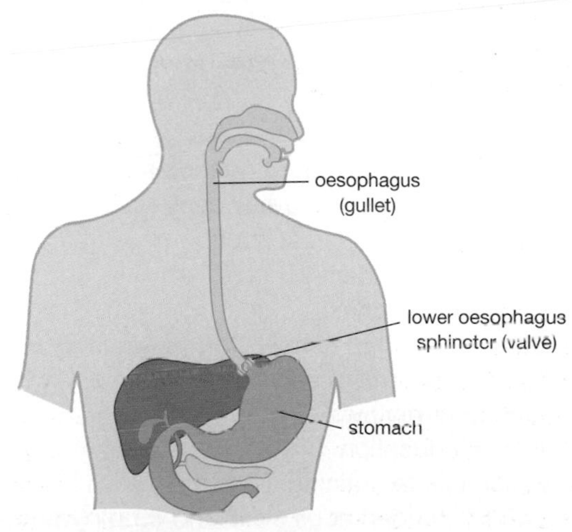

The oesophagus.

oestrogen
A female **hormone**. Produced mainly in the **ovaries**, it has an important role in maintaining

A B C D E F G H I J K L M N O P Q R S T U V W XYZ

female characteristics and **menstruation**. At the **menopause**, the production of oestrogen falls and results in the loss of **skin** elasticity, **vaginal** dryness, mood swings, hot flushes and other menopausal **symptoms**.

offence
A crime or other action that is outside the **law**.

offending behaviour
Behaviour that results in a crime or **offence**. Offenders are considered adults when they are 18 or older. Young offenders are between the ages of 10 and 17. Behaviour may not be criminal in itself, but can make it difficult for someone to break away from the criminal **culture**. **Anti-social behaviour** such as being in gangs, being involved in rowdy or drunken behaviour, being abusive or **aggressive** or causing a neighbourhood nuisance can make it more likely that the person involved will commit a crime.

Office for National Statistics
A national **organisation** that produces **data** and **reports** about all aspects of **society** in the UK. Much of the **information** comes from the **census**, and also from other information provided by public organisations. The information is used by **government** and many other organisations for planning purposes.
More information can be found at www.ons.gov.uk

Ofsted
The Office for Standards in Education, Children's Services and Skills. Originally just responsible for the **inspection** of **schools** in England, since April 2007 it has also been responsible for inspecting and regulating:

- **childminders**
- full and sessional day-care **providers**
- **out-of-school** care
- crèches
- **adoption** and **fostering agencies**
- residential schools, **family** centres and homes for children
- all state-maintained schools
- some independent schools
- pupil referral units
- the Children and **Family Courts** Advisory Service
- the overall level of services for children in **local authority** areas (these are called **joint area reviews**)
- further education
- initial teacher training
- publicly funded adult skills and **employment**-based training.

More information can be found at www.OFSTED.gov.uk

old age
The **life stage** that begins around 65 years of age, although there are some suggestions that it should be regarded as beginning at 70 as people are now living longer. The **government** view of old age is that it begins at **retirement** and on receipt of a **pension**; that is, 65 years for men and presently 60 years for women, but due to rise to 65 for women too over the next few years.

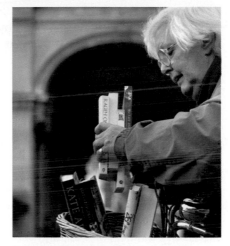

Intellectual activity is part of staying active, fit and well in old age.

older people
People who are in the **life stage** defined as **old age**. People age differently, and some people will always seem 'young' because of a positive and interested mental attitude to life.

olfactory
To do with the sense of smell. Humans detect smells through the olfactory epithelium, a patch of sensitive yellow **tissue** located at the top of the nasal cavity roughly level with the eyes. The epithelium contains several types of **cells**, which relay messages via **neurones** into the olfactory bulb in the **brain**.

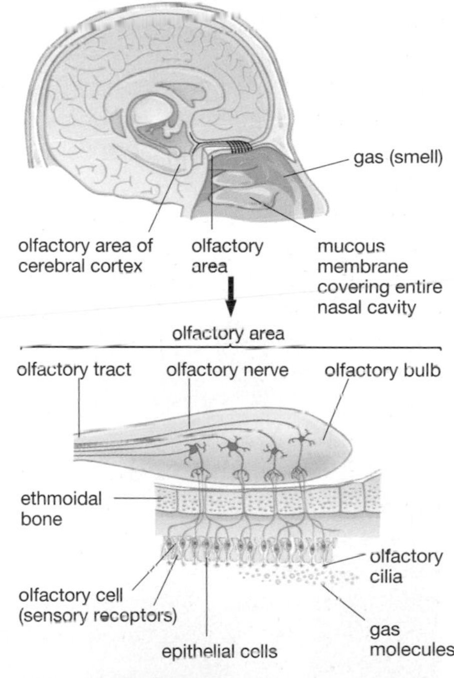

The olfactory system.

ombudsman
A public officer who investigates **complaints** about poor **service** or unfair or improper actions from **public services**. There are two different types of ombudsmen: the Parliamentary and Health Service Ombudsman investigates complaints about **government** departments and the **NHS**, and the **Local Government** Ombudsman investigates complaints about local councils.

oncology
The study, **diagnosis** and **treatment** of **cancers**. **Health professionals** specialising in working with cancers are usually based in specialist regional units.

open question
A question that cannot be answered by just 'yes' or 'no'. This type of question usually begins with questions such as 'what sort of…', 'how do you feel about…' or 'how should we…'. Questions like this encourage people to talk, as they need to be able to **communicate** the answers.

opiate
A substance based on opium. Originally it came from opium poppies, but it is also manufactured synthetically. Is the base for many drugs, particularly **painkillers** such as **morphine** and diamorphine. It is also the base for cocaine and **heroin**.

opinion poll
A **survey** carried out to find the views of a **sample** of the **population**. The results of the sample are multiplied to give a result for the general population. There are always margins of error, and various influencing factors must be taken into account. Opinion polls are used by **governments** and political parties to judge the views of the public about policies, candidates and important issues. Manufacturers can also use them to help make decisions about new products under development.

oppression
The exercise of authority and dominance by one person or **group** over another, bringing about hardship, injustice and exploitation.

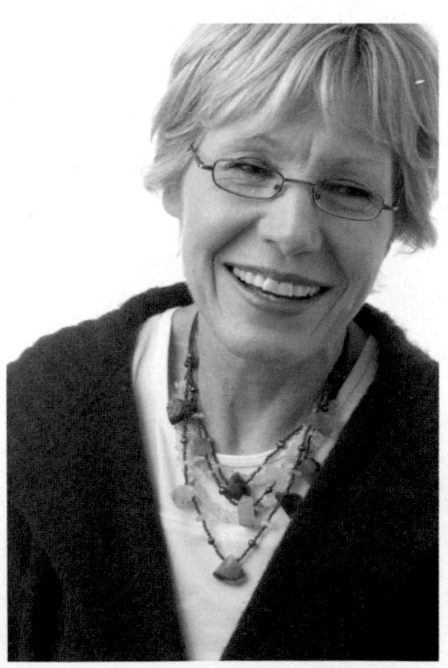

Opticians help correct sight problems.

opticians
Services that help to correct sight problems. There are two types: an ophthalmic optician is qualified to test and prescribe **treatment** including spectacles and contact lenses; a dispensing optician is qualified to measure, fit and supply spectacles and contact lenses.

optional unit
A part of an **S/NVQ** that candidates can choose to take if it is relevant for their **work**. A given number of optional units must be taken for a full **qualification**, but there is usually a wide selection to choose from.

oral questioning
A verbal interview that plays an important part in assessing candidates for **S/NVQs**. This gives a good opportunity for assessors to ask about

underpinning knowledge and is helpful for those candidates who find it difficult to explain things in writing.

organ
A part of an **organism** with a specific function, for example, the **heart** and the **liver**.

organisational systems
The structures of an **organisation** covering, for example, its **governance**, how the organisation is managed, how finances are dealt with, how **communication** and **information** are shared, and how people in the organisation receive training.

organisations
Entities that have a purpose and that structure themselves to pursue and achieve aims. The purposes of organisations can include business, finance, delivering **services**, providing **charitable** help, **lobbying**, campaigning, **teaching** or **learning**. There are many different types of organisations, from huge multi-national corporations to tiny voluntary organisations with two or three employees.

organism
A form of life that has, or could develop, the ability to function independently, for example, a **cell** or a **virus**.

orientation
Becoming familiar with surroundings. In **health** and **social care**, the term can be used to describe the **process** of encouraging people with **dementia** to recognise familiar day-to-day features such as the weather and the day of the week. It is also usually part of the **induction** process when starting a new job.

orthodontics
A specialist area of **dentistry** that is concerned with the identification, prevention and correction of problems and irregularities in the **teeth** or jaw.

orthopaedics
The study, **diagnosis** and **treatment** of **disease** or **injury** to **bones** and **joints**.

osmosis
A special type of **diffusion** involving water molecules. The movement of water molecules from a region of high concentration (of water molecules) to one of low concentration through a partially permeable membrane. The membrane is usually the cell membrane. It is vitally important that the cell contents neither lose or gain too much water. Concentration of urine occurs through osmosis.

osteopathy
An **alternative** approach to **diagnosis** and **treatment** of problems with the **muscles** and **joints**. Osteopaths train for several years and treat problems through

manipulation and massage. Many **patients** are referred to osteopaths through **medical practitioners** when traditional medicine has been unable to help.
More information can be found at www.osteopathy.org.uk

osteoporosis
Literally, 'porous **bones**'; a disorder where bones lose density and become porous and thinner, thus making them much more prone to **fractures**. It is commonest in **older people**, particularly women after the **menopause**, but also found in people who take particular types of **medication** or who have digestive **diseases** that affect **food** absorption.
More information can be found at www.nos.org.uk (National Osteoporosis Society)

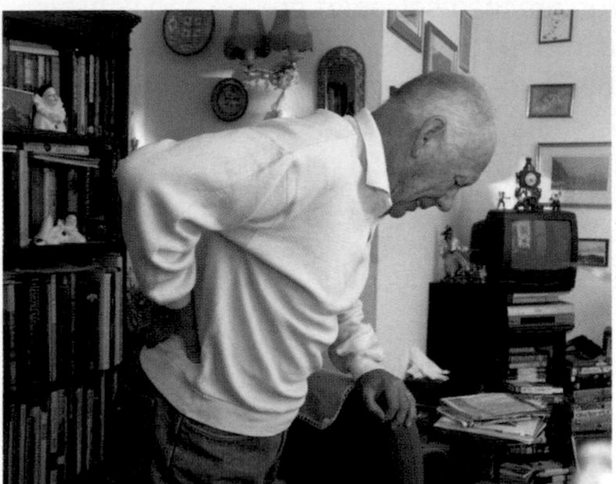

Osteoporosis is commonest in older people.

normal bone matrix

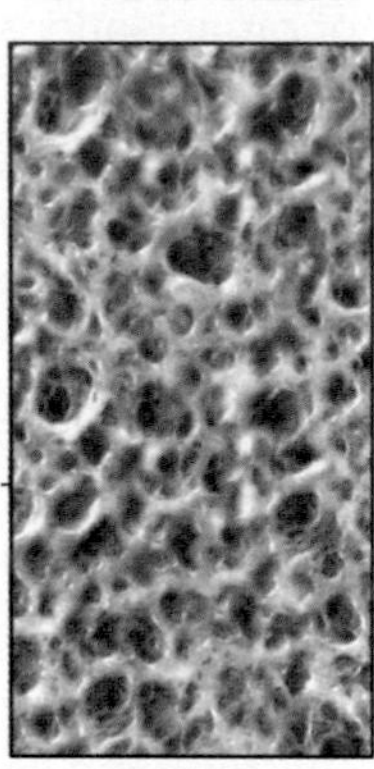

osteoporosis

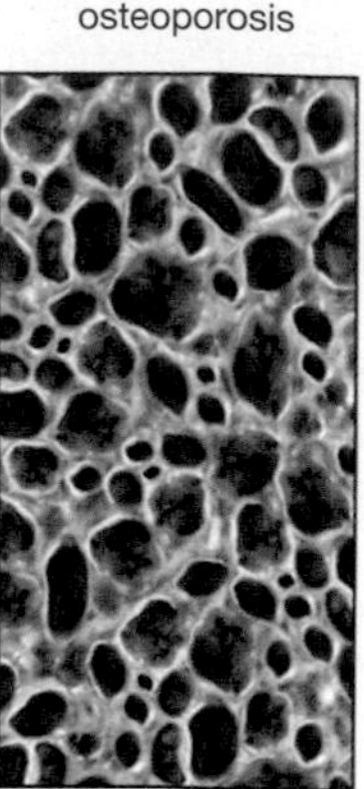

other persons
This phrase refers to everyone covered by Health and Safety at Work Act including visitors, members of the public, colleagues, contractors, clients, customers, patients, students, pupils.

out-of-school clubs
Supervised settings for children to socialise and **play**. These can take place either before or after **school** and are usually held on school premises or very close by. They provide children whose **parents** are working with a safe **environment** until parents can collect them.

outcome
The result to be achieved by an action, for example the desired outcome from providing someone with a **prosthetic** limb is that he or she will be able to participate fully in activities; the desired outcome of a **re-ablement** programme is that someone will be able to undertake daily living tasks without assistance within a specified period of time. **Services** are usually **commissioned** on the basis of outcomes.

outdoor play
Opportunities for activities in the fresh air. These are very important for children's **physical development**. All early **education** settings and **schools** must have **facilities** for children to **play** outside.

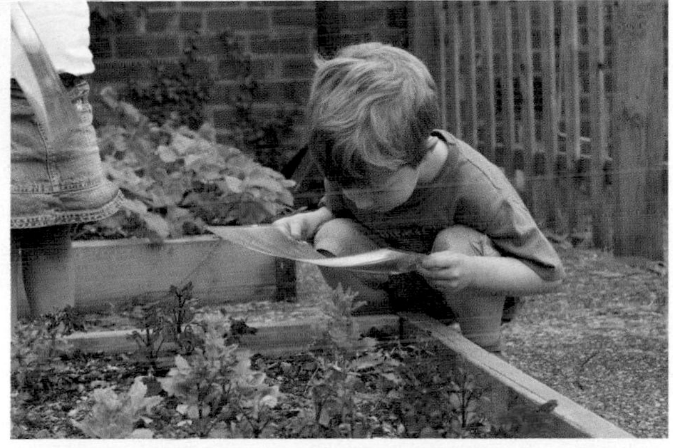
Outdoor play is important for children's physical development.

outpatient
A person receiving a medical diagnosis, or treatment, without being admitted to a hospital.

ovaries
Two small oval **organs** in the female **pelvis** (lower abdominal area). When a female **baby** is born, her **ovaries** already contain about half a million eggs. The function of the ovaries is to produce one of these unfertilised eggs (ovum) each month at the start of the reproductive cycle. Ovaries also produce the **hormones oestrogen** and **progesterone**.

ovulation
The release of an unfertilised egg (ovum) from the follicle on the outside of the **ovary** each month. *See* **menstruation**.

oxygen
A colourless, odourless, tasteless gas that makes up about 20 per cent of the air. It will combine with almost all **elements** to make other compounds and dissolves in water. It is essential to human life. It is taken into the body through the mouth and nose and into the **lungs**, where it passes into the bloodstream by **diffusion** and delivered to cells.

oxygenated
Combined with **oxygen**, or containing dissolved oxygen.

oxytocin
A **hormone** produced by the pituitary gland that causes the **uterus** to contract during **labour** and also stimulates milk production following **birth**.

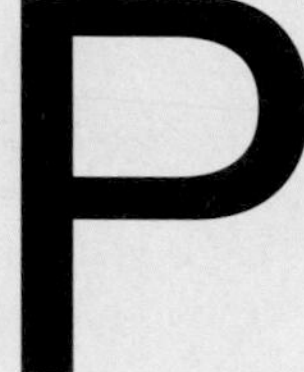

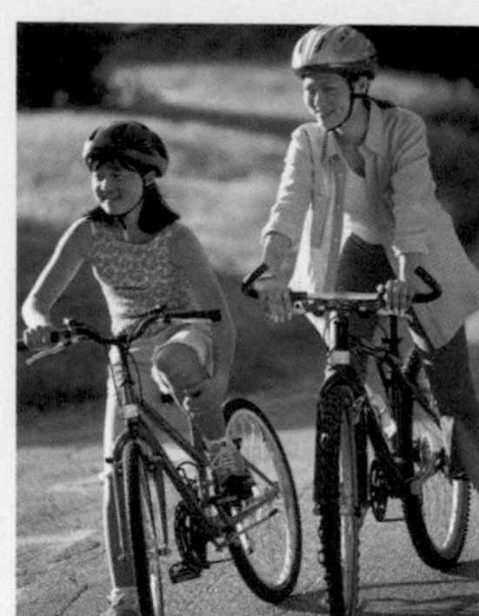

paediatrician
A doctor who specialises in the medical care and treatment of children.

pain
An unpleasant physical sensation that can result from **injury** or illness. It can range from discomfort to agony, and can be short lived or a **chronic** state. Managing pain is now a specialised area of nursing **practice**, and there are specialist pain **clinics** for people with long-term pain and no prospect of improvement.

painkiller
An analgesic drug, such as codeine or paracetamol, given for the purpose of relieving **pain**.

palliative care
An approach to providing care that is available to people in the later stages of a **terminal illness**. The purpose is to provide the best possible **quality of life** for people approaching the end of life. The approach is **holistic** and includes all aspects of the person's life, and also **supports** the **family**. The aims of palliative care are to:

- affirm life and regard **dying** as a normal **process**
- provide relief from pain and other distressing **symptoms**
- integrate the psychological and spiritual aspects of **patient** care
- offer a support **system** to help patients live as actively as possible until **death**
- offer a support system to help the family cope during the patient's illness and in their own **bereavement**.

More information can be found at www.ncpc.org.uk (National Council for Palliative Care)

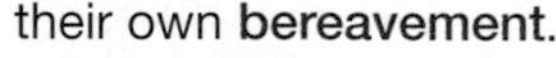

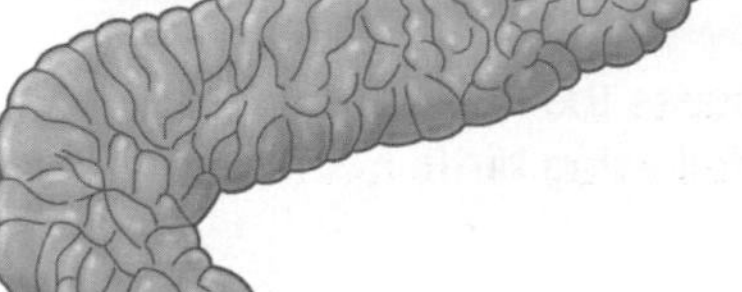

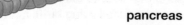

The pancreas.

pancreas
A **gland** situated near the **stomach** that secretes **digestive** juice containing salts and major enzymes and also produces **insulin** from the **Islets of Langerhans**. *See* **diabetes**.

paralysis
Loss of the ability to move one or more parts of the body. There are many, complex causes for paralysis, but it results from damage to the motor **neurones** (**nerves**) that send messages about movement from the **brain**. The damage can be caused through a **stroke**, **tumour**, **multiple sclerosis** or severe **trauma** or **injury**. Paralysis of one limb is called monoplegia. If two limbs on the same side of the body are involved it is hemiplegia. If both legs are paralysed, the term is paraplegia, and if all four limbs are paralysed the term is **quadriplegia**.

paranoia
A **mental disorder** that results in **delusions** where people are suspicious of others and believe that they are under **threat** from, or persecuted by, people around them. Someone with paranoid delusions will misinterpret the motives of others and believe them to be threatening and **harmful**. Delusions can also be about objects; for example, radio waves or advertising hoardings can be believed to be sending threatening messages.

paraplegia
Loss of movement and sensation in both legs.

parasite
An **organism** that lives on another organism (the host) without giving it any benefit or killing it, but usually causing some degree of **harm**. Well-known parasites with human hosts are tapeworms, hookworms, fleas and bed bugs. Some parasites also introduce **diseases** into human hosts. This is a particular problem in developing countries where there may be poor sanitation and drinking water is not clean. Female mosquitoes can introduce the **pathogen** that causes malaria, and sleeping sickness is caused by a pathogen from the tsetse fly.

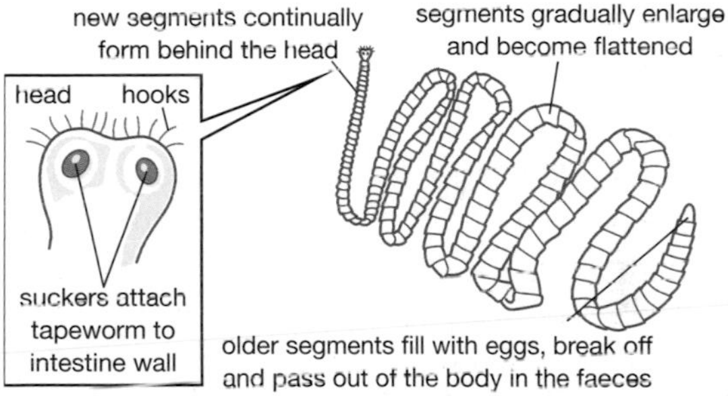

A tapeworm.

parent
A child's main carer, and the holder of **parental responsibility** in respect of the child. Regardless of whether parents are the natural father or mother of a child or the **adoptive** parents, the **responsibilities** and legal requirements are the same.

parental responsibility
The legal requirements of **parents** with regard to children, such as ensuring that children are provided with warmth, **food** and shelter, that they have a loving home

where they feel safe and secure, and that they are protected from **harm**. Parents are also responsible for maintaining the **health** and **education** of their children by ensuring, for example, that they have all necessary health checks, **vaccinations** and **dental** care, and that they attend **school**. Parental responsibility is shared equally between two parents if they are married, but is vested only in the **mother** where parents are not married. Since December 2003, however, **putative fathers** can have parental responsibility if the child's **birth** is jointly registered by both parents. Same-sex partners in a civil partnership can also share parental responsibility for children.

parenting order

An order that can be made by a **court** in respect of the **parents** of a child who has offended, or who has been persistently **truanting**, or who has received an **anti-social behaviour order**. The order usually requires parents to attend parent **education** sessions, and may include other conditions such as meeting with teachers or **social workers**. A parenting order does not result in a criminal record, but failure to comply with its conditions may do so.

parole

A period towards the end of a prison sentence when prisoners can be released into the community, but will be recalled to prison if they fail to comply with specific conditions.

Parliament

The democratically elected **law**-making and governing body of the UK. Scotland, Wales and Northern Ireland have separate parliaments with law-making powers. England does not have a separate parliament, but is governed by the UK Parliament.

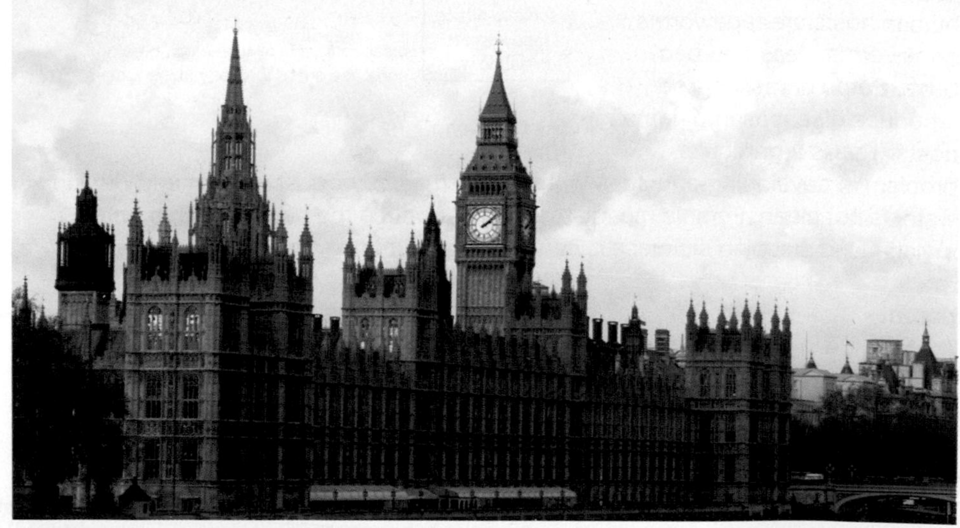

Parliament.

A B C D E F G H I J K L M N O P Q R S T U V W XYZ

participant observation
A **research method** where the researcher takes part in the events that are being researched. Examples include a consumer affairs researcher may 'infiltrate' an **organisation** to find out about concerns over **standards**, or a researcher may spend time living on state **benefits** to look at how it is possible to survive on the sums available.

participation work
Providing ways for children and **young people** to have a voice in policies and decisions that affect their lives. Many different projects are run by children's **organisations**, and specialist participation workers try to ensure that children and young people are able to influence developments and **decision makers**.
More information can be found at www.participationworks.org.uk

partnership
Care workers, professionals, the service user and families working together for the benefit of the client. More generally, people or organisations working together towards a common goal.

passive
Being accepting and unresisting; taking no active part in events. People who are passive will not raise objections or try to influence others. Traditionally, people using **health** and care **services** have been viewed as the passive receivers of services or **treatment**. This is no longer the case, and the role of people using these services has moved through being regarded as active participants to the current **model** of being in control.

passive immunity
When an individual receives **antibodies** from another person or animal such as a baby in the first few months of life from the mother or antisera prepared from another individual or animal.

passive smoking
Inhaling **toxins** from breathing in the **smoke** of other people's cigarettes. There is clear evidence that non-smokers living or working in smoky atmospheres have a higher than normal **incidence** of smoking-related **diseases** than would be expected in a non-smoker. This was a key factor in the passing of **legislation** across the UK to ban smoking in all public places.

pathogens
Organisms, such as **bacteria** or **viruses**, that cause **disease**. The entry of a pathogen into the human body **triggers** a response from the **immune system**.

pathology department
A department comprising mainly scientists offering **diagnostic laboratory** services.

patient
A person making use of the medical attention, **diagnosis** or **treatment** offered by **health care services**. Patients were traditionally seen as **passive** receivers of treatment, but current thinking puts them, rather than medical staff, at the centre of **health** services.

Patient Advice and Liaison Service (PALS)
A **service** provided in all **NHS** trusts in England. PALS staff are employed by the **NHS**, although volunteers also **support** the service in some areas. The service provides a source of advice and **information** for **patients**, and a means of resolving concerns about services or **facilities**. Although it is not a formal **complaints procedure**, PALS staff may liaise with **hospital** staff to try to resolve immediate issues or conflicts to avoid escalation into a formal complaint.
More information can be found at www.pals.nhs.uk

Pavlov, Ivan
A Russian **physiologist** (1849–1936) who developed one of the very earliest **learning theories: classical conditioning**, which is essentially 'learning by association'. He demonstrated that dogs would salivate when **food** was produced; a nearby church bell sounded at the same time as the dogs were fed, and he noted that after a time the dogs salivated at the sound of the bell regardless of whether the food was produced. This effect is commonly experienced when we hear a piece of music that arouses physical or emotional responses associated with a different time, or notice a particular smell that brings about responses not connected with current circumstances.

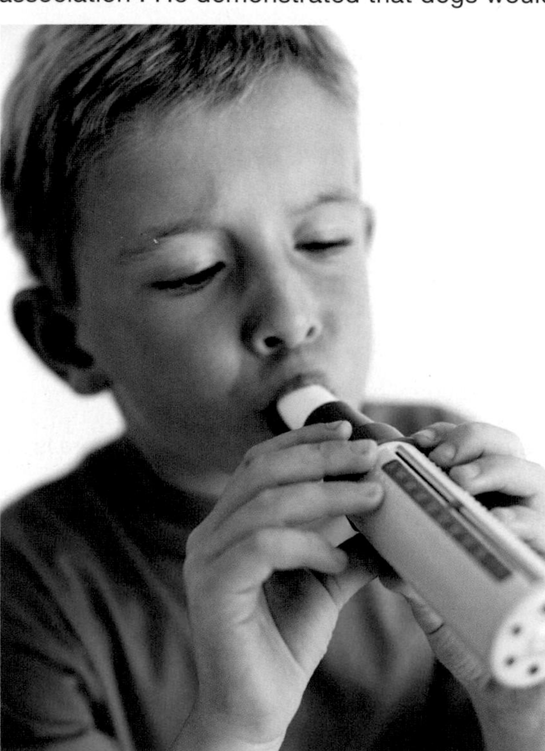

Peak flow readings indicate how open the airways are and this helps to determine any airway or lung changes.

peak flow
A **measurement** of how quickly air can be expelled from the **lungs**. This shows how well airways are functioning. Peak flow is measured through a peak flow meter in litres of air per minute. Expected peak flow rates vary between men

and women and with age and height, so there are significant variations between individuals. People with **asthma** are likely to have a lower peak flow, and regular measurements can be a useful part of managing asthma.

peer group

A group of people who share at least one identifying characteristic. This could be, for example, age group, **gender**, job role, level of **education**, living **environment**, aspirations or social circumstances. There is strong pressure on people to conform to the expectations of their peer group about behaviour, dress or preferences. **Young people** in particular are usually strongly influenced by their peer group.

pelvic cavity

The lower **abdomen** between the hips. It contains reproductive **organs** such as **uterus** and **ovaries** (in women) and also the **bladder**.

pelvis

The bony arch that supports the lower body. The hip **joints** are attached to the pelvis and its structure protects the **pelvic cavity**. Several **bones** make up the pelvis: the sacrum, the coccyx (also called the tailbone) and the hip bone (made up of the ilium, pubis and ischium). The male and the female pelvis are slightly different shapes, because the female pelvis has to accommodate the **uterus** and have enough room for a **foetus** to develop.

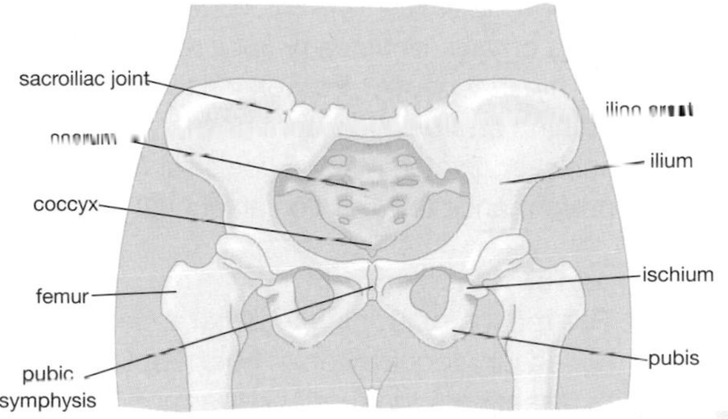

The pelvis.

penis

The male **organ** used for **reproduction** and urination. The opening of the **urethra** is at the tip of the penis and this is the route for releasing **urine** from the **bladder**. During sexual stimulation, the organ becomes infused with **blood** and becomes stiff and erect, and able to penetrate the **vagina** to deposit **semen**, which contains the **spermatozoa** necessary for **fertilisation**.

pension

Money saved throughout someone's working life in order to provide an **income** in **retirement**. Everyone who has paid National Insurance contributions is entitled to a pension from the **state**, called the state pension, commonly known as the old age pension. People may also have contributed to an occupational pension through their employer, and some people will have chosen to contribute to a private pension which is arranged through an insurance company and invests contributions on the stock market. Pensions are usually paid monthly, although the state pension can be weekly. Some occupational and private pensions include a lump sum of **cash** in addition to regular payments.

percentage
One-hundredths of a whole, often shown by the % sign, for example if there are 100 people in a **group** and 42 of them have brown eyes, then it can be stated that 42 per cent (42%) of the group are brown-eyed; out of a **population** of 1,000 people, if there are 890 people who have been **vaccinated** against **meningitis**, then 89 per cent of the population have been vaccinated.

percutaneous endoscopic gastrostomy (PEG feeding)
A method of tube feeding directly into the **stomach** through the abdominal wall. The tube can be used to provide liquid nourishment for people who are unable to **swallow**.

performance
The way in which a person or **organisation** has met **targets** and **goals** for their **work**. Most organisations carry out a **review** of employees' performance on a regular basis to ensure that people are working to the best of their ability and to identify any additional **training and development needs**. Organisations are also judged on how well they have achieved the targets and goals set for them; **local authorities** and **NHS** trusts have their performance reviewed on an annual basis against a clear set of targets.

performance criteria
The means of judging whether a person or **organisation** has achieved the necessary requirements. For people being **assessed** for **S/NVQs**, these are used by assessors to identify performance that is satisfactory and shows **competence**. **Local authorities**, **NHS** trusts and other organisations will have their performance judged by **inspectors** using performance criteria.

peripheral nervous system
The parts of the **nervous system** that connect the **central nervous system** (the **brain** and **spinal cord**) to other parts of the body. Peripheral nerves may carry sensory, motor fibres or both (mixed) and include the autonomic nerves that carry out the involuntary functions such as regulating the heartbeat.

peristalsis
Wave-like contractions of two antagonistic sheets of **muscle** that force movement along tubes or similar structures in the body. Examples include peristalsis pushes **food** along the **alimentary canal** in the digestive process, and in the **fallopian tubes** the egg is pushed towards the **uterus**.

permanency
Focus on promoting secure, stable and fulfilling relationships for children and young people whether they are living with their birth families, in foster, adoptive or

residential homes. Permanency planning uses this criterion to underpin work to meet the short-, medium- and long-term needs of children and young people, i.e. until they are 21, or 25 if still in education.

personal and professional development
Practice of any type that will enable you to develop within your job as a person and as a practitioner.

personal care
Tasks that are non-medical, but important parts of daily living. They include **bathing**, dressing, going to the **toilet** and personal **grooming**. People may wish to have **support** to carry out these tasks for a range of reasons including illness or **disability**. Personal care can be provided by **professional carers** over the age of 18. Personal care may be provided by **family** and friends of any age.

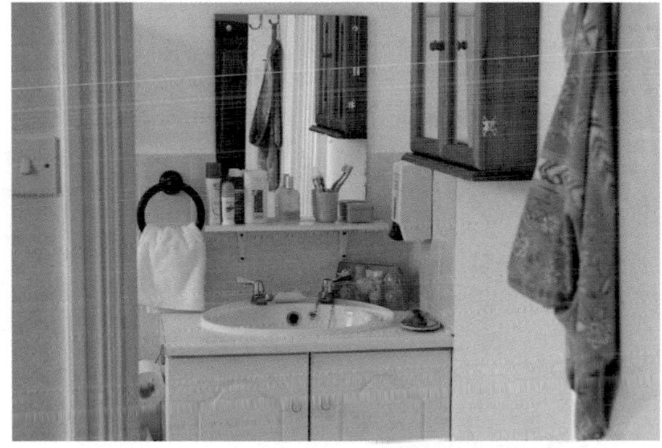

Keeping everything neatly and to hand will make personal care easier.

personal clothing and fashion items
Includes outer clothes worn from home to work, jewellery, acrylic nails, nail varnish and false eyelashes.

personal constructs
A psychological theory of **personality** which suggests that people behave like scientists. A scientist will have a **hypothesis** and will then carry out **experiments** and **research** to confirm or deny it. This theory suggests that people develop 'constructs' about what they anticipate will happen, then test them. If what they have anticipated happens, their behaviour is confirmed; if it does not, they will incorporate the new **information** into an adjusted 'construct' and go on to test that. A five-year-old on his first visit to the zoo may have formed ideas from television and stories about what the animals will look like and that they will be fun to **touch**. When he gets to the zoo, many of the animals are very big and scary, some are smelly, a lot are behind glass and none of them can be touched. He re-thinks his **understanding** of what zoos are like based on his experience.

personal development plan
An individual plan developed jointly between a practitioner and supervisor, or line manager, that identifies personal and professional goals and targets, and gives plans and time-frames for how and when these will be met.

personal finances
The money that a person receives as income and spends on regular items such as **food**, clothing, **rent**, household bills, holidays and savings. Sometimes people need advice and **information** to help them to manage personal finances.

personal hygiene
Keeping the hair and body clean by **bathing** or showering daily, regular hair washing and cleaning the **teeth** and mouth at least twice daily. Some people may need **support** to manage personal hygiene.

personal presentation
This includes: personal hygiene; use of personal protection equipment; clothing and accessories suitable to the particular workplace.

personal protective clothing
Includes items such as plastic aprons, gloves – both clean and sterile, eyewear, footwear, dresses, trousers and shirts and all-in-one trouser suits and gowns. These may be single-use disposable clothing or reusable clothing.

personal safety
To keep yourself safe from any type of danger, abuse, harm, neglect or exploitation.

personal space
The physical distance between people that is considered comfortable. This is partly a cultural matter, as people from Arab **cultures**, for example, tend to stand far closer to each other than many from European cultures. Everyone has their

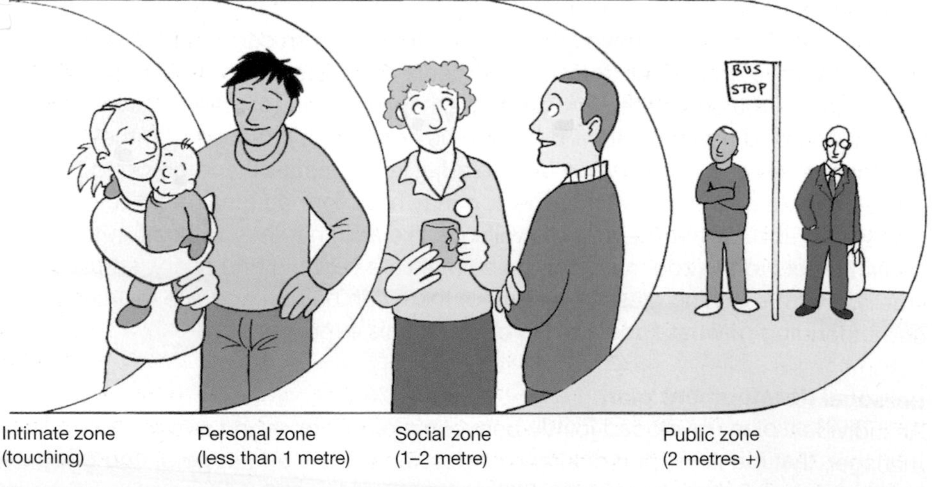
BUS STOP
Intimate zone (touching)
Personal zone (less than 1 metre)
Social zone (1–2 metre)
Public zone (2 metres +)

Zones of personal space.

own 'comfort zone' and it will vary depending on the nature of the contact. The picture on the previous page gives an idea of the distances within which people are usually comfortable.

personal support needs
The needs of people relating to their personal activities such as going to the toilet, bathing, dressing or grooming.

personalisation agenda
The process of putting people in control of the services they receive by giving them control over how the budget for their support is spent. People in receipt of Direct Payments, or who have an individualised budget, are able to decide the service that they want, the provider they wish to purchase it from and how they want it to be delivered.

personality
The **interaction** of the behaviour, character features, attitudes, emotional and social **traits** of a unique individual. **Understanding** someone's personality makes it possible to predict behaviour and responses.

personality disorder
A condition involving ways of behaving that are anti-social, possibly **violent**, **aggressive**, irresponsible or **harmful** to the individual or others, but that is not the result of a **mental health problem**, and is not treatable. People with a personality disorder are classed as having a **mental disorder** and can be hospitalised for their own **safety** and the safety of others.

personality trait
An aspect of a person's character that is a consistent response to particular circumstances, for example some people are **resilient**, while others are prone to despair easily; some people are extrovert, and others are more **introverted** and reserved; some people always take a positive view, and others are often negative and pessimistic.

person-centred planning
An approach to provision of care that began in the **learning disability** sector but is now being used more widely; it puts the person at the centre of all planning and always has a positive focus. Plans are made around what people can do, not what they cannot do. Rather than the traditional **social care** approach of looking at what people's **needs** are and then encouraging them to do as much as possible for themselves, person-centred planning involves looking at what people can do and then seeing whether there are areas where extra **support** might be needed. Support is then made available to fill the gaps.

A B C D E F G H I J K L M N O **P** Q R S T U V W XYZ

person specification
Part of the **information** supplied for a job vacancy. It describes the type of personal qualities that are needed for the job, rather than details of **qualifications** and experience, which are listed in the **job description**.

phagocytosis
The **process** of **white blood cells** (neutrophils) overwhelming invading **bacteria** and **parasites**, then removing the remains. They do so by consuming the invaders in a self-contained vesicle within the **cell** called a phagosome. The cell then kills off the bacteria by 'digesting' them so that they disintegrate and the debris is then 'spat out' by the cell and cleared away in the bloodstream.

pharmacist
Qualified in the development and use of **medicines** and in understanding their effects on the body and **disease**. Pharmacists dispense drugs and give advice. Pharmacologists do the discovery, research and development.

phenotype
The **observable** qualities and characteristics of an **organism** or individual, such as its development or behaviour, as opposed to the genotype (the inherited instructions it carries, which may or may not, be outwardly expressed).

phenylketonuria (PKU)
A **genetic metabolic** disorder that prevents the normal breakdown of **protein** because of a defective **enzyme**. If untreated, the disorder can cause **brain** damage. PKU can be treated very successfully if **diagnosed** soon after **birth**. The heel-prick test (Guthrie test) is carried out on all **newborn babies** to identify PKU. The condition is then controlled by **diet**.

pheromones
A type of **hormone** produced in tiny quantities that attracts and identifies suitable mating partners. The hormones have a smell that subconsciously attracts some people and repels others. They are thought to be located in the **sweat glands** of the armpits and groin.

philosophy
A belief, or view of the world, that guides how a person thinks or behaves.

phobia
A debilitating and irrational **fear** of an activity, event, object, **food** or living creature. To be classified as a phobia, the fear must be so strong that it interferes with normal living – for example, a fear of going outside the house so that someone has to stay indoors, or a fear of using public **toilets** meaning that someone

cannot go out very far or travel any distance. **Symptoms** include fast heartbeat, shortness of breath, palpitations, sweating, dizziness and a feeling of dread. People with phobias can be helped through counselling or de-sensitisation therapy.

phototherapy
Treatment with ultraviolet light, which is effective for various **skin** conditions and for **neonatal jaundice**.

pH scale
The degree of alkalinity and acidity based on the concentration of hydrogen ions in a substance measured on a scale ranging from 1.0 (strongly acid) to 14.0 (strongly alkaline), with 7.0 being neutral. The pH of the skin is 4.0–5.5 and the eyes have a pH of 7.4–7.6.

physical
To do with the body.

physical abuse
The deliberate **harming** of a **child** or **vulnerable adult** by hitting, slapping, punching, kicking, scalding, burning or hitting with an object such as a stick or a belt. Any **disclosure** or suspicion of abuse must be **reported** immediately, according to the protection procedures for the **organisation**, or to the **police** or **local authority**. *See* **abuse**.

physical activity
Bodily **exercise**. It is essential for **health** and **well-being**; it is vital for children's development and for maintaining health in adults. Activity does not have to be in organised sports or games. It can be walking or simply climbing stairs rather than using lifts. Physical exercise uses calories, strengthens **muscles** and **bones** and improves cardiovascular and **respiratory** health.

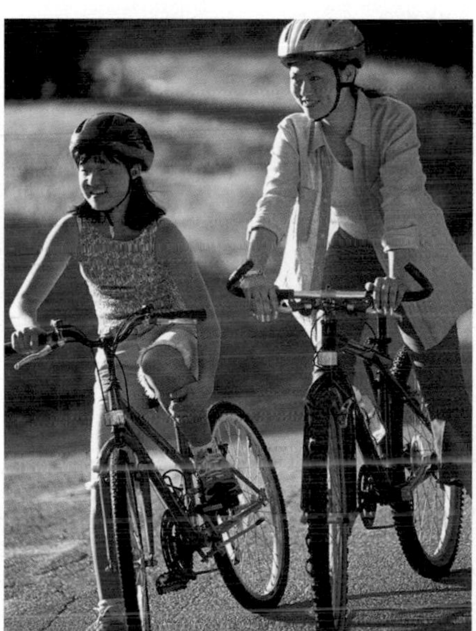
Physical activity is essential for health and well-being.

physical development
Growth and development of body **systems** and physical abilities such as walking, jumping, hopping, kicking balls, lifting, carrying and **hand–eye co-ordination**. A healthy, balanced **diet** and **physical activity** are both important for **promoting** physical development.

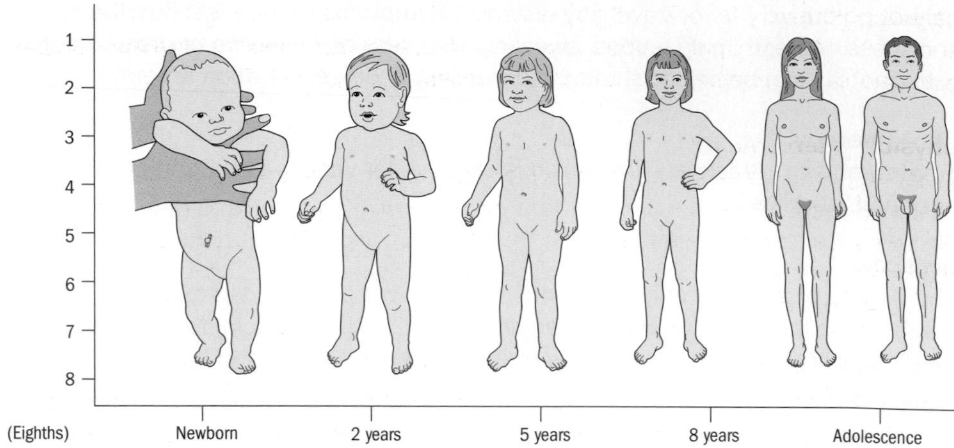

■ Growth profiles from birth to the end of adolescence.

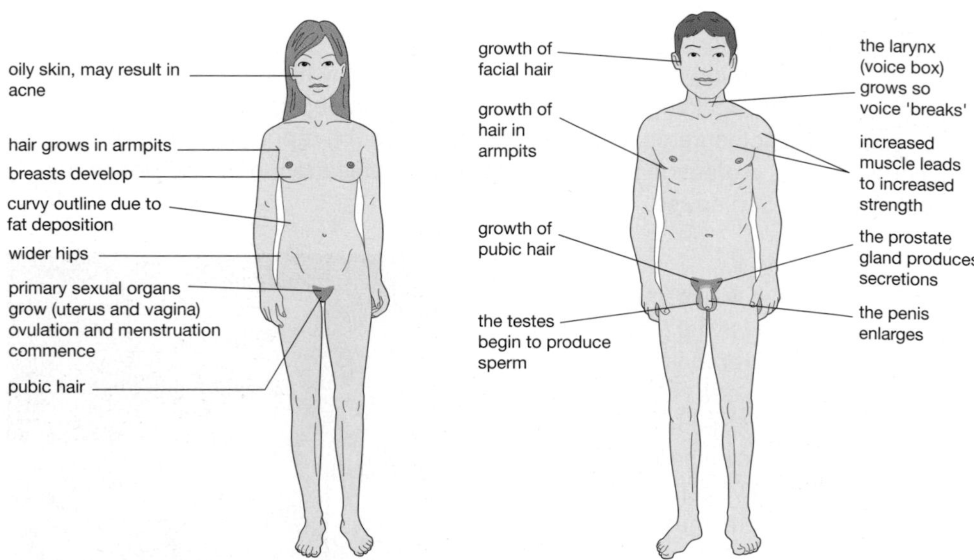

■ Body changes at puberty in males and females.

physical difficulties

Problems with walking, lifting, maintaining **personal hygiene** or any **physical activity**. These can be the result of illness, **injury** or the **ageing process**, where some **muscles** lose strength and **bones** can become porous and fragile.

physical health

The state of wellness that is mainly the absence of illness, but also a state where all body **systems** are functioning properly.

physical illness
A **disease** or **injury** that can be **diagnosed** through **symptoms** that are measurable and can be tested chemically or through scans or **X-rays**.

physical intervention
Where a professional worker makes physical contact with an aggressive or potentially **violent** person in order to prevent harm or injury. It is to be used only as a very last resort when managing **conflict** or **challenging** situations and is restricted to the minimum contact necessary to prevent harm to the individual, the worker or others.

physical risks
Risks of damage, **illness** or injury as a result of **behaviour** or **lifestyle**. This could include risk of damage from substance abuse or the risks to a **vulnerable** person living with a person with a history of violence.

physiology
The biological study of the normal functions of living **organisms**.

physiotherapist
A health professional who treats the physical problems caused by **accidents**, **illness** and **ageing**.

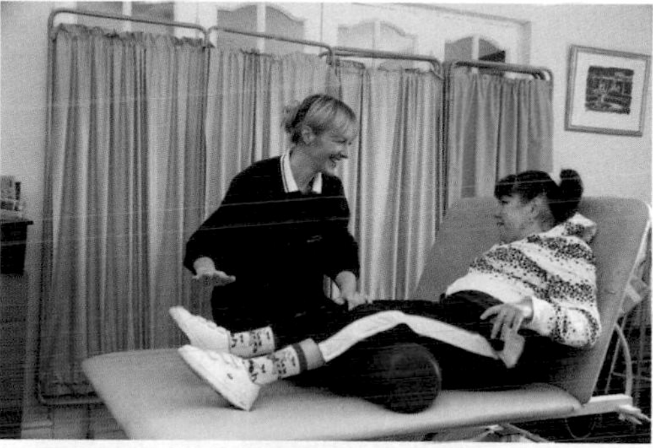
Physiotherapist.

physiotherapy
A **health** profession that aims to maintain and/or restore the maximum potential functions and movement for people using the **service**. A range of **treatments** are used including **exercises**, massage and manipulation, and the use of electronic devices to improve movement and flexibility. It is mainly **hospital** based, but there are some physiotherapists working in the **community**.

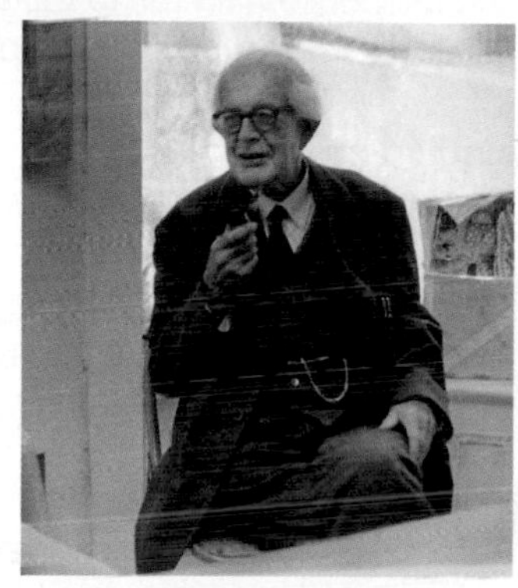
Jean Piaget.

Piaget, Jean
A Swiss **psychologist** (1896–1980) who developed one of the most influential models of children's **learning** and development. Piaget suggests that children, from **birth**, actively choose and make sense of **information** from the **environment** and have the ability to adapt and learn.

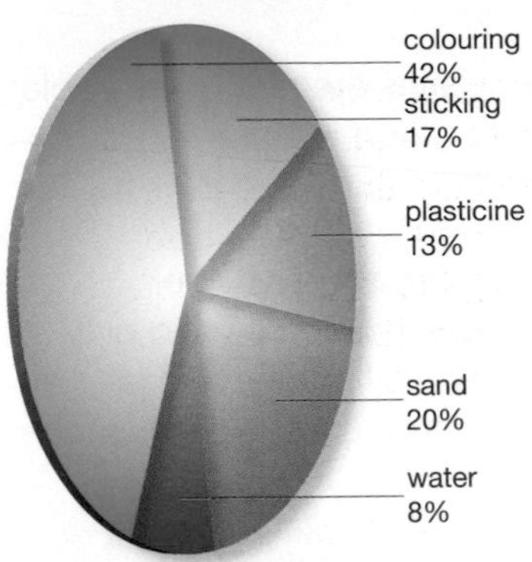

This pie chart shows activities engaged in by children over a period of time.

pie chart
A way of representing **research data** that shows the proportionate size of different parts of the data by showing them as segments of a circle.

pilot survey
An initial **survey** before starting a main piece of **research** work which tests the materials and methods. Changes may be made to methods or materials following the pilot survey.

pituitary gland
The main **endocrine gland**. It is a small oval **gland** at the base of the **brain** and it secretes the **hormones** that regulate the hormonal activity of many other glands in the body. It is largely governed by the hypothalamus in the brain.

placebo
A 'dummy' or 'pretend' drug that is used in clinical trials. Some people are given the real drug and others the placebo, but they are not told which group they are in. The drug being tested must produce results measurably better than the placebo for it to be considered successful. The reason that people are not told whether they are receiving the real drug is that psychological factors, such as expectations of recovery or of side effects, could affect the results of the trials.

placenta
A temporary **organ** attached to the wall of the **uterus** that develops in **pregnancy**. The **blood** supply of the **mother** and the **foetus** lie close enough together (they do not join) so that **nutrients** can pass from the mother to the foetus and waste products pass from the foetus to the mother. The placenta supplies hormones to establish pregnancy and anchors the foetus to the uterus wall via the umbilical cord. The placenta detaches from the wall of the uterus and is expelled during the third stage of **labour**.

plagiarism
The unauthorised copying of someone else's work without acknowledgement of the source. This practice is common among students, but educational establishments use special software program to detect plagiarism in essays, assignments and **examinations**. If plagiarism is found it will usually result in a fail mark. Where authors believe their work to have been plagiarised by another person, they can sue for damages.

plan
A detailed proposal for doing or achieving something and the process of organising an activitity.

plasma
The yellowish, liquid part of **blood**, in which cells are suspended (hanging). It makes up to 50 per cent of the total volume of the blood and contains vital proteins, including: fibrinogen, which helps with blood clotting; globulins such as antibodies; and serum albumin (which helps body fluid move into body tissues). Plasma is a means of transport for glucose, lipids (fatty chemicals), amino acids, hormones, the end products of metabolism, dissolved carbon dioxide and oxygen.

platelets
Bodies in the **blood** that assist with clotting. They are fragments of larger cells made in bone marrow.

play
Activities that are an essential part of children's development. Children learn through play, they **experiment** and develop creative **skills** and **imagination**. Children also need to be able to take assessed and well-managed risks when they play in order to provide them with challenges and opportunities to try out new things.

playgroups
Groups for pre-**school** children, organised by local **communities** on a not-for-profit basis. They usually run for 2- to 3-hour sessions; some are available five days a week and others just two or three days. The emphasis is on **play**. They usually accept children from 2–5 years of age.

playworkers
People who work with children, usually from 5–15 years of age, to provide opportunities for child-directed **play**. This is usually delivered through after-**school** clubs and holiday play-schemes. Playworkers may **support** children's play but do not direct it; children have a free **choice** of play within the **facilities** available and there is no set **curriculum** or framework to follow.
More information can be found at www.playwork.org.uk

pneumonia
A **respiratory disease** resulting in **inflammation** of the **lungs** and congestion. It can be caused by a **virus** or by **bacteria**. The condition is particularly serious in those who are already ill or in very young children.

police
A series of local services throughout the country whose role is to maintain **law** and order and to gather evidence against any people thought to have broken the law. Local police services are led by a Chief Constable.

police authorities
Local bodies, made up of elected **councillors**, local **magistrates** and independent members, which have the **responsibility** to deliver policing in an area. In Scotland and Wales, policing is the responsibility of the devolved **parliaments**. The police authority has the **power** to determine policing **priorities**, to provide a **strategic** plan and to set the budget, all of which must be within **government targets** set by the Home Secretary. However, the operational delivery of policing is the responsibility of the Chief Constable.

policies and procedures
Plans for action or statements outlining underlying **values and principles**, along with the instructions for carrying out all the necessary activities to achieve the policies. An **organisation** may have a policy about **safeguarding vulnerable adults** which states that the organisation is fully committed to protecting people from risk of **harm** and to taking prompt action in the event of any concerns. This will be **supported** by a set of procedures that provide detailed **information** about how to assess risks, the person to whom concerns are to be **reported**, the information that must be **recorded**, and the limits of **confidentiality**. **Political parties** will have policies that they offer to the people when they are seeking to be elected as a **government**.

political party
An **organisation** that **promotes** and publicises a set of **beliefs** and proposals about how the country should be governed. These are presented to the voters at election time as a manifesto outlining how the party would govern if its members were elected. The political party that wins the most seats in **Parliament** will be invited to form a **government** by the Queen.

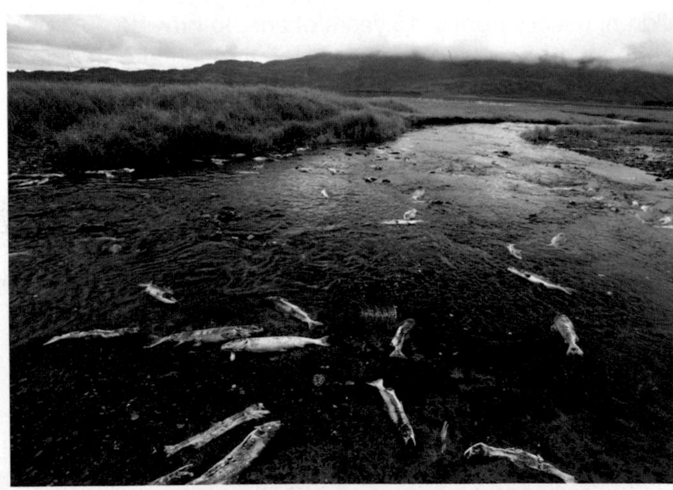

Contamination of the environment by human activity.

pollution
Contamination of the **environment** by human activity. The environment can be earth, water, air or atmosphere and can be local, national or global.

Poor Law
The system of taking care of people living in **poverty** in England and Wales from the sixteenth century

until the establishment of the **Welfare State** in the twentieth century. The first major piece of **legislation** was in 1601 when the poor were divided into the 'impotent poor' (**older people**, **disabled** people, widows and the very young) and the 'able-bodied poor' (those who refused to work, alcoholics, criminals and beggars). Each parish was required to make **provision** for the poor. In 1834 a further major piece of legislation grouped parishes together as people began to live in towns and cities. The Poor Laws were not abolished until 1930, but the notion of the 'deserving' and 'undeserving' poor is still evident in some attitudes towards poverty.

population
The people who live in a particular place. Term also used in research to refer to people in a sample group.

portfolio
A collection of evidence for an **S/NVQ**, another **vocational qualification** or a piece of coursework for other qualifications.

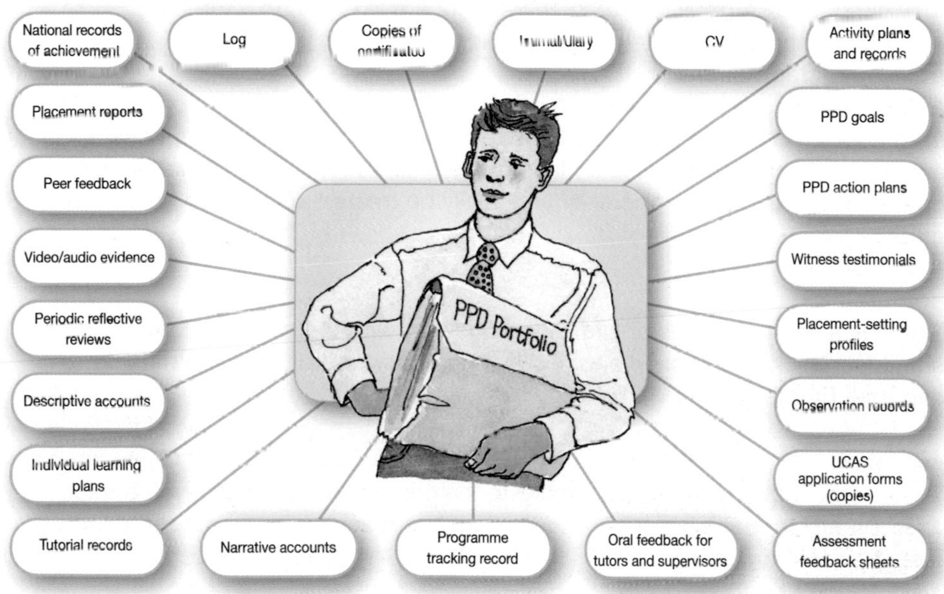
National records of achievement
Log
Copies of
CV
Activity plans and records
Placement reports
PPD goals
Peer feedback
PPD action plans
Video/audio evidence
Witness testimonials
Periodic reflective reviews
PPD Portfolio
Placement-setting profiles
Descriptive accounts
Observation
Individual learning plans
UCAS application forms (copies)
Tutorial records
Narrative accounts
Programme tracking record
Oral feedback for tutors and supervisors
Assessment feedback sheets

Potential sources of evidence for personal development for health and care practice.

positive action
Procedures aiming to ensure that **under-represented groups** are included in those employed in an **organisation**. This can be done through targeted advertising, checking that any **barriers** are removed, and providing additional training where needed. This is part of an equal opportunities approach to **employment**.

positive discipline
An approach that rewards behaviour which is being encouraged rather than punishing unwanted behaviour. An example is where some children may be given star charts, where they receive a star each time they do something they have been asked to do. Children respond well to this approach, which is based on social **learning theories.** However, it does not address the underlying reasons for behaviour; it simply changes it.

positive discrimination
Planned actions to promote the interests of a particular group of individuals, usually ones who have been previously under-represented.

postal questionnaire
A technique used by **researchers** to obtain answers to questions from a wide audience. **Questionnaires** asking for views and opinions can be distributed widely by using the postal service. Researchers do not expect everyone to return questionnaires distributed in this way, and so they will send out many more than they need for a **sample**; less than 10 per cent are likely to be returned.

post-natal depression
A common condition in women after they have given **birth.** Many women suffer from **depression**, as opposed to the 'baby blues' which happen to most women a few days after birth and usually last for a day or so. This is a **mental disorder** and requires help and **support**. It can usually be treated with a combination of **medication** and counselling.

posture
The way a person stands or sits. Good posture, with the back straight, shoulders back and relaxed and head up, is important for avoiding **muscle** and **joint** problems.

potential
The very best that a person can achieve; there is no set **target** or level, but for an individual to reach his or her potential means reaching the very best **standard** possible for him or her.

poverty
There are two definitions of poverty. **Absolute poverty** is defined by the United Nations as living on the equivalent of less than US$1 a day, with a shortage of the basic essentials of life. **Relative poverty** occurs where people have a very small share of the **resources** that are usual in the **society** in which they live.

power
The ability to exercise control and influence over people or events. Power can be evident at all levels: in **relationships**, **families**, **organisations**, local **communities**, nationally and globally. Power can be used positively or negatively.

practice
The day-to-day delivery of **professional services** and **expertise**. Professionals must keep their practice up to date by ensuring that they are aware of current thinking and developments.

practice nurse
A **health professional** attached to a **GP practice**.

pre-conception
The time before a **pregnancy** is established. Advice is offered by **midwives** and other **health professionals** to people who are considering becoming pregnant. Advice may be about the best ways to become pregnant and the actions to take to keep healthy. The **health** of the potential **mother** is important so that the best possible conditions for a successful pregnancy are in place.

pregnancy
The state of having an **implanted foetus** growing in the **uterus**.

prejudice
Judgements made about **groups** of people or individuals based on generalised negative views and **feelings** of **fear** or ignorance rather than facts, **information** or knowledge of individuals. This leads to **stereotyping** and **discrimination**.

premature
Early; of a **baby**, born before developing for 36 weeks in the **uterus**. Some babies are able to survive from 25 weeks, but face significant risks of **brain** damage or **disability** and are also very much at risk of illness and **infection** in the early weeks, as some of their **organs** are not fully developed. Premature babies are looked after in special units with specialised **equipment** while they complete the development **process**. They can take up to 2 years to catch up on developmental **milestones**.

prescription
An order for drugs or other medical supplies that can be written only by certain **health professionals**: **doctors**, **dentists**, **midwives** and **nurse** practitioners.

presentation
The sharing of **information** with others, usually a **group**, in an interesting and informative way. This is an important **skill** and is a requirement of many **learning** programmes for **health** and care **professionals**.

presentation methods
Ways of communicating and sharing **information**. Technology, including software program such as PowerPoint, is often used, but information can also be presented using charts or **handouts** or simply by delivering a **lecture**.

pre-speech
The sounds made by children before they are able to speak using words. Children make sounds and 'speak' in sentences in preparation for speech.

pressure ulcers/sores
Skin breakdown, usually caused by friction or pressure. This usually occurs when someone has restricted movement, and is in bed or in a chair. If the person is not moved frequently, pressure on areas such as heels, buttocks and shoulder blades can result in skin breakdown due to poor local circulation. In order to limit the risk of pressure sores, good **nutrition** is essential, along with regular movement and ensuring that friction (such as being pulled along a bed) is minimised.

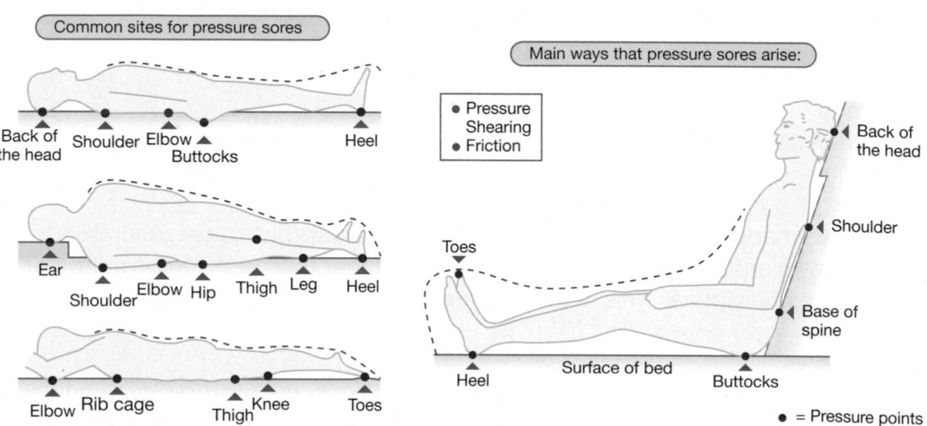

Common sites for pressure sores – lying on back, front, side and sitting.

preventive action
Contingency action to leave a situation for the safety of an individual or others. If there is a direct risk which may escalate if staff leave a situation, the risk needs to be reduced through team working or other actions. It may be beneficial if the risk of escalation is assessed at the time by competent staff who are familiar with the individual.

preventive measures
Actions that are taken to avoid something happening, rather than dealing with issues after the event. For example, if there are concerns that someone is at risk of falling, the provision of a stair lift and handrails is better than having to deal with a hip **fracture** resulting from a fall.

Primary Care Trusts (PCTs)
Bodies set up after 1999 to commission services from hospitals and other agencies to deliver care.

primary data
First-hand **research information** collected directly from the sources. This means information gathered through **interviews** or **questionnaires**, not taken from **surveys** or research that have been reported by others (**secondary data**).

primary health care
The first port of call for **health services** in the **community**. This includes **GPs**, community **nursing**, community **midwives** and **clinics**. If specialist **diagnosis** and **treatment** is needed, **referrals** can be made to **secondary health care providers**.

primary information
A term used in research to describe information obtained by asking someone directly and recording what they say, rather than found in books, articles or other research carried out by someone else.

primary socialisation
The **process** of a child **learning** to **understand** the roles and **norms** that are expected, and how to integrate into **society**. In the first five years this happens within the **family**. Children learn about **gender** roles and acceptable ways of behaving before they reach school age, but after this they are exposed to **secondary socialisation** in **school** and among their **peer group**.

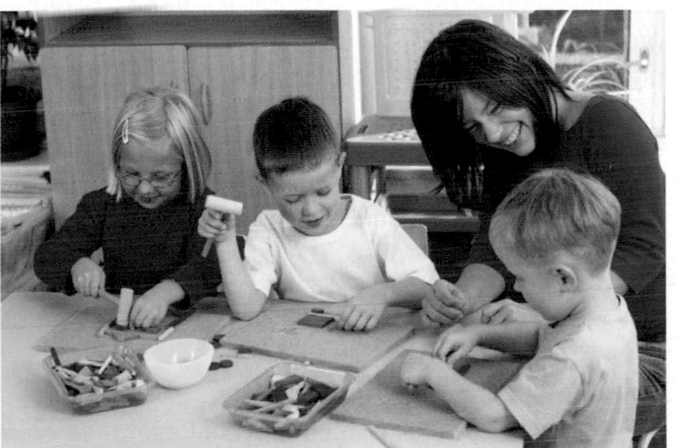

Children learning to socialise.

primitive reflexes
Reflexes that a **baby** presents before and at **birth**. They appear and disappear at expected stages in development. Primitive reflexes that remain beyond the time when they are expected to have disappeared may be a sign of damage to the **central nervous system**.

principle
A basic belief as to how to behave. There are basic principles that underpin work in health and social care.

priorities
The factors that are most important in a situation; the key areas where **resources** will be targeted. Priorities may be set by an **organisation** or by another body such as the **government**.

prison sentence
The length of time a person will spend in prison as a punishment handed out by a court after being found guilty of a crime.

privacy
Personal space and the ability to be alone, particularly when undertaking personal tasks such as **bathing** or using the **toilet**. People also need space and privacy to see friends and **family** or just to be alone.

private hospital
A **hospital** that delivers **health care** and charges a fee to the **patient**. Most people using private hospitals are insured, and the costs are met by the insurance company.

private sector
Companies that deliver **social care** or **health services** as a business that makes a profit. Much of the social care that is delivered in **residential** and **domiciliary care** is provided by the private sector and **commissioned** by **local authorities**.

Probation Service
The **service** that provides **supervision** and **rehabilitation** for **offenders**. Probation officers complete pre-**sentence reports** for the **courts** and supervise people carrying out **community sentences**. The service works with about 175,000 offenders each year, 90 per cent of whom are male. Probation is the **responsibility** of the **Home Office**. More information can be found at www.probation.homeoffice.gov.uk

problem solving
An important key **skill** that employers look for when recruiting staff. People need to be able to look at a range of solutions to a difficult situation and be able to select the best way to approach a difficulty in a calm and reasoned way.

procedure
A list of steps to follow to complete a particular task in the correct way.

process
The steps that need to be taken in order to get something done or to achieve an aim.

professional
A person who has completed a recognised training and **qualification** for the job he or she is doing.

professional body
An organisation that sets standards for and looks after the interests of its members, who all do one type of job. An example in the health sector is the Royal College of Nursing. A professional organisation has to have a specific body of knowledge.

professional boundaries
The limits of professional **expertise**. An important **skill** for all **professionals** is to recognise when to refer a situation to another professional whose expertise is more appropriate. There are also **protocols** and agreements about when it is possible to move across professional boundaries in the interests of the person using **services** or when working in an integrated way.

professional development
Ongoing training and updating to ensure that knowledge and **skills** are current. Professional development gives people the opportunity to learn new skills and acquire further knowledge in order to extend and improve their abilities and **expertise**.

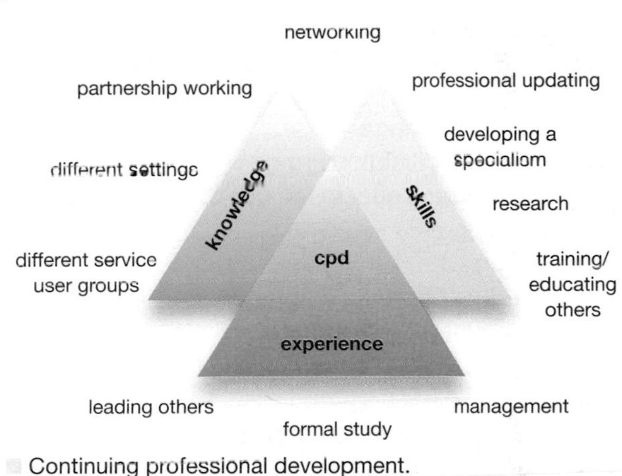

Continuing professional development.

professional misconduct
Behaviour that does not comply with the standards set out by a regulatory body.

professional relationships
Working **relationships** with colleagues who may work within the same **organisation** or for other organisations. Working relationships are based on agreed arrangements about sharing **information**, **confidentiality** and **consultation**.

profoundly deaf
With little or no hearing.

progesterone
A female **hormone** produced by the **ovary** and the adrenal **gland**. The **placenta** produces large amounts during **pregnancy**. Its function is to maintain a pregnancy and to regulate the **menstrual** cycle. It also contributes to **libido**.

A B C D E F G H I J K L M N O **P** Q R S T U V W X Y Z

promote
Encourage and take forward an issue.

properties
The features and factors that are key parts of something, for example some of the properties of a successful support plan are:
- it has been designed by the person it is about
- it identifies the outcomes the person has identified
- it is providing support in the way that the person wants
- the support can be monitored and changed if necessary.

Some of the properties of a good residential home are:
- the people who live there can have a say in how it is run
- it is run in the interests of the people who live there, not of the staff
- people have choices about day-to-day aspects of their lives
- there are plenty of activities for people to be involved in.

proposals for change
May include modifications to goals or objectives, such as the individual deciding not to reduce or cease substance use, or changes in the methods or strategies used.

prosecution
The procedure of bringing someone before a **court** to answer charges that he or she has committed an **offence**.

prostate
A gland associated with the male reproductive system that surrounds the urethra as it emerges from the bladder. Prostate secretions form part of semen. With increasing age, the prostate may become enlarged and hard-making urination more difficult. Eventually, without treatment, the flow of urine may stop and the resulting condition known as uraemia is life-threatening. Treatment can be by catheterisation and/or surgery.

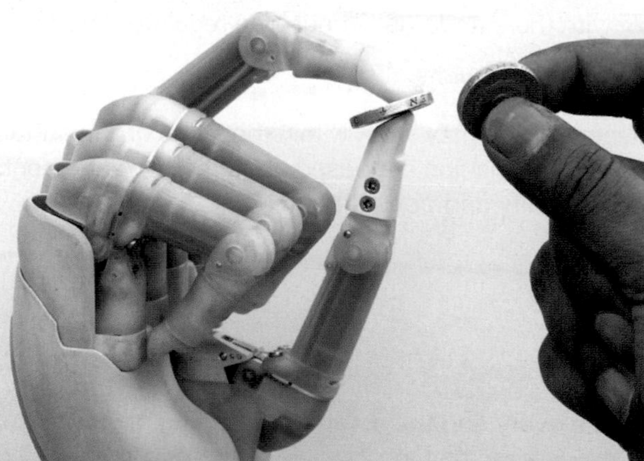
An example of a prosthesis.

prosthesis
An artificial substitute for a missing part of the body, such as a limb, hand, eye or breast.

Protection of Vulnerable Adults scheme (PoVA)
The **vetting and barring** system that provides for a work ban on people who have harmed **vulnerable adults** in their care. All potential employees must undergo a **Criminal Records Bureau** check including a check of the scheme register. All employers are required to advise the scheme of any employees who have been found to have harmed those in their care. **Local authorities** must have procedures in place for protecting vulnerable adults, and regulations require **agencies** to work together to offer effective protection from **harm**.

protective clothing
Clothes worn as a means of reducing the risks of **infection** and cross-infection. Protective clothing includes latex **gloves**, plastic aprons, full-length gowns, masks and hats. The appropriate clothing should always be used when carrying out any personal or invasive contact with people.

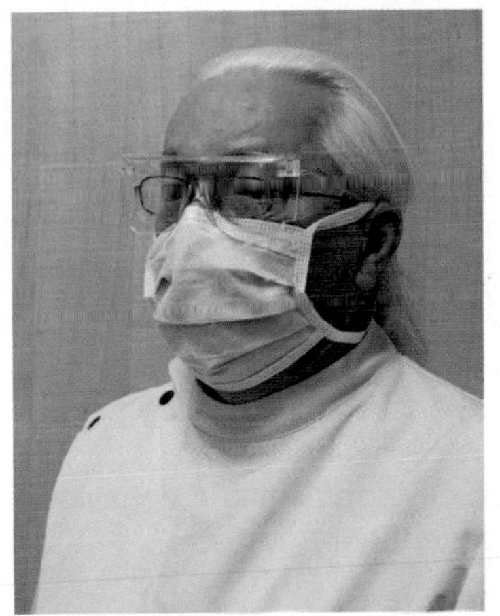

Protective clothing reduces the risk of infection and cross-infection.

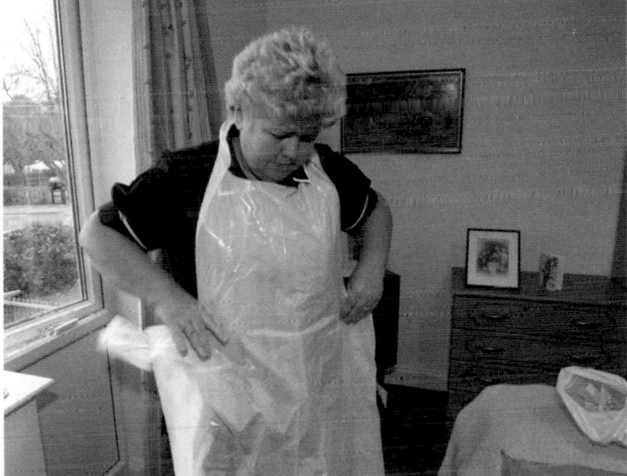

Protective aprons help to reduce infection.

protective factors
The aspects of someone's circumstances that balance the risks, for example a **risk factor** could be that a young **mother** with a history of substance **abuse** has the care of a small **baby**. The protective factor could be that the maternal grandmother lives in the next street, visits daily and often takes care of the baby overnight.

protein
An essential **macronutrient** found in meat, cheese, eggs, nuts and fish. It is used by the body for growth and repair. Proteins are broken down to their chemical units (amino acids) during digestion.

protocol
An agreement about how matters should be handled in particular circumstances. In an agreement about **joint working**, there may be a protocol about when and under what circumstances one **organisation** can act alone. In **health** settings, protocols are also **treatment** regimes that are used when **patients** meet a given set of criteria.

protozoa
Organisms consisting of a single **cell** with a **nucleus**. There are many different shapes and types. About 10,000 are **parasites** and cause many **diseases** including malaria, sleeping sickness and bilharzia. Numerically, they are by far the largest group of living organisms on the planet.

provider
An **organisation** that delivers **social care services**. These are usually **commissioned** by **local authorities**.

provision
The delivery of **services** by **providers**. These can include **domiciliary care, residential care, nursing homes,** meals services, transport services and practical **support**.

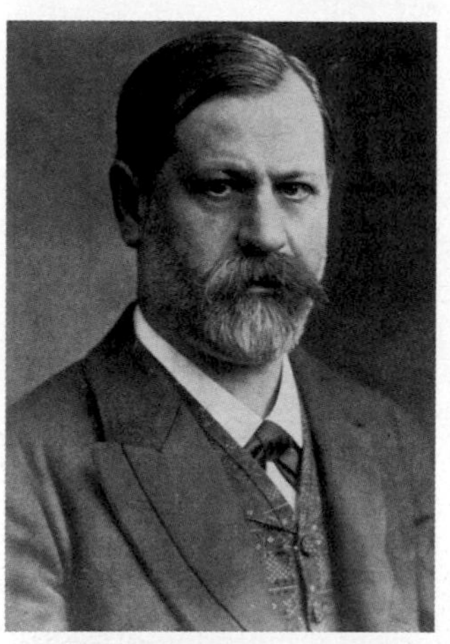
Sigmund Freud.

psychoanalytic theory
A theory of personality developed by Sigmund **Freud**. The id (instinct, seeking pleasure, avoiding pain), ego (seeks reality between the id and super ego) and superego (conscience, morals) are prominent influences on development and behaviour. Relates to **psychodynamic theory**.

psychodynamic theory
A theory of **human behaviour** developed by Sigmund **Freud**, and still widely used and very influential. It suggests that human behaviour is strongly affected by experiences from childhood and also that all behaviour is the result of **interaction** between the conscious and the **unconscious**. For instance, when someone uses a word by mistake that could be interpreted as showing his or her true **feelings**, it is called a 'Freudian slip' because Freud would argue that this shows that the unconscious is making the person say the word that expresses a genuine feeling, despite the conscious intention to say something else.

psychologist
A qualified **professional** trained in the study of **human behaviour**.

puberty
The beginning of physical **hormonal changes** as the body starts to mature. This stage normally takes place around 10–12 years of age.

public health
The **health** of a **community** or a nation. This is promoted by health programmes such as **vaccinations** and screening, also **education** and **health promotion**. Public health officials are also responsible for preventing and dealing with **epidemics** and the spread of **disease** within a community.

public services
Central or **local government**-funded **services** delivered by public bodies such as **NHS** trusts, the fire service, ambulance service, **police**, and **social services**.

puerperal
Relating to childbirth, or immediately following childbirth.

pulmonary artery
The artery that carries venous de-oxygenated **blood** from the right **ventricle** of the **heart** to the **lungs**

pulmonary veins
The veins that carry **oxygenated blood** from the **lungs** to the left **atrium** of the **heart**.

pulse
The local expansion of an artery caused by the contractions of the left **ventricle** of the **heart** that can be felt at the wrist, neck and groin where the artery passes over bone.

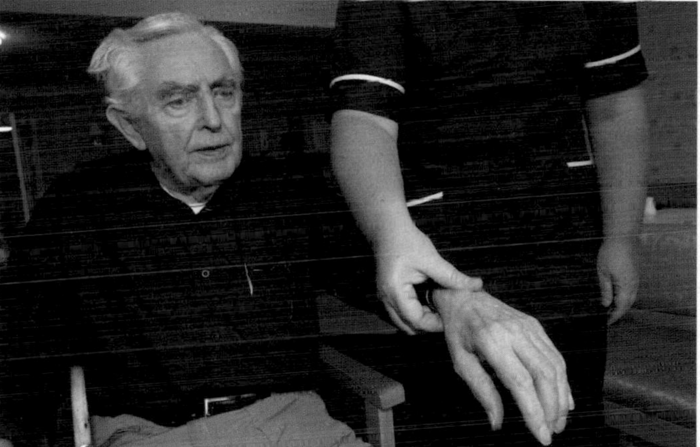

Taking a pulse from the wrist.

putative father
The unmarried father of a child. For children born before 2003, all **parental responsibility** was vested in the **mother**, unless it was established in **court**. Since 2003, putative fathers can share parental responsibility if they jointly register the **birth** along with the mother.

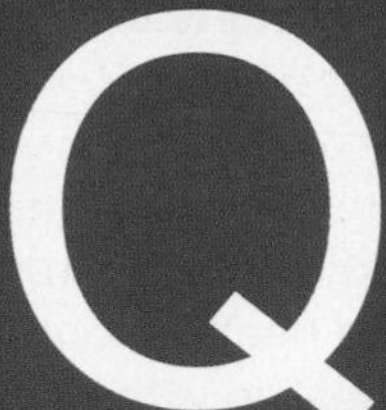

Question	Range of answers available
1 Are you male or female?	Male/Female
2 Please circle your age: [15–19] [20–24] [25–29] [30–34] [35–39] [40–44] [45–49]	Only one age range can be chosen
3 Do you smoke?	Yes/No
4 Are you a heavy smoker?	Yes/No
5 Do you smoke cannabis?	Yes/No
6 Do you smoke cannabis often?	Yes/No

quadriplegia
Loss of use of all four limbs. This is usually the result of **disease** or **injury** to the **central nervous system.**

qualifications
The proof of having successfully undertaken a **learning** or training programme and having completed the **assessment process**. People are usually given a certificate to confirm that they hold the qualification. Many jobs in **health** and **social care** require people to hold particular qualifications.

qualitative data
Information about people's views, opinions and **feelings**. This is a **research** approach commonly used in **health** and **social care**. Information is usually collected by **interviewing** people and **recording** their views in answer to **open questions.**

quality assurance
A **process** of checking to make sure that goods or **services** reach the expected **standards.** Quality criteria are developed on the basis of the standards of service expected, and then delivery is measured against them to ensure that standards are as high as expected.

quality of life
The ability to experience enjoyment, pleasure and satisfaction from life. Judgements about a person's quality of life are very difficult for others to make, and there are no clear **guidelines** about what constitutes a 'good' quality of life. It very much depends on the personal experience of an individual.

quantitative data
Statistical information about numbers, quantities, **incidence**, frequency or anything else that can be measured by counting.

quarantine
The **process** of keeping a person (or animal) isolated, either because of an **infectious disease** or because the **immune system** is not functioning. This involves a person being cared for in a separate room, and anyone providing care or medical attention must take full precautions and wear **protective clothing.** Some specialised **hospital** rooms have 'air scrubbers' that change and clean the air in the room.

questioning
Asking questions is an essential **skill** for all **professionals** working in **health** and **social care.** There are two types of questions: **open** and **closed.** Open questions begin with words like How? What? When? and require at least a sentence to answer. Closed questions can be answered with a yes or no, and they begin with words such as Do you? or Have you? After asking questions it is important to listen to and **record** the answers.

questionnaire
A **research** tool used for asking questions and gathering **data**. Questionnaires have to be very carefully put together so that they will gather the appropriate data, be straightforward to complete, not give the opportunity for contradictory answers, and not influence people to choose particular answers. Questionnaires can be completed in writing by people on their own, or can be used by **interviewers** to ask the questions and **record** the answers.

Question	Range of answers available
1 Are you male or female?	Male/Female
2 Please circle your age: [15–19] [20–24] [25–29] [30–34] [35–39] [40–44] [45–49]	Only one age range can be chosen
3 Do you smoke?	Yes/No
4 Are you a heavy smoker?	Yes/No
5 Do you smoke cannabis?	Yes/No
6 Do you smoke cannabis often?	Yes/No

quota sampling
A **research method** where specific numbers of particular **groups** of the **population** are identified to be included in a **sample.** This method is used when it is important that all groups making up a specific population are sampled.

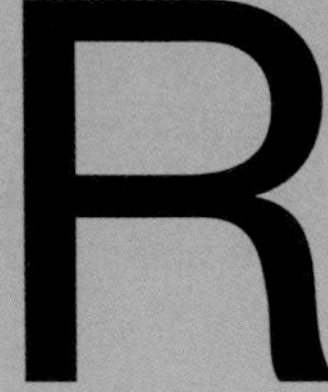

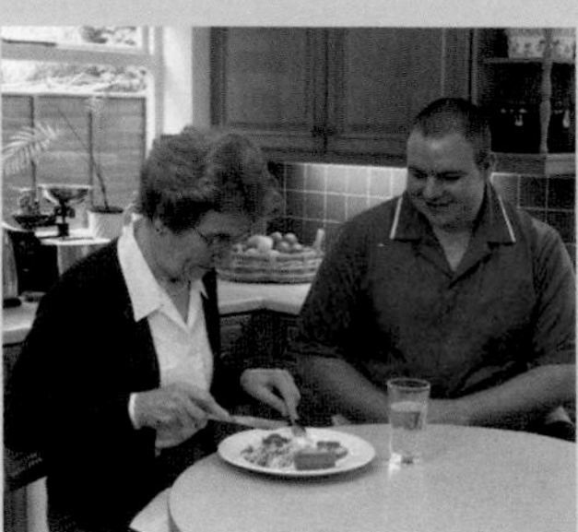

race
This term was used to describe the biological groupings of people. It is now known that 'race' is not the primary determinant of human traits amongst groups of people and there are as many biological differences within a group as there are between different **racial groups.** The preference is now to refer to an individual or groups **ethnicity**.

racial group/community
A **population group** with physical characteristics distinct enough to be identifiable. A group or **community** may also share the same **ethnicity** and **cultural** background.

racism
Negative or **oppressive** attitudes and behaviour towards people based on their **race.** Such behaviour can lead to discrimination and is **illegal** in the UK.

radiographer
A **health professional** responsible for undertaking **X-ray** procedures. Usually working in **hospitals**, radiographers will undertake **diagnostic** procedures such as X-rays, **computed axial tomography (CAT) scans, magnetic resonance imaging (MRI)** and **ultrasound.** They may also undertake **therapeutic** radiography such as **radiotherapy.**

radiologist
A **medical practitioner** who **diagnoses** and treats illness or **injury** using **X-rays** and other **processes** involving radiation.

radiology
The study of the use of radiation for **diagnosis** and **treatment** of **disease.** Diagnosis involves interpreting the results of **X-rays** and scans, and treatment involves the use of **radiotherapy**.

radiotherapy
Use of radiation to reduce or control the progress of **cancers**.

Randomised Clinical Controlled Trial (RCCT)
A research method involving more than one sample group. One group receives a specified treatment, the other doesn't (it either receives another treatment, a placebo or no treatment at all) and the results are compared.

rape
Penetration by a **penis** of a person's **vagina**, **anus** or mouth without **consent**. Most rapes are committed against girls and women, but boys and men can be the **victims** of **homosexual** rape. Consent must be a free **choice** and must be actively given.
More information can be found at www.rapecrisis.org.uk

rash
An eruption or **inflammation** of the **skin**. It can take the form of spots, blotches, blisters, pustules or patches and be the result of a viral or **bacterial infection**, an **allergic reaction** or external factors such as excessive heat. Rashes should always be investigated.

rationale
The reasoning or explanation behind something, especially for the carrying out of a piece of **research**. A clear and well-understood rationale is helpful for both those participating and those carrying out the research.

rationing
In **health** and **social care**, the term describes an approach to allocating scarce **resources**. Decisions can be made that rationing will be universal (i.e. everyone gets a bit less) or targeted, so that some people get less and others continue to get the same.

raw data
Information that has been collected, but not yet processed, organised or **analysed**.

re-ablement
An approach to homecare/ **domiciliary care** that is **outcomes**

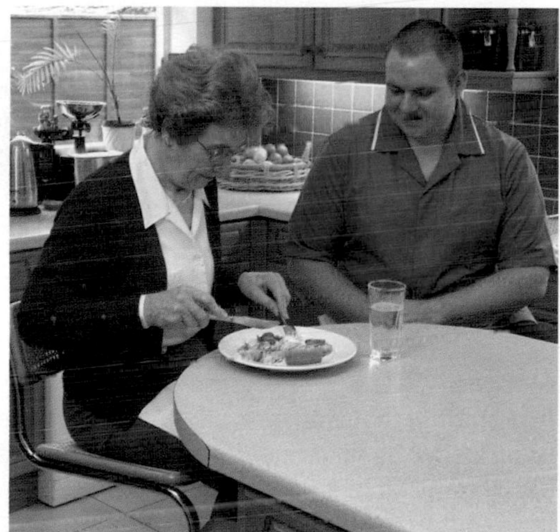
Re-ablement.

based, lasts for a short time period (usually around six weeks), and has a guiding principle of helping people to re-learn the **skills** of daily living rather than carrying out tasks for them.

reaction
A response. People can have a negative or **allergic** physical reaction to many factors such as **medication**, **food**, clothing, atmosphere or light. Some reactions can be minor, such as a mild **rash** following a change in soap powder. Others can have very serious effects, such as the **anaphylactic shock** that can result from some allergic reactions.

reasoning
The **process** of considering options and reaching thought-out conclusions. In order to be able to reason, people have to be able to **understand** the issues involved and also to understand the **choices** available.

recall
The ability to remember and call to mind things such as facts, events, people or places. The ability to do this can deteriorate for a range of reasons such as **injury**, **disease** or the **ageing** process. *See* **memory**.

reception class
The first class for **statutory education** in a primary **school**. Children who are due to reach their fifth birthday during the school year will be admitted to a reception class. The class is the **transition** from **nursery**, **playgroup**, **childminder** or home into school, and needs careful planning and management to ensure that children are able to cope with the **changes**.

re-constituted family
A **family** consisting of **parents** who already have children from previous **relationships**, who then set up a home with both sets of children.

recording
The **process** of making written notes, or recording verbal notes that will be transcribed later, in line with an organisation's policies and good **practice**.

records
Information that is written and retained, either electronically as a computer record or on paper as hard copy. Records must be **accessible**, stored securely and be easily retrievable if necessary.

recovery position
The safest position for an **unconscious** person to be placed in if, after checking the **ABC of resuscitation**, he or she is found to be breathing with no **injuries**. This prevents the **tongue** from blocking the airway and allows fluids to drain from the mouth.

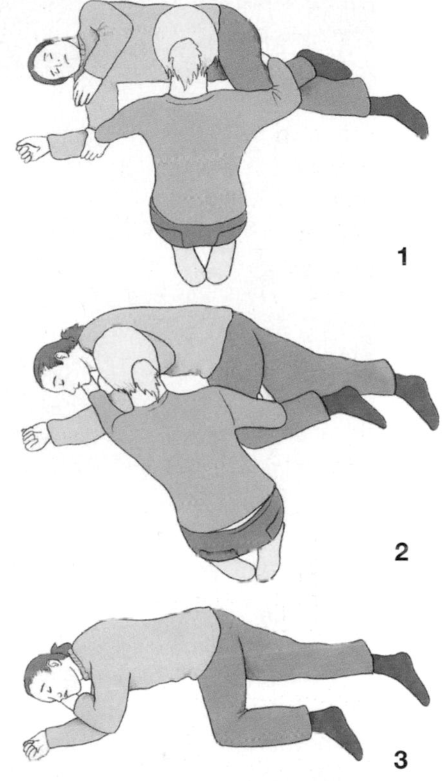

The recovery position.

recreational activities
Leisure, sport or hobby activities that people take part in during their spare time.

recreational drugs
Illegal drugs that are taken for pleasure in social situations. Such substances can include **cannabis**, cocaine, ecstasy and amphetamines.

rectal examination
Also known as DRE (digital rectal examination), an examination carried out by a **doctor** inserting a lubricated, gloved finger into the **rectum**. The rectum is very elastic and has thin walls, so it is possible to feel other **organs** in the **pelvis** from a rectal examination. It is used to examine the rectum itself, but also the prostate, the appendix and the lower **abdominal** area.

rectum
The last part of the colon that links it to the **anus**. **Faeces** are stored in the rectum until they can be expelled from the body through the anus.

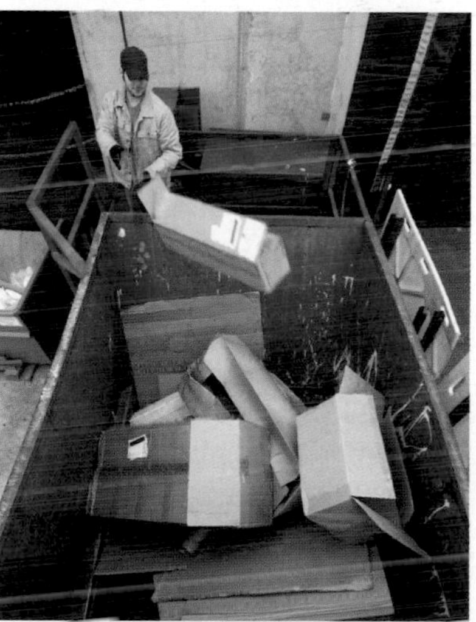
The recycling of waste is important.

recycling
Re-using waste materials. This is done in order to reduce the amount of carbon emissions and the amount of **energy** required to process the disposal of waste.

red blood cells
Cells made in the **bone** marrow, which are red because of **haemoglobin**. They carry **oxygen**, and the haemoglobin carries some **carbon**

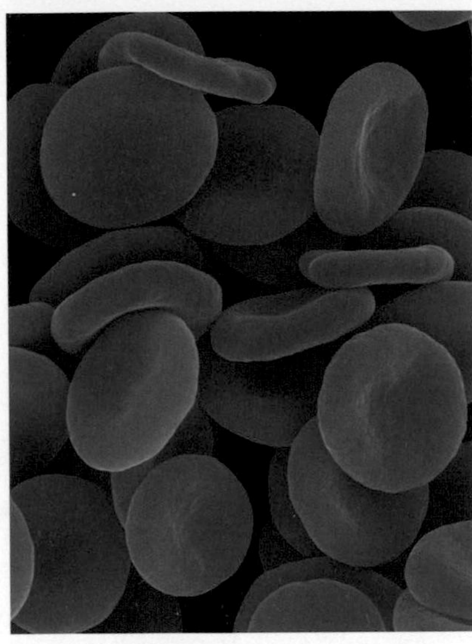
■ Red blood cells.

dioxide, around the bloodstream. There are about a million red blood cells (also known as **erythrocytes**) per cubic millimetre of **blood**. They have no nucleus and are bi-concave in shape to maximise surface area for exposure to oxygen.

redundant
No longer needed. The term is commonly used to describe the loss of a job. People are 'made redundant' if an **organisation** is closing, merging or reducing the size of its business operation. Losing a job can be very hard for some people to cope with and help is often provided to assist people to find other jobs. There is a high **incidence** of **depression** among people who have been made redundant and who have been unable to find other **work**.

reference
A means of acknowledging the work of others that has been used as evidence in a **research** project or in a piece of writing such as an assignment, an essay or an article. There are various methods of referencing, but they all include acknowledging and **recording** the author, the name of the book, research project or article, and the date. *See* **Harvard referencing system**.

referral
The passing on of a request for involvement to another **organisation** or **professional**. The **consent** of the individual or **family** concerned is required, and appropriate **information** is shared between the organisations.

referral order
A **court** order made for a **young person** where an **offence** is admitted and is not sufficiently serious for a custodial **sentence**. The order requires the young person to go before a Youth Offender Panel consisting of two people from the local **community** and a panel advisor from the **Youth Offending Team** (**YOT**). The panel, the young person, his or her **parents** and the **victim** (if they wish) decide an appropriate **contract** to repair the **harm** done and to address the causes of the **offending behaviour**. The contract will last between 3 and 12 months.

reflective listening
The **process** of clarifying **understanding** by listening carefully and then repeating the sense of what the other person has said, as a way of demonstrating understanding.

reflective practice
The essential **professional skill** of thinking about **practice** and considering what is going well, what can be improved and why. It is also important for professionals to work out how the improvements can be achieved; this is often done in consultation with a line manager.

reflexes
Rapid automatic involuntary reactions to a stimulus without control by the individual, such as blinking in bright light, the knee jerk when the **tendon** just below the knee cap is tapped, and the rapid withdrawal of a hand from a hot object. Reflexes are protective as they limit damage to the body with minimum energy expenditure. Human **babies** are born with **primitive reflexes** that disappear as they grow and develop. Autonomic reflexes maintain body functions such as **digestion** and **blood pressure** levels without the conscious awareness of the individual.

reflexology
An **alternative** therapy involving the massage and manipulation of pressure points in the feet. These are said to link to specific areas of the body, and the massage and manipulation can improve problems in these areas.
More information can be found at www.reflexology.org

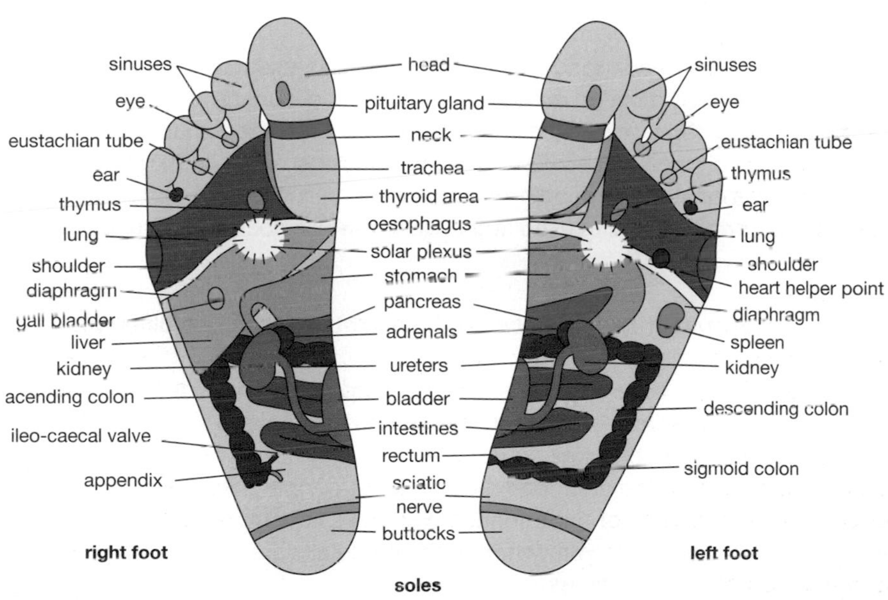

Reflexology is an alternative therapy involving the massage and manipulation of pressure points in the feet.

A B C D E F G H I J K L M N O P Q R S T U V W XYZ

regulation
An enforceable guideline that must be followed by people and **organisations** delivering **services**, for example there must be a certain number of qualified staff in any social care setting.

regulator
An **organisation** that **monitors** a **professional** area. The regulator will usually hold a register of those people who are eligible to practise because they have achieved the appropriate **qualifications** and maintained continuing **professional development**. The regulator will also lay down **codes of practice** to set out the expected conduct of people in the profession. For **social care**, the regulators are the **General Social Care Council** (England), the Scottish Social Services Council, the Care Council for Wales and the Northern Ireland Social Care Council. There are different regulators in **health** depending on the profession; **doctors** are regulated by the General Medical Council and **midwives** and **nurses** by the **Nursing and Midwifery Council**. Regulators are responsible for checking that people are appropriately qualified to be on the register and also for removing people from the register who are guilty of **negligence**, professional misconduct or who fail to maintain their professional development.
More information can be found at www.gscc.org.uk, www.sssc.uk.com, www.ccwales.org.uk, www.niscc.info, www.gmc-uk.org, www.nmc-uk.org

rehabilitation
The **process** of people re-adjusting to everyday living and resettling into **society**. Rehabilitation can follow a period in **hospital** or **residential care** as the result of illness, **injury** or **addiction**, or follow a prison **sentence**. The process is about people regaining as much physical or emotional **health** as possible and adjusting to living in an independent **environment**. For people who have been in an institution for many years, the process also involves getting used to the ways in which society has changed.

relationships
The ways people **interact** and associate with each other. There are different types of relationships.

- **Family** relationships: **parent**, child, **sibling**, grandparents and extended family members. These relationships provide emotional stability and **security** for most people and continue throughout life.
- Friendships: these can be at different levels. Most people have a few close friends and a wider circle of other friends who are a little more distant. Close friends are usually the ones with whom intimate details are shared and who provide support in difficult times.
- **Sexual relationships**: these can be permanent or short term and can involve emotional commitment or not. Most people will have a long-term sexual

partner with whom they maintain a relationship for many years. Many sexual relationships are formalised by marriage or a civil ceremony, although large numbers of permanent relationships do not have any formal status.

- **Professional relationships**: these occur in the **workplace** with colleagues, managers and individuals who use **services**. There are accepted **boundaries** and ways of conducting professional relationships with users of services that are designed to protect **vulnerable** people and to discourage personal involvement. Some people will develop close friendships with work colleagues, while others prefer to keep personal and **professional** life separate.

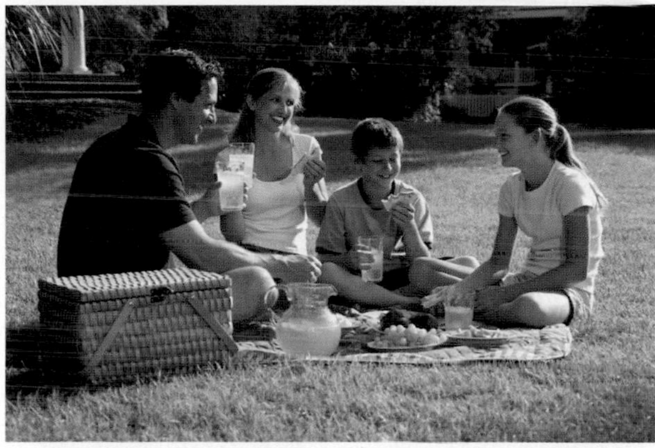

Family relationships provide emotional stability and security.

relative poverty

The term used to describe a lack of **resources** or **income** in relation to the average for the **society** in which people live. For example, someone in the UK may have a home, but may not be able to heat it adequately; he or she may have enough **food** not to starve, but may struggle to afford to travel by either public or personal transport.

relaxation

In **physiology**, the gradual lengthening of **muscles** or muscle fibres. In general use, the term also means reducing mental and emotional activity by slowing down and eliminating **stressful** thoughts. There are various techniques for relaxation including muscle tensing and releasing, breathing **exercises**, massage, music, and flotation in buoyant water at **body temperature**.

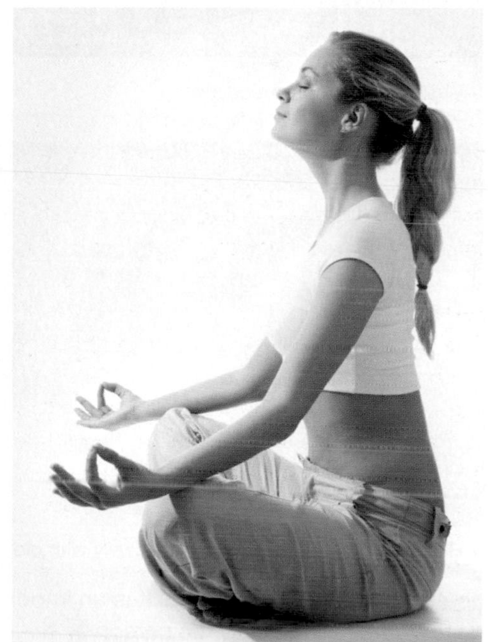

Yoga helps to relax and reduce stress.

A B C D E F G H I J K L M N O P Q **R** S T U V W XYZ

relevant national bodies
Includes voluntary and independent organisations who are of national importance.

relevant people
People to whom a particular issue or incident is important or who are affected by it, or people who are important to an individual.

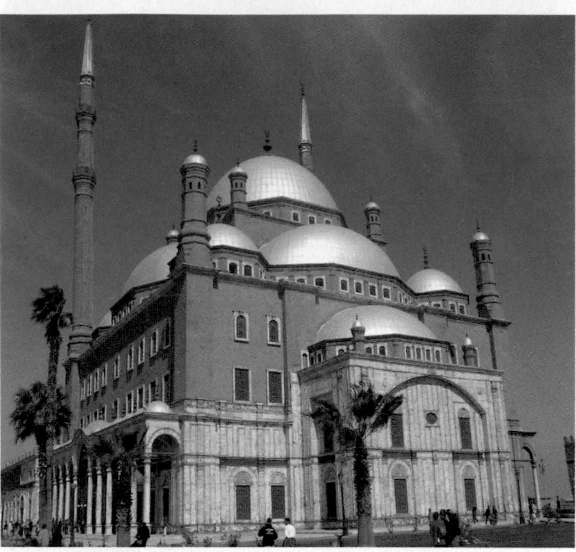

Muslims worship in a mosque.

religion
A **system** of **beliefs** and **values** that attracts large numbers of followers to worship a higher being, creator or god. Religions are some of the most significant influences in global developments and conflicts. Most religions have an **organisation**, hierarchy and infrastructure of buildings. Religious belief is of great importance to many people and is a key **cultural** influence. Major world religions include Christianity, Islam, Hinduism, Judaism, Sikhism and Buddhism.

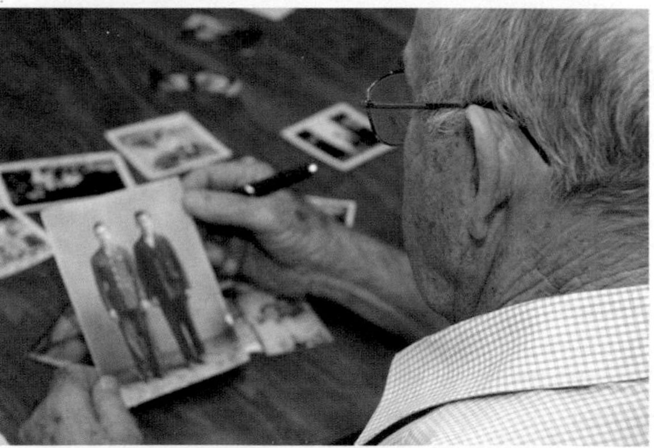

Reminiscence work is used extensively with older people.

reminiscence
Recalling and talking about past experiences. Reminiscence work is used extensively with **older people**. It is beneficial in several ways. For the person recalling the past, it can help to make a link to the present; it can also encourage people to **communicate** as **memories** are sparked by someone else's past. For the **health** and care **professional** it is an important way of **understanding** someone's history and recognising the person as an individual with a unique and interesting life experience.

renal artery
A short branch of the aorta on each side carrying blood to the left and right kidneys.

renal system
The system that maintains the composition and volume of all body fluids by filtering the **blood**. The **kidneys** are the major **organs** of the renal system. Blood passes into the kidneys from the renal **arteries** and after filtration it is returned via the renal **veins**. Waste products that have been filtered out are **excreted** from the kidneys as **urine**, and this passes down the **ureters** into the **bladder**, where it is held until it is passed out of the body. Each kidney contains about a million microscopic filtering units called nephrons.

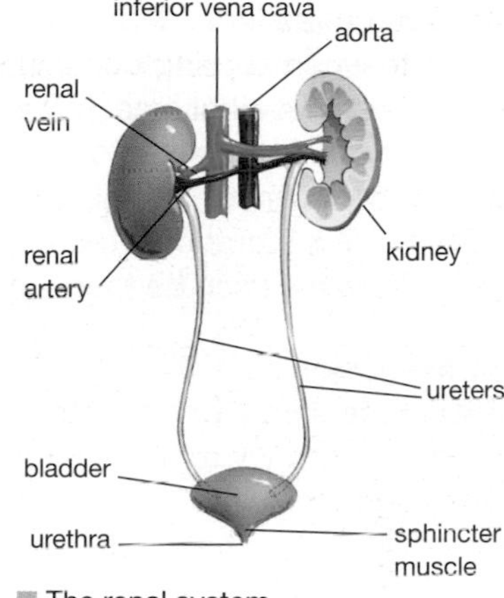

The renal system.

rent
A regular payment to a **landlord** for living in a property owned by that landlord. Rent does not give ownership, but the right to live somewhere for the length of the tenancy agreement. People can be **tenants** of a **local authority**, a private landlord or a **housing association**.

reparation order
An order made by a **court** in respect of a **young person** who has committed an **offence**. The purpose is to make young people understand the effects of their crimes and take **responsibility** for their actions. They may have to make reparation directly to the **victim**, if the victim agrees, or to the **community** as a whole by making a **supervised** contribution.

report
A written document or verbal **presentation** which has a specific purpose and contains specific **information**. Reports may be of any length and for any purpose. **Courts** will require reports so that they have information before **sentencing** offenders. **Social workers** or other **professionals** may prepare reports for **case conferences** or **reviews**, and professionals may use reports to share information when working together.

Reporting of Injuries, Diseases and Dangerous Occurrences Regulations 1995 (RIDDOR)
Regulations that list **workplace** incidents and diseases that must be reported by **employers**, the self-employed or those in control of **premises**. The list is very

long, but includes **deaths** and major injuries, and any injury which results in an employee being absent from **work** for more than three days. Work-related diseases that must be reported include certain poisonings, some **skin** diseases such as occupational dermatitis, skin **cancer**, chrome ulcer, oil folliculitis/acne; **lung** diseases including occupational **asthma**, farmer's lung, pneumoconiosis, asbestosis, mesothelioma; **infections** such as leptospirosis, **hepatitis**, **tuberculosis**, anthrax, legionellosis and **tetanus**; other conditions such as occupational cancer; certain **musculo-skeletal** disorders; decompression illness and hand-arm vibration syndrome.
More information can be found at www.hse.gov.uk/riddor

re-possession
A legal **process** by which a **landlord** can regain possession of a property if a **tenant** breaks the tenancy agreement by failing to pay the **rent** or damaging the property. A similar process applies if a bank or building society wishes to gain control over a property where someone has failed to make mortgage repayments.

reproduction
The act of creating new individuals of the same species.

reproductive systems
The **female reproductive system** is located in the **abdomen**, and consists of the group of **organs** and parts of the body that enable the reproductive **process** to work. It includes the following.
- The vulva: the entrance to the **vagina**.
- The vagina: the canal leading to the **uterus**. During **sexual intercourse** the male penis is inserted into the vagina and semen is **ejaculated**. During **birth** the vagina is part of the birth canal through which the **baby** passes.
- The **cervix**: the entrance to the uterus. Normally tightly closed, it opens during **labour** to allow the baby to move out of the uterus into the birth canal.
- The uterus: the **womb**, the organ where a fertilised egg grows and develops until the baby is ready to be born.

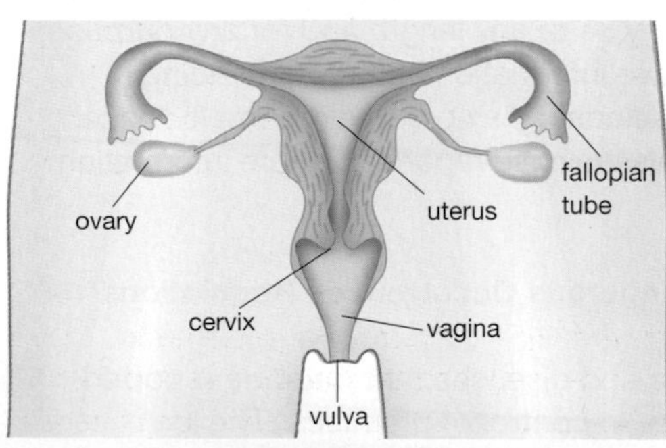

The female reproductive system.

- The **fallopian tubes**: these provide the route for the egg to travel from the **ovary** to the uterus.
- The ovary: the female **gonad** covered in follicles that produce eggs in a regular cycle.

The **male reproductive system** consists of three primary organs: two **testes** and the **penis**. The testes are situated in the **scrotum**, which hangs between the legs, below the abdomen, in order to provide the necessary conditions for **spermatozoa** production at below **body temperature**. Within the testes are coils of tubes which produce spermatozoa. The penis is a soft, spongy organ consisting of erectile **tissue** with many tiny **blood** vessels that fill with blood during sexual arousal, causing the penis to become stiff. This is called an erection. When the penis is erect, it is able to penetrate the female vagina and deposit spermatozoa through the ejaculation of a fluid called **semen**, which contains millions of spermatozoa.

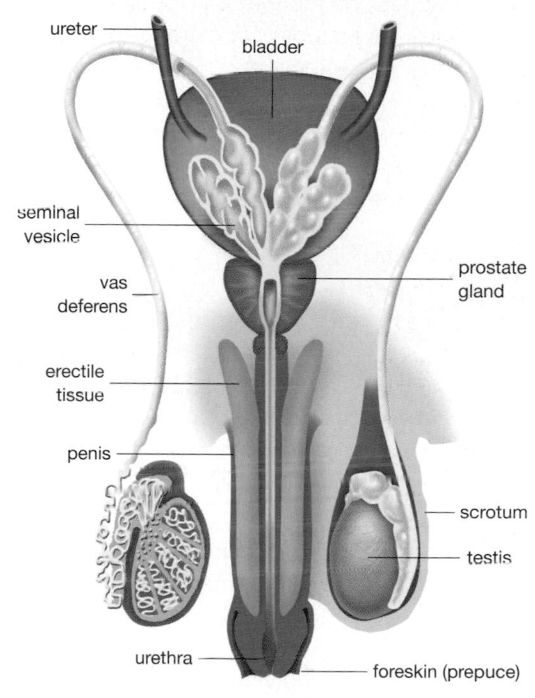

The male reproductive system.

research

A **process** of enquiry that sets out to prove or disprove a **hypothesis**.

research methods

The ways in which **research** can be undertaken. These are divided into **quantitative** research, where the **data** collected is factual and numerical (this can be collected using **questionnaires** with tick boxes, or as **secondary data** from other **reports**); and **qualitative** research, where **information** is gathered about **feelings** and opinions. Qualitative research is more often carried out by **interview**, where there may be structured questions designed in advance, or there may just be a narrative of people's views.

resettlement

A **process** of readjusting to living in the **community**. This term is often used to describe the process put in place to **support** people when they come out of prison or out of a long stay in **hospital**. It is about practical as well as emotional adjustment;

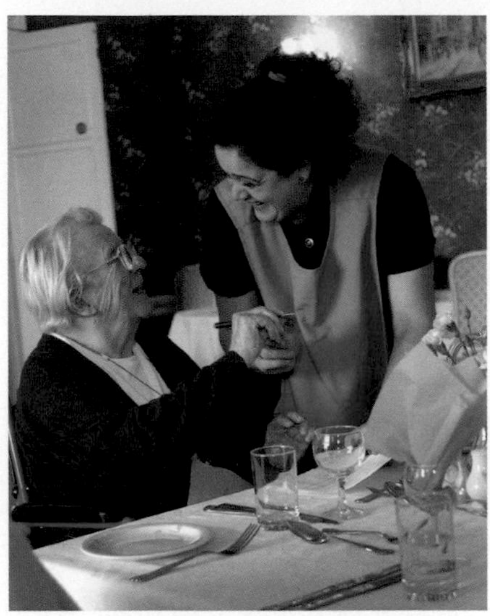
Support may be needed at meal times.

managing money and **budgeting**, finding **work**, finding somewhere to live, relating to neighbours, making decisions and **learning** to make **relationships** are all parts of readjusting to life in a different **environment**.

residential care
Group accommodation where people can receive any additional **support** they may need for daily living.

resilience
The ability to overcome setbacks and disappointments without giving up and becoming demoralised. Children who have had a safe, secure and stable upbringing are most likely to be resilient as they grow and develop.

resources
The financial and physical items necessary to carry out planned actions. Resources can include money, **equipment**, people, time, **skills** and knowledge.

respect
Valuing people as individuals with life experience, views and opinions worth listening to. Respect can be shown by ways of addressing people, the attitudes displayed towards people, maintaining **privacy** and ensuring **confidentiality**.

respiration
The process of releasing energy inside cells by the oxidation of glucose. Water and carbon dioxide are waste products of respiration.

respiratory system
The body system involved in **gaseous exchange**, which begins with the nose, where air is breathed in. Once warmed, filtered and moistened in the nasal passages, the air passes down the pharynx, larynx and trachea until it reaches the bronchi (left and right). Once inside the **lungs**, the bronchi

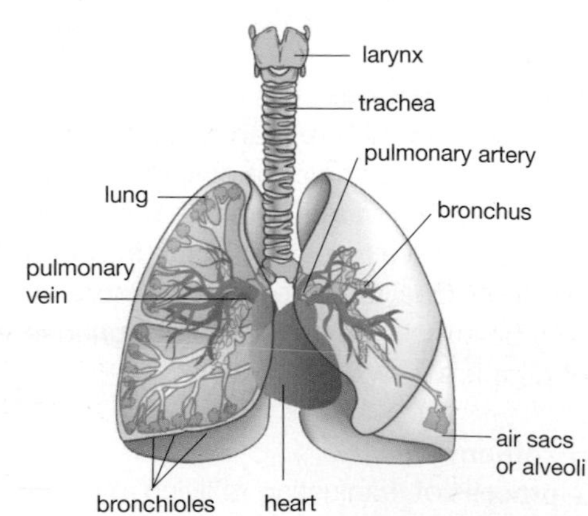

The respiratory system.

divide into further branches, called bronchioles, and further into alveoli. There are about 600 million alveoli in an adult human, giving an area of about 100 square metres for the exchange of gases which takes place through the alveoli, where **oxygen** dissolves and diffuses into the **blood**. The pulmonary blood vessels take blood to and from the lungs and heart.

respite care
This term is no longer used. *See* **short breaks**.

responsibility
Accepting and being prepared to deal with the consequences of personal actions.

responsible persons
In terms of **health and safety** or **child protection** this is a person, or persons, to whom workers report any concerns or issues.

restorative justice
Making amends directly to the **victim** or **community** that has been **harmed** by an offence. The approach tries to encourage offenders to accept **responsibility** for their actions by agreeing with the victim and/or the community on what the appropriate reparation may be.

resuscitation
The **process** of restoring life through medical **intervention**. It is a controversial area and surrounded by ethical issues, as some people would want the right to refuse resuscitation, for example, if they were **terminally ill**. In other circumstances, **doctors** may follow agreed **protocols** and make decisions about resuscitation despite the views of relatives.

retina
The light-sensitive lining at the back of the eye that converts images into electrical impulses, which are sent to the **brain** through the optic **nerve**. The brain interprets the nervous impulses into images.

retirement
The time of life when a person no longer works, but receives a **pension**, which usually happens at around 60–65 years of age. For many people this is an opportunity to do many things for which they have not previously had the time.

review
A regular meeting, usually held every six months, to look at an individual's circumstances and discuss with him or her and other **relevant people** whether

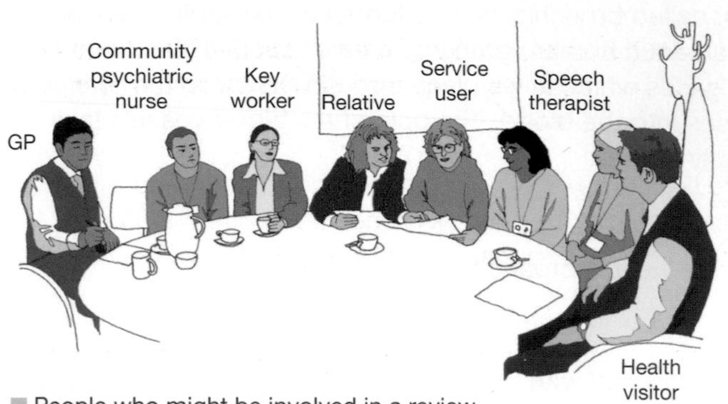

People who might be involved in a review.

the current **provision** is the best option or if there may be better ways of achieving the **outcomes** an individual has identified as desirable.

rewards and recognition
Used in **behaviour management** programmes, based on social **learning** theories, these are normally used with children and **young people** and work by rewarding wanted behaviour and ignoring unwanted behaviour. They can be very successful in altering behaviour, but do not always deal with the underlying reasons for it.

rhesus factor
A **blood group** antigen in the **blood** of rhesus-positive people. The biggest impact can be between a **mother** and her **baby** where the mother is rhesus negative (RH-) and the **foetus** is rhesus-positive (RH+), and is prevented by an injection of 'anti-D' (rhesus antibodies) shortly after the birth which neutralise the rhesus antigens.

ribonucleic acid (RNA)
Ribonucleic acid. Found in the nucleus and cytoplasm of a cell, it transmits genetic information from DNA to the cell.

ribs
The **bones** that form a protective cage around the **heart** and **lungs**.

rickets
A **disease** that affects children and causes poor **bone** development. It was common in Victorian times, but better **nutrition** has made it very rare today except in communities who wear garments that cover more of the skin and consume little fatty foods and in countries with long winters.

rights and responsibilities
What people are entitled to, and what others are entitled to expect of them. People have the right to **services** and to be treated lawfully, but along with rights go responsibilities to make contributions to **society** as a citizen, for example there is a right to free **medical treatment** from the **NHS**, but there is also a responsibility to follow a healthy **lifestyle** and take care by participating in **screening programmes** and having check-ups as requested.

right to enter

Those people who have a right to be on the property, it excludes people who may have a court order against them and those who have no need to be on the premises.

risk

A risk is the likelihood of the hazard's potential being realised; it can be to individuals in the form of infection, danger, harm, violence and abuse and/or to the environment in the form of danger of damage and destruction.

risk assessments

The investigation and identification of the likelihood of an undesired **outcome** or event happening.

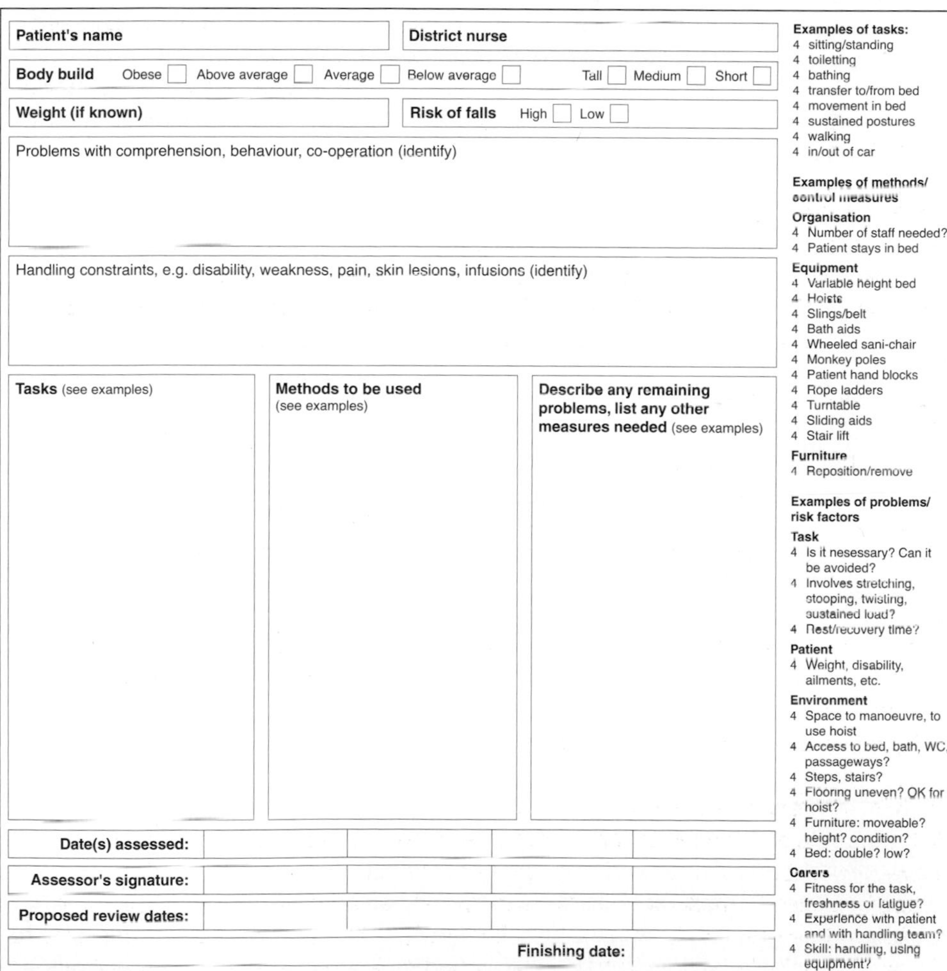

Patient's name | **District nurse**

Body build Obese ☐ Above average ☐ Average ☐ Below average ☐ Tall ☐ Medium ☐ Short ☐

Weight (if known) | **Risk of falls** High ☐ Low ☐

Problems with comprehension, behaviour, co-operation (identify)

Handling constraints, e.g. disability, weakness, pain, skin lesions, infusions (identify)

Tasks (see examples)	**Methods to be used** (see examples)	**Describe any remaining problems, list any other measures needed** (see examples)

Date(s) assessed:				
Assessor's signature:				
Proposed review dates:				
			Finishing date:	

Examples of tasks:
4 sitting/standing
4 toiletting
4 bathing
4 transfer to/from bed
4 movement in bed
4 sustained postures
4 walking
4 in/out of car

Examples of methods/control measures

Organisation
4 Number of staff needed?
4 Patient stays in bed

Equipment
4 Variable height bed
4 Hoists
4 Slings/belt
4 Bath aids
4 Wheeled sani-chair
4 Monkey poles
4 Patient hand blocks
4 Rope ladders
4 Turntable
4 Sliding aids
4 Stair lift

Furniture
4 Reposition/remove

Examples of problems/risk factors

Task
4 Is it nesessary? Can it be avoided?
4 Involves stretching, stooping, twisting, sustained load?
4 Rest/recovery time?

Patient
4 Weight, disability, ailments, etc.

Environment
4 Space to manoeuvre, to use hoist
4 Access to bed, bath, WC, passageways?
4 Steps, stairs?
4 Flooring uneven? OK for hoist?
4 Furniture: moveable? height? condition?
4 Bed: double? low?

Carers
4 Fitness for the task, freshness or fatigue?
4 Experience with patient and with handling team?
4 Skill: handling, using equipment?

A risk assessment form for manual handling.

A B C D E F G H I J K L M N O P Q R S T U V W XYZ

risk factors
The aspects of a person's circumstances that make a poor **outcome** more likely.

risk management
The **process** of identifying ways to reduce the likelihood of each of the identified risks making an impact.

ritual
A prescribed or established rite, ceremony, proceeding or service.

role model
A figure who is well known, either on a personal level or as a 'celebrity', and in whom people can identify similar characteristics or background to their own, so feel that they are able to have similar ambitions.

rough sleeper
A person who is **homeless** and living on the streets. There are sometimes **hostel** beds available, but these are short term.

routine
The **process** of doing things in the same way, in the same order and/or at the same time each day. Routines are important for children and they add to a feeling of **safety** and **security**. They can also be beneficial for **older people**.

rubella (German measles)
Very infectious viral illness that can have serious effects on a **foetus**, especially in the first 12 weeks. *See* **MMR**.

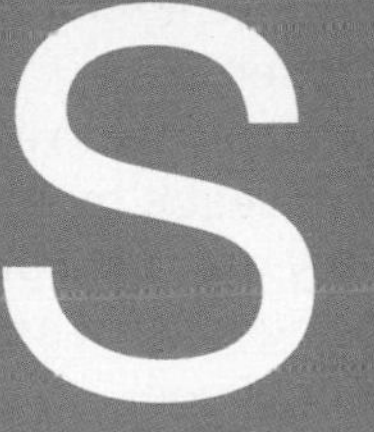

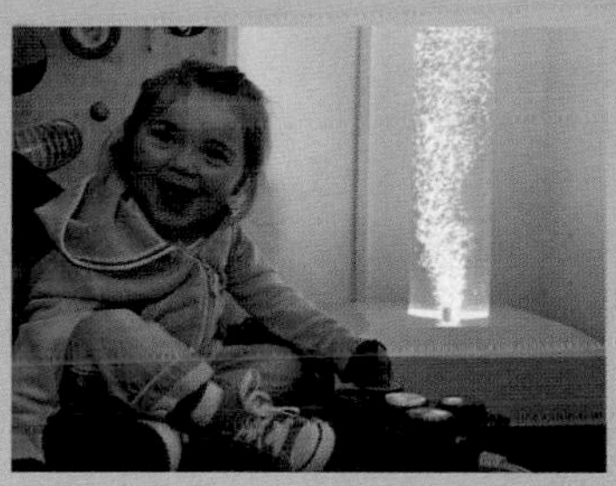

safeguarding
Keeping someone, especially a child, safe from any sort of **harm**, such as illness, **abuse** or **injury**. This means all **agencies**, **parents** and **families** working together and taking **responsibility** for the **safety** of children, whether it is by **promoting** children's **health**, preventing **accidents** or protecting children who have been abused. Safeguarding Vulnerable Adults refers to the policies relating to vulnerable people.

saliva
This is the first digestive juice to break down food. Secreted by salivary glands close to the mouth, it softens food and lubricates the mouth for swallowing. Saliva contains water, mucus, salts and the enzyme salivary amylase which breaks down cooked starch.

Salmonella
Group of **bacteria** that cause **food poisoning**, **vomiting** and **diarrhoea**. It is commonly found in raw poultry, which requires thorough cooking to ensure the removal of Salmonella. If frozen poultry is not properly thawed before cooking this can mean that the **temperature** is not high enough to kill the bacteria. Salmonella can also be transferred from preparation surfaces that have not been properly cleaned after being used for raw meat, and from unwashed hands. Other types of Salmonella are responsible for serious food-borne illnesses such as typhoid fever.

sample
A collected specimen of body fluids or exudates for **laboratory** testing, for example, **blood**, **urine**, **faeces**, or **sputum**. In **research**, a representative **group**. *See* **sampling**.

sampling
The **process** of selecting a representative **group** for **research** purposes. Sampling can be:

A B C D E F G H I J K L M N O P Q R S T U V W XYZ

- random – there is an equal chance of any of the target **population** being selected
- selective – specific types or groups of people are chosen
- stratified – non-overlapping groups are identified and then samples are chosen from each group (for example, stratification could be by age, **gender**, geographical location or any characteristic that clearly defines a group)
- quota – selection is made by the interviewer after being given a set quota to complete (for example, 25 young men under 25 years of age).

scabies
A highly infectious **skin disease** caused by a parasitic mite. It causes redness and itching. **Treatment** is with anti-parasitic ointment, but all bedding, towels and clothing of the infected person must be washed and all other people who live with the person must also be treated.

scapegoating
A behaviour where someone moves blame and **responsibility** away from himself or herself and on to another person or **group**.

scattergram
A diagram that shows how different sets of **data** relate to each other. An example is if a **research** project collected data about people's height and ages, it could plot the two sets of data on a scattergram and show if there were any links between them.

schizophrenia
A serious **mental disorder** in which people can lose touch with reality. People experience very distressing **symptoms** and can have **hallucinations** and **delusions**; they may feel **paranoid** and very muddled, with great difficulty in concentrating. Schizophrenia most commonly starts between the ages of 15 and 35 and it affects about 1 per cent of the **population**. During a schizophrenic episode people may need to be hospitalised for their own **safety** or the safety of others.

school
A centre providing **education** for children. Education is compulsory in the UK from the age of 5 to 16.

SCOPE
A national charity that represents the interests of people with cerebral palsy. The organisation lobbies on behalf of people with cerebral palsy and provides advice and information.
More information can be found at www.scope.org.uk

Scottish Social Services Council
Established in 2001 by the Regulation of Care (Scotland) Act. The Council is responsible for registering people who work in social care and social work and regulating their education and training.

screening programme
A national programme based on screening all, or large proportions of, a target **population** in order to identify **disease** in early stages. Examples are cervical screening and breast **cancer** screening.

scrotum
The **skin** sac that contains the male **testes**. It hangs between the legs outside the body as **sperm**, stored in the testes, need to be just below **body temperature**.

scurvy
A gum **disease** caused by lack of **vitamin** C. It used to be very common among sailors in the days when there was no **access** to fresh fruit and vegetables during long sea voyages, but it is also found in people with a poor **diet**.

secondary data
Information or statistics that have already been collected in other people's **research**, or gathered through **census** or other **government** returns.

secondary health care
Health care provided in general, acute **hospitals**. This can include inpatient and outpatient **diagnosis** and **treatment**.

secondary information
Information gained from second-hand sources, such as books, other people's research, government statistics or the Internet.

secondary socialisation
The **process** of socialisation that children experience outside the home. **Peer groups**, teachers and other influences will help children to develop behaviour that is acceptable and conforms to **norms** and expectations.

sector
A division, for example in the care industry, is divided into sectors that are responsible for different aspects of the care and support of people, such as the social care sector and the health sector. Those are further divided into the public sector: **local councils** and the **NHS** and the private sector: private hospitals and care providers.

sector skills councils

Government-appointed bodies responsible for **workforce** development and training for a particular sector. The Skills for Care and Development is the sector skills council for **social care**. Skills for Health is the sector skills council for **health** and the Children's Workforce Development Council is the sector skills council for children and young people.
More information can be found at www.cwdcouncil.org.uk, www.skillsforcareanddevelopment.org.uk, www.skillsforhealth.org.uk, www.sscalliance.org

security

Measures to ensure safety, especially making **vulnerable adults** and children safe from intruders. Methods include identity cards, security-coded entry systems, **CCTV** cameras and **retina** or fingerprint scanning. Security can also mean emotional comfort and a feeling of **safety** within a **family** or a **relationship**.

seizure

A sudden and uncontrolled electrical activity in the **brain** commonly known as a fit. The electrical activity may result in a sudden change in senses or a movement. An individual experiencing a pattern of seizures is said to have epilepsy. Infants and young children can have seizures as a result of high body temperature.

self-assessment

The **process** of people working out for themselves what their current progress is and what they need in order to achieve the **outcomes** they want to reach. This can happen when people are deciding on the **services** they want and the best ways for them to be delivered.
The term is also used in **education** and training, where candidates can undertake self-assessment of their knowledge or **performance**; and in **inspection**, where many **organisations** will complete a self-assessment process if they have a history of receiving high grades for inspections.

self-awareness

Knowing who you are and why you do what you do. People with self-awareness **understand** what makes them 'tick', are aware of what influences their own behaviour, and know how **values**, **culture** and **beliefs** affect what they do.

self-concept

How you see yourself and how you feel about yourself, your identity, self esteem and self image; all of the features that you would mention if you had to describe yourself. Much of someone's self-concept is formed around **gender**, age, **culture**, role and **personality** type.

self-confidence
A measure of how much you believe in yourself and your ability to achieve. Someone with low **self-esteem** will have low levels of self-confidence. People with good self-esteem will have a greater belief in their own capacity and achievements.

self-esteem
Part of **self-concept**. How you value yourself, and therefore how you believe the rest of the world sees you. People who have a poor opinion of themselves will not see themselves as likeable, attractive, clever, or good at what they do. People with good self-esteem will like themselves and believe that other people like them too.

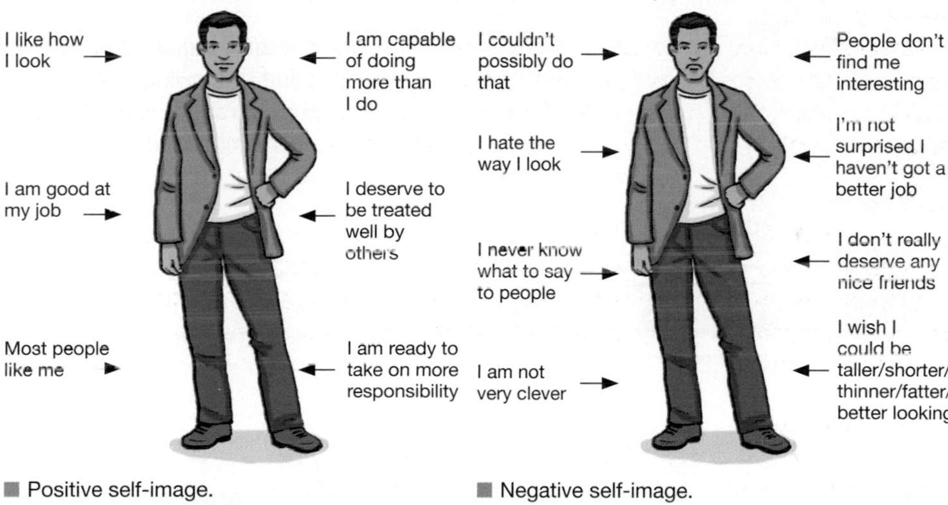

■ Positive self-image.

■ Negative self-image.

self-fulfilling prophecy
A belief in an **outcome** which is then brought about by the behaviour resulting from that belief. A child who believes that new foster carers will soon reject him or her may consequently present very **challenging behaviour** and eventually – just as predicted – the placement breaks down, thereby in the eyes of the child 'proving' that he or she was right.

self-help
People **supporting** and helping themselves without the **intervention** of **professionals**. There are **groups** and **organisations** that support people to help themselves such as AA (Alcoholics Anonymous). Many people find it easier to work in a group to overcome difficulties. There are many self-help groups for people with **mental disorders**, and for people who have had particular types of **surgery** such as mastectomy or colostomy.

semen
The fluid, containing **spermatozoa**, and the **secretions** of glands associated with the male reproductive system. It is ejaculated during sexual excitement.

Senco
Special Educational Needs Co-ordinator, a specially trained, designated teacher within a **school** who takes **responsibility** for arranging all its special **education**.

sense
How different conditions are perceived such as pain, hunger, thirst. The special senses are taste, smell, sight, hearing and touch.

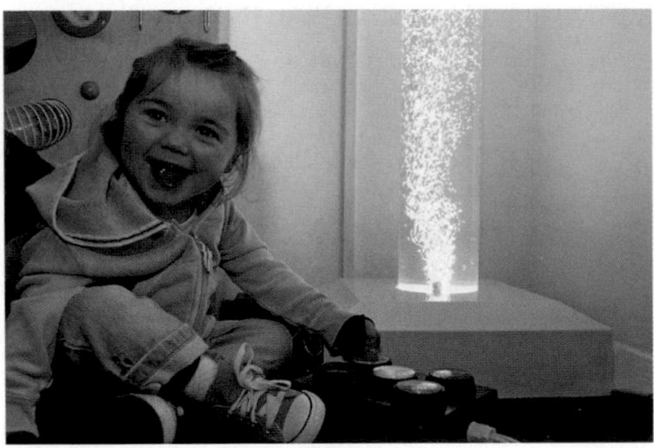
■ A sensory room is a therapeutic area.

sensory
Relating to sensations. A sensory room is a therapeutic area with specialised technology that stimulates particular senses, for example music, lights and aromas.

sensory impairment
Loss of or reduction in response to stimulation in any of the senses, such as vision or hearing.

sentence
The punishment that the **courts** decide on for those convicted of a crime. Decisions about sentences are made by **magistrates** or **judges**. Sentences can be custodial or a **community** sentence, where people will have to make **reparation** to the local community for their crime.

separation
A term usually used to refer to a child being apart from its **mother**. The **bonding** and **attachment** of the time immediately following **birth** are important in establishing long-term **relationships** between mother and child. The term can also refer to the situation where the two partners in a marriage are no longer living together, but have not legally **divorced**.

service level agreements
The basis of agreement between a **commissioner** and a **provider** specifying how **services** will be provided. The agreement/specification usually includes details of the nature, quantity, quality and **outcomes** of services to be provided, and the period between **reviews**. A service provider for domiciliary care, for example, will have to achieve all the outcomes set out in the service level agreement, provide sufficient staff to undertake the work and ensure that there are always sufficient staff available to provide a service to everyone who wants to use it.

service provider
An **organisation**, either from the **statutory**, **voluntary** or **independent sectors**, that is commissioned to provide care **services**. The **providers** can be small businesses or **charities** or national, multi-million pound businesses.

services
The **support** that is provided to meet the requirements of those people who need additional support with daily living or with maintaining or improving their **health**. Services can be aimed at health or care and can be delivered in someone's home or elsewhere. They can range from something very simple such as **provision** of a small aid, to a complex package of 24-hour care.

service users
People who make use of the **services** that are available or who use the opportunity to have **direct payments** and commission their own services.

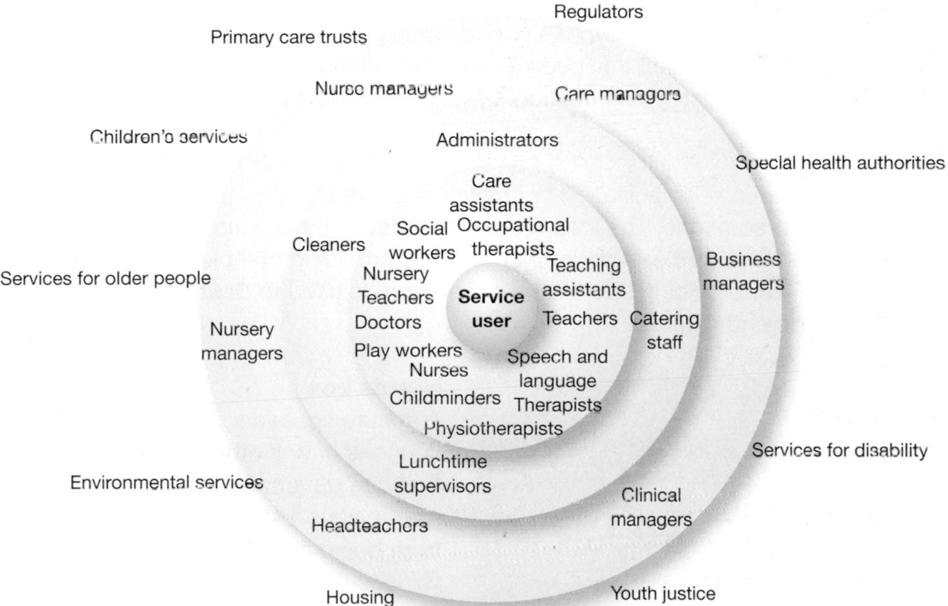

■ The service user is at the centre of a care organisation's activities.

sexism
Discrimination on the basis of a person's **gender**.

sexual abuse
The exploitation of children or **vulnerable adults** for the sexual gratification of the **abuser**. Children and vulnerable adults cannot give **informed consent** to sexual activity, and it is a criminal **offence**.

sexual intercourse
Sexual activity where an erect **penis** is inserted into the **vagina** and **semen** is **ejaculated**.

sexual offence
A criminal act including **rape**, sexual assault, viewing or purchasing child pornography, 'grooming' **young people** for sex, engaging in child prostitution, sexual activity with a person under the age of 16, or **sexual** activity with someone who has not given, or is not able to give, **consent**.

sexual orientation/sexuality
Sexual preference for either **heterosexual** or **homosexual relationships**.

sexual relationship
A relationship where sexual activity takes place.

sexually transmitted infection
A **disease** such as gonorrhea, syphilis or chlamydia passed on through unprotected sexual activity. It is important that people take precautions when engaging in sexual activity to avoid contracting an **infection**. Wearing a condom is a necessary protection.

shared care
Where more than one organisation or individual come together to provide care and support for someone. The idea recognises that all those who contribute are of equal importance regardless of whether they are providing complex medical care or are a volunteer providing short breaks. The term is used to describe sharing care with family or friend carers.

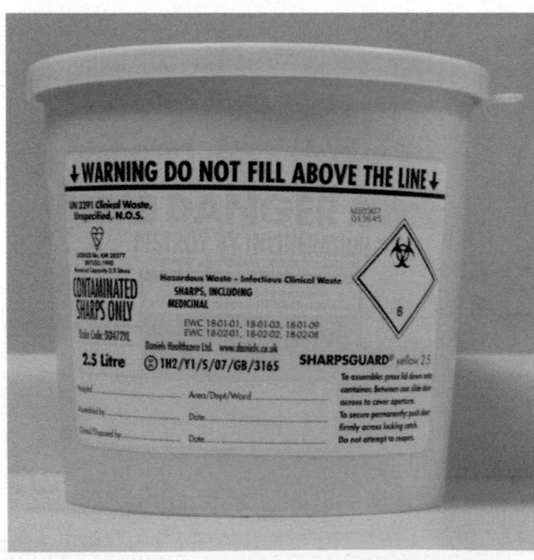

■ Sharps box.

sharps box
A secure container for used **needles**, venflons or any other instruments that can puncture the **skin**. This is an essential part of protecting people from being exposed to **blood-borne viruses** through **accidental injuries**.

sheltered housing
Accommodation where people live in their own unit, but with the option to meet up with others in communal areas. Additional **support** is available on site in case of emergencies. This option works well for people who are able to manage with limited

assistance. People in sheltered housing can retain their **independence**, but have the option to have company if they wish.

shock

A physical **reaction** that causes a sudden drop in **blood pressure** and consequently a lack of circulating blood volume as fluid leaks into the tissues. The reaction can happen as the result of an emotional or physical **trauma**, such as an **accident**, the sudden onset of an illness or serious emotional distress. **Symptoms** include becoming pale and clammy with shallow, rapid breathing, a rapid weak **pulse** or feeling faint. Shock has the potential to be a very serious condition and medical help must be sought immediately.

short breaks

The term now used to describe periods when carers make other arrangements for the person they care for and have a break. Breaks can be for a day, overnight, a week or longer periods. This used to be referred to as respite care, but this is no longer used because of the implication that the cared-for person is a burden.

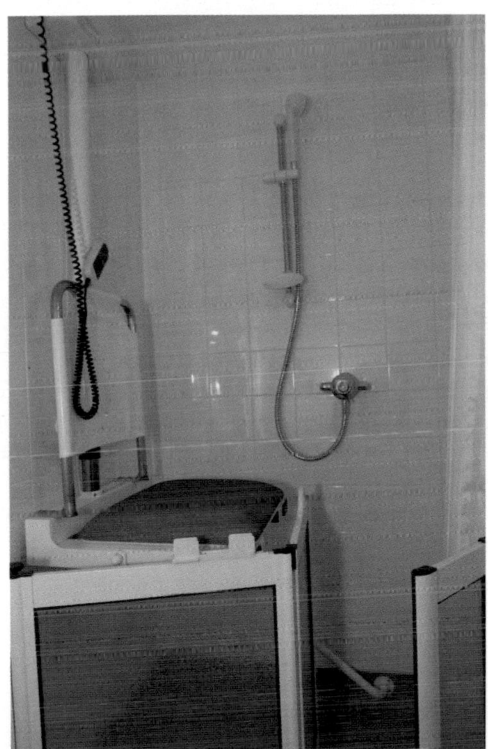

■ Shower chairs are used by people who need to be able to sit down in the shower.

short-term memory

Information stored and **recalled** after a matter of minutes or hours. Some conditions such as **dementia** will result in the loss of short-term memory, although people will often have excellent recall from their long-term memory of events that happened years ago.

shower chair

A waterproof chair that allows water to drain away, used by people who need to be able to sit down in the shower.

siblings

Brothers and sisters within a **family**.

sickle-cell disorders

A group of **genetic disorders** that affect the **haemoglobin** in the **red blood cells.** People with sickle-cell disorders have a different type of haemoglobin (sickle haemoglobin) that becomes rigid and sickle-shaped after giving up **oxygen** to the **tissues**. Usually red blood cells remain flexible and can move freely around the body; the rigid sickled cells can prevent **blood** flowing freely, and as a result can deprive vital areas of blood and cause intense pain.

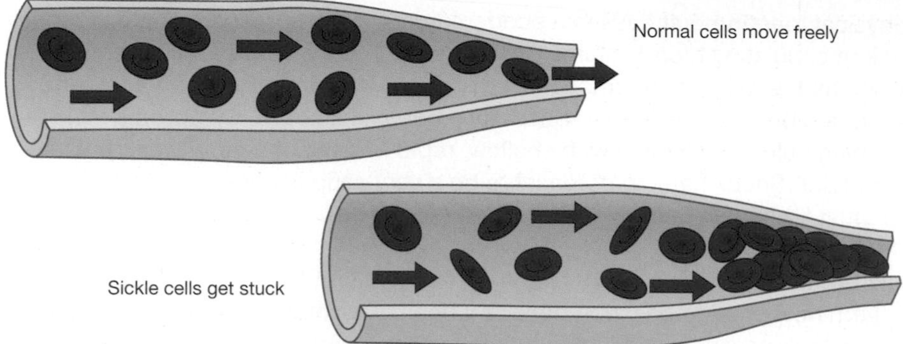

■ People with sickle-cell disorders have a different type of haemoglobin (sickle haemoglobin) that becomes rigid and sickle-shaped after giving up oxygen to the tissues.

significant adult
A person who is important to a child. This is usually a **parent**, but could equally be a grandparent or other relative, or a foster carer.

significant harm
There are no clear legal criteria to define significant harm, but the **risk** of such harm triggers **statutory intervention** in a child's life. **Professional** judgement is required in order to determine the harm that could be caused to any individual child. In some cases, one instance of **violent abuse** is enough to justify intervention; in other circumstances it may be a gradual build-up of verbal abuse and **intimidation** over a period of time, or it may be the persistent failure of **parents** to **support** the achievement of positive **outcomes** for the child. Significant harm can also be caused to children if they **witness** harm being caused to others within the same household.

significant other
Anyone who is important to someone and whom they wish to be involved in their life. This may include partner, relative and/or friend but also could include members of the community or other workers such as volunteers, other care practitioners, advocate, interpreter, police or prison officer.

signing
Communicating using **British Sign Language**. *See* **British Sign Language**.

signs
Objective indications of a disorder noticed by a doctor or nurse. *See* **symptoms**.

signs and symptoms of abuse
There are signs and **symptoms** that may indicate **abuse**, but they must be considered alongside other **information**.

Physical	Unexplained or regular **bruises**, fractures or cuts, round burns (from a cigarette), straight burns (from an electric fire), scalds with straight edges, black eyes, bruised ears, mouth **injuries**, restraint marks, 'fingermark' bruises, reluctance to get changed or take off long sleeves
Emotional	Unexplained change in **personality**, becoming withdrawn, expressing **fear** about being 'in trouble', fear of going home, fear of a particular person, loss of **confidence**
Sexual	**Rectal** or **vaginal** bleeding or bruising, urinary **infections**, marked and stained underwear, inappropriate or unusual sexual behaviour or comments
Financial	Unexplained shortage of money, unexplained withdrawals from bank accounts, inability to locate **pension** or **benefit** books
Neglect	Appearing unkempt, dirty, hungry or thirsty, wearing the wrong clothing for weather conditions, wet or soiled clothing

single assessment process (SAP)
The **process** of undertaking one **assessment**, and all the **organisations** involved in working with the individual using this rather than repeating the assessment process many times. This approach **supports** the concept of **person-centred planning** and a **holistic approach** to assessment and delivering **services**.

sitting next to Nellie
Popular name for 'on the job' **learning** gained by watching or shadowing an experienced colleague. This way of learning suits some people. The potential risk of this method is that 'Nellie' may not be doing the job properly and bad habits can be picked up.

skeleton
The hard, jointed structure of **bones** and cartilage that supports the shape of the body is able to resist the force of gravity and protects the **muscles, soft tissues** and **organs**. The skeleton is capable of movement at the joints due to the action of muscles attached across the joints. There are 206 bones in the human skeleton. *See* **musculo-skeletal system** for diagram.

skill
The ability to undertake practical tasks. The skills needed to provide **health** or **social care** usually need to be learned on the job, and it is difficult to learn them in the classroom. It is also important that people understand not only what to do,

but the reasons why it needs to be done, so skills alone are not sufficient; the knowledge underpinning the skills is also important.

1 Watch
The student nurse or midwife watches a trained member of staff read the prescription, gather together the equipment, draw up the injection, check the client's identification, give the injection, sign the prescription and dispose of the needles. She may watch this procedure many times before being confident enough to try giving an injection on her own.

2 Copy
Student nurses or midwives often copy giving injections by injecting into oranges before trying it on clients. Oranges don't mind so much when it goes wrong! Then when they feel confident, they will proceed onto real clients.

3 Practise
With practice, the student nurse or midwife will become more confident with her new skill.

4 Do
Finally, the student nurse or midwife will become competent at giving injections. She will have the skills to reassure the patient, give injections and clear away safely afterwards.

■ How the student nurse or midwife learns the skill of giving an injection.

skin

The largest **organ** of the body, providing a protective covering for the body. It also contains **nerve** endings that serve the sense of **touch**, sweat **glands**, pores and hair follicles. Skin exposed to the sun manufactures vitamin D and it has an important role in temperature regulation.

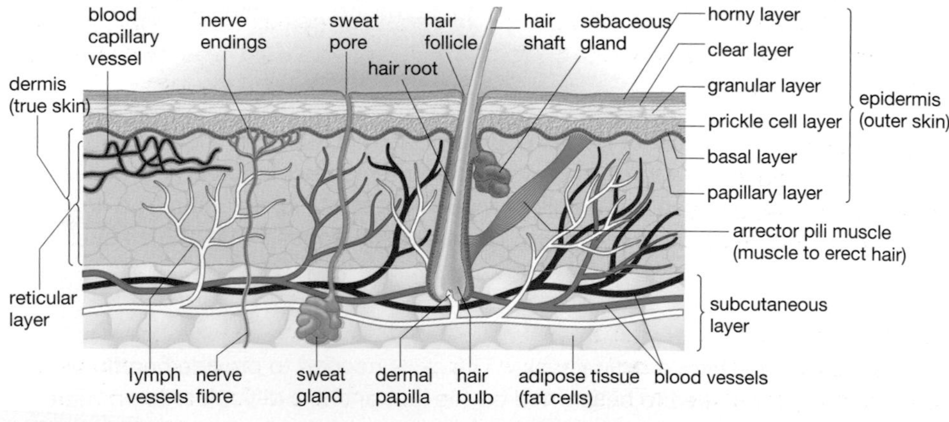

■ Structure of skin.

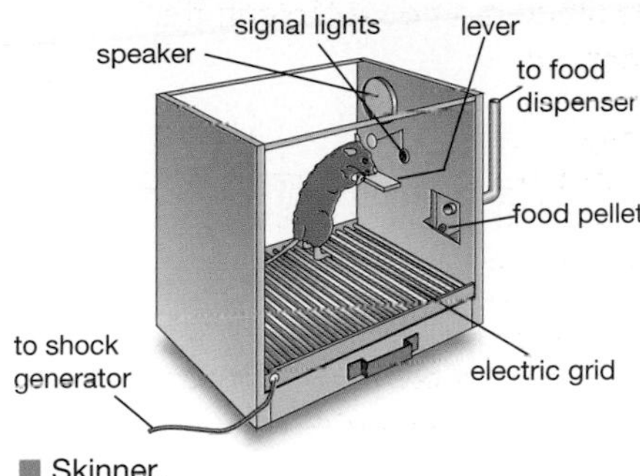

■ Skinner.

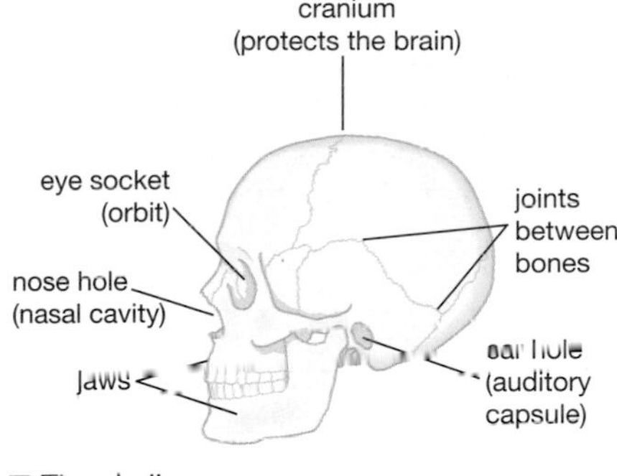

■ The skull.

Skinner, Burrhus Frederic
An American **psychologist** (1904–1990) who developed the work done by **Pavlov** on **learning theory** and behaviour modification. He developed the concept of 'operant conditioning'. Basically he found that if behaviour has good consequences it will be repeated, and if behaviour has negative consequences it will happen less often and eventually stop.

skull
The bony part of the **skeleton** that covers the **brain** (cranium) and forms the shape of the head and face.

sleep
A state of rest where **consciousness** is suspended. For people to function effectively they need 6–8 hours of sleep every 24 hours. People who are deprived of sleep lose concentration and become confused, and the ability to perform some functions is reduced.

smacking
The act of adults hitting children. It is **illegal** in most countries of Europe, but is permitted in the UK.

smoking
The highly **addictive** and **harmful** habit of using cigarettes or other tobacco products. Smoking tobacco is legal in the UK outdoors and in private homes, but it is not permitted in any public places or **workplaces**. Smoking causes **diseases** for those who smoke and for people around them who inhale the smoke. *See* **passive smoking**.

smooth muscle
The type of muscle that performs involuntary tasks, such as expanding and contracting airways and **blood** vessels, and moving **food** along the **alimentary canal**. Also known as involuntary, plain and unstriated muscle.

SVQ
Scottish Vocational Qualifications based on **National Occupational Standards**. Work-based **learning** where **performance** in the **workplace** is assessed along with underpinning knowledge. SVQs are the standard **qualifications** for **work** in **health** and **social care**.

social
Making connections and communicating with people.

social care
Practical **support** with personal and daily living tasks and emotional support where necessary.

social class
A method of differentiating between different **groups** in **society** based on occupation.

1	Higher managerial and **professional** occupations	
	1.1	Large employers and higher managerial occupations
	1.2	Higher professional occupations
2	Lower managerial and professional occupations	
3	Intermediate occupations	
4	Small employers and own-account workers	
5	Lower **supervisory** and technical occupations	
6	Semi-routine occupations	
7	Routine occupations	
8	Never worked and long-term **unemployed**	

social enterprise companies
Not-for-profit companies that work in a similar way to a commercial business, but the basis of their existence is to provide benefit to the **community** they function in. Social enterprises can make a profit, but it must be re-invested in the **organisation**. Social enterprises may be contracted by a local authority, for example, to provide an advocacy service for looked-after children, or the nursing staff of an NHS Trust may form a social enterprise company and have a contract to provide nursing services to the Trust.

social exclusion
A situation where **groups** or individuals are not able to join in **society** or function as citizens. The government's Social Inclusion Unit defines social exclusion as 'what can happen when people or areas suffer from a combination of linked problems such as **unemployment**, poor **skills**, **low income**, poor **housing**, high crime, bad **health** and **family** breakdown'.

socialisation
Learning the values and normal behaviour of a social group or culture in becoming part of it. Primary socialisation usually takes place in the family. Secondary socialisation takes place with other adults and children at school, clubs and other influences from society. *See* also **primary socialisation**.

social isolation
A situation where a **group** or individual has limited or no contact with other people. This can be because of physical or emotional **barriers**.

social learning theory
The view that learning has a very significant influence on behaviour and that any behaviour can be changed by the ways in which others respond to it.

social mobility
The ability to move through the socio-economic groupings as a result of **employment**.

social model
An approach to **disability** that considers which aspects of the **environment** are disabling someone. There may be nothing stopping a wheelchair user from preparing his or her own meals except the inability to reach the kitchen units; therefore the answer is to change the height of the units. The social model recognises that **society** and the environment are what disable people.

social norm
Behaviour that is expected by a **family**, social or cultural grouping in any given situation.

social risks
Includes risks related to legislation (such as possession, driving with excess alcohol) and to relationships (such as the effects of the individual's substance use on others).

social services
The **statutory local authority** directorate, responsible for the **commissioning** of **social work** and **social care services**.

social stratification
The identification of social groupings that are based on **power**, wealth and influence. In the UK this is evident in the **social class system**, whereas in some countries, such as India, it is seen in the caste system.

Social Trends
A national **reference** source using **data** from a range of **government** departments. There is coverage of the following different aspects of social policy: **population**, households and **families**, **education** and training, labour market, **income** and wealth, **expenditure**, **health**, social protection, crime and justice, **housing**, **environment**, transport, **lifestyles** and social participation.
More information can be found at www.statistics.gov.uk/socialtrends/

A
B
C
D
E
F
G
H
I
J
K
L
M
N
O
P
Q
R
S
T
U
V
W
X
Y
Z

social work
A method of working in partnership with people to help them find ways to overcome **barriers** and participate fully as citizens.

social worker
A **qualified** and registered **professional** who provides **social work services** for **statutory**, **independent** or **voluntary organisations**. Social workers in statutory organisations have **responsibilities** to **safeguard** and protect children and **vulnerable adults**.

society
A collection of people living together in an organised way with **norms**, rules and expectations of behaviour, and structures in place to ensure that they are followed. There are also **values** and generally held **moral standards**, along with **processes** for bringing up children so that they will **understand** and follow the rules and expectations.

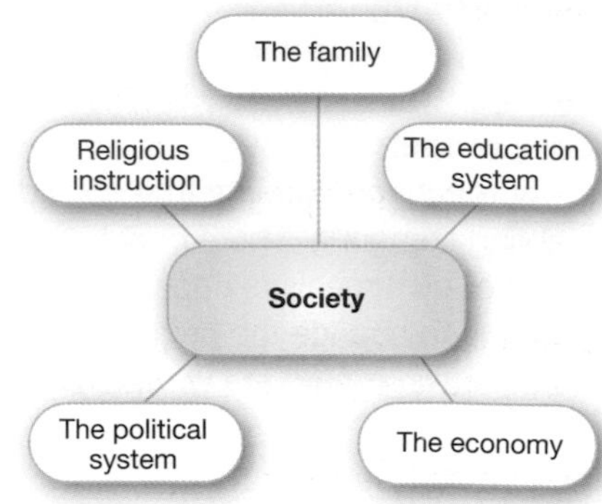

■ Key institutions in our society.

socio-economic
A mix of social considerations and income issues such as employment, living conditions, education and social activity that are used to define social class.

sociogram
A diagram showing **relationships** between people. It can show how people are linked together much more clearly than a written **report**.

sociology
The study and **analysis** of **society**.

sodium
A **mineral** that is needed in small amounts for a healthy, balanced **diet**. The main source of sodium is salt.

soft tissues
Muscle, **fat** and **skin**. These soft tissues of the body are supported and protected by the hard bony **skeleton**.

solicitor
A qualified lawyer who is available to work with the general public. Solicitors can provide legal advice, undertake legal **processes** or can act as **advocates** in lower **courts**. They can also instruct **barristers**, who can act as advocates in all courts.

soluble
Able to be dissolved in a liquid to form a solution.

solvent
A liquid that dissolves other substances to form a solution. Some solvents are misused or **abused** because they have similar effects on the body to alcohol or some drugs. In these cases, solvents such as aerosols, dry cleaning fluid, paint stripper or butane gas are usually sniffed, a **harmful** process that can result in **death**.

special care baby unit (SCBU)
Units in **hospitals** that care for **newborn** babies who are **premature** or have other problems at **birth**. Highly specialised **equipment** is used to treat and support the babies.

special constable
A volunteer **police** officer who has the same **powers** as regular police.

special education needs
The **needs** of children for whom the **education system** is required to respond with an additional level of **provision**. All children with special education needs have a

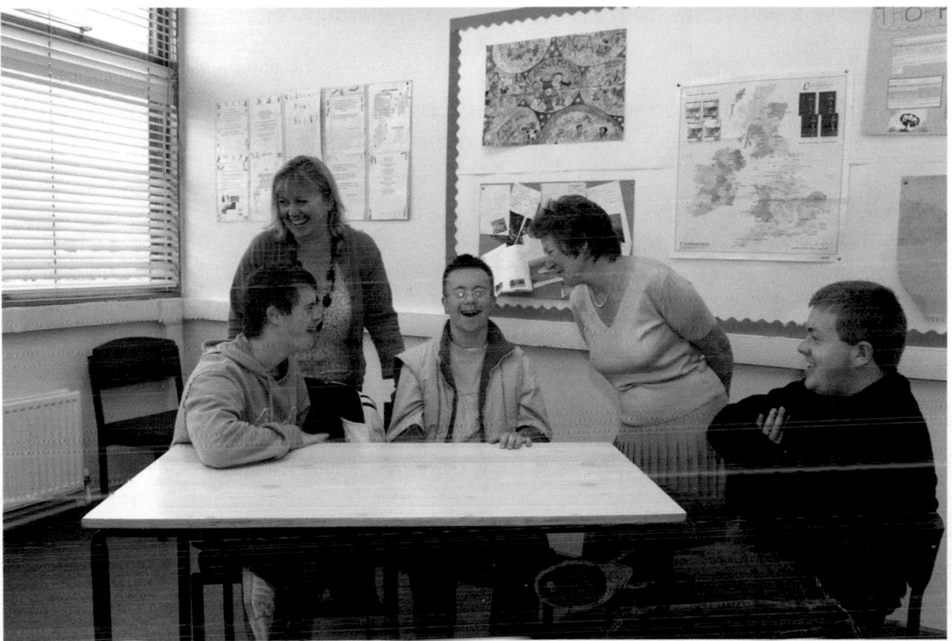

■ Special education needs.

right to **access** education at a local **school**. The school is required to be accessible for all children.

Specialist Diabetic Team
A healthcare team specialising in diabetes and consists of doctors, nurses, dieticians, podiatrists and administration staff.

specific aids
Specific aids that will enable individuals with speaking, sight or hearing difficulties, additional needs or learning difficulties, to receive and respond to information.

speech therapist
A **professional** who works with people who have language and **communication** disorders.

sperm (spermatoza)
The male reproductive **cell** that fertilises the female egg (ovum).

sphincter
A circular muscle that constricts (narrows) a body passage, for example the anal sphincter around the anus and the pyloric sphincter at the lower end of the stomach, which allows food to pass from the stomach to the duodenum.

sphygmomanometer
An instrument for **measuring** and **recording blood pressure** in the **arteries**. Most instruments are digital, but some are still operated manually.

spina bifida
A **genetic** condition that develops before **birth**. Some of the **vertebrae** do not develop properly and so leave the **spinal cord** exposed to damage. This can result in walking difficulties; sometimes **hydrocephalus** can develop and this can lead to a **learning disability**.

spinal cord
The column of **nervous tissue** that is located within the **vertebral** column and directly connected to the **brain**. The brain controls **muscles** of the body through spinal nerves leaving the spinal cord at intervals through spaces between vertebrae. For this reason the spinal cord gets narrower the further away from the brain.

spine
The backbone, vertebral column or a pointed projection on a bone.

spiritual needs
These encompass hope, a quest for meaning and inner peace, a need to be valued and to receive assistance to cope with anxieties and fears.

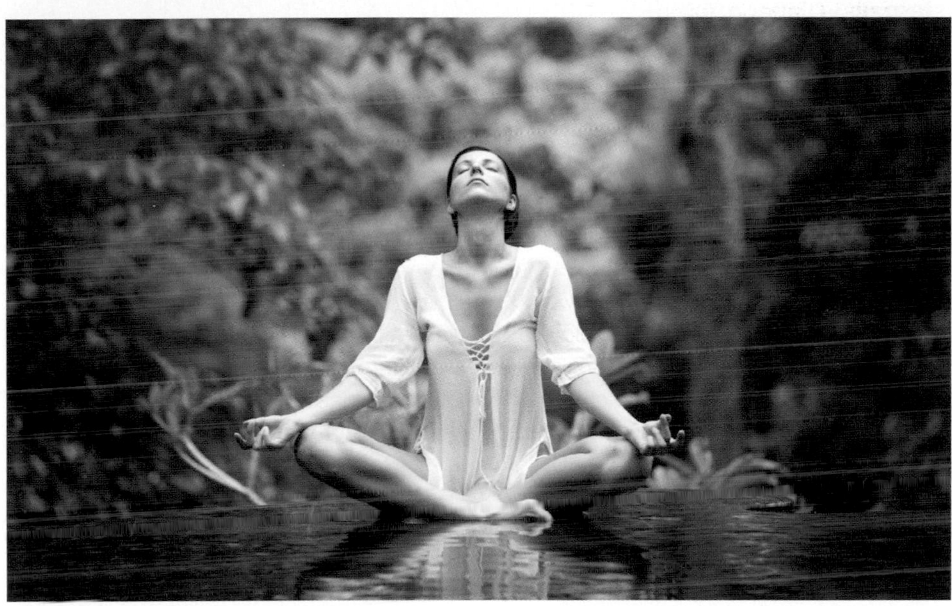

Spiritual needs.

spiritual well-being
State of wholeness when every aspect of life is in balance.

spleen
A dark-red sponge-like **organ** located in the upper abdominal area behind the stomach. It filters **blood** and destroys old **red blood cells**. It is also part of the body's defence mechanism and makes lymphocytes, as well as providing a reservoir of blood. It is not an essential organ as other organs also filter blood, but people are more at risk of **infections** if it is removed.

sputum
Mucus and saliva coughed up from the **lungs** and respiratory passages.

squint
A condition caused when eye **muscles** are not co-ordinated, leading to one or both eyes turning inwards or outwards. This results in a problem with vision.

stages of development
May be age-related and/or related to the individual's mental health or developmental stage.

stakeholder
Someone who has a share or an interest in an organisation or a policy.

stamina
Enduring strength and energy.

standard precautions (health and safety measures)
Recommendations, guidelines and procedures set down for staff with the purpose of reducing/preventing accidents and infection and maintaining a safe environment, e.g. hand washing, protective clothing, safe disposal of soiled equipment, bed linen, tissue, correct use of equipment, chemicals, drugs etc.

standards
Statements about how tasks should be carried out and the minimum acceptable quality of **service** or **practice** that should be delivered. National **minimum standards** are set by **regulators** and checked by **inspectors**. **National Occupational Standards** form the basis for **qualifications** including SVQs and **NVQs**.

starvation
Where there is insufficient **food** to sustain life.

state, the
A general term referring not only to the **government** and the civil service, but also other institutions such as the monarchy or the armed forces.

state benefits
See **benefits**

statementing
The **process** of **assessing** the **needs** of and the **services** that are required for a **disabled** child, in order for the child to participate fully in **education** and **society**. Following assessment, a statement of the child's needs is provided.

statistics
Numerical **data** that has been **analysed** to provide **information**. In **health** and **social care**, statistics are important in helping to plan future **service** requirements, looking at the **incidence** of **diseases**, and for identifying social trends and changes in behaviour.

status
Position in **society**, usually as a result of **power**, influence, and commonly wealth. A high status can also be gained as a result of outstanding ability.

statutory
Required by **law** and governed by **legislation. Local authorities**, **health authorities**, primary care trusts and **hospitals** all have statutory requirements to deliver certain **services** and to meet **targets**.

stereotyping
Making negative or positive judgements about whole **groups** of people based on **prejudice** and assumptions, rather than facts or knowledge about individuals, for example the stereotype of women as the main carer.

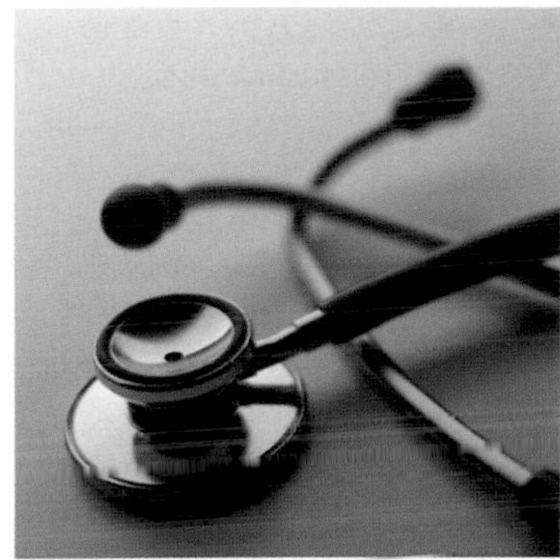

■ A stethoscope is used to listen to the internal organs.

stethoscope
A listening instrument to hear the sounds made by internal **organs** such as the **heart** and **lungs**.

stillbirth
The **birth** of a **baby** born after the 24th week of **pregnancy** who showed no signs of life at any time after birth. The delivery of a **foetus** born without signs of life before 24 weeks is called a **miscarriage**.

stoma
An artificial opening in the intestine through the abdominal wall. This is usually made to allow **faeces** to be removed from the body and collected in a special bag without passing through the large bowel or through the **anus**. It can also be to allow feeding directly into the **stomach**. Stoma sites have to be given very careful care and bags must be changed regularly to ensure that **skin** irritations are kept to a minimum.

stomach
The pouch for holding **food** during the early part of the **digestive process**. Food is churned in the stomach and mixed with acid and **enzymes** ready to pass on to the next stage of the digestive process.

strategic health authorities
Regional bodies (there are 10 in England) responsible for:

- developing plans for improving **health services** in their local area
- making sure local health services are of a high quality and are performing well
- increasing the capacity of local health services – so they can provide more services
- making sure national **priorities** are integrated into local health service plans.

Strategic health authorities manage the **NHS** locally and are a key link between the Department of Health and the NHS.

strategy
A plan to deliver **services** or to reach **targets**. Strategies provide an overall direction and **guidelines** for an **organisation**.

strength
The body's physical power and ability to exert force.

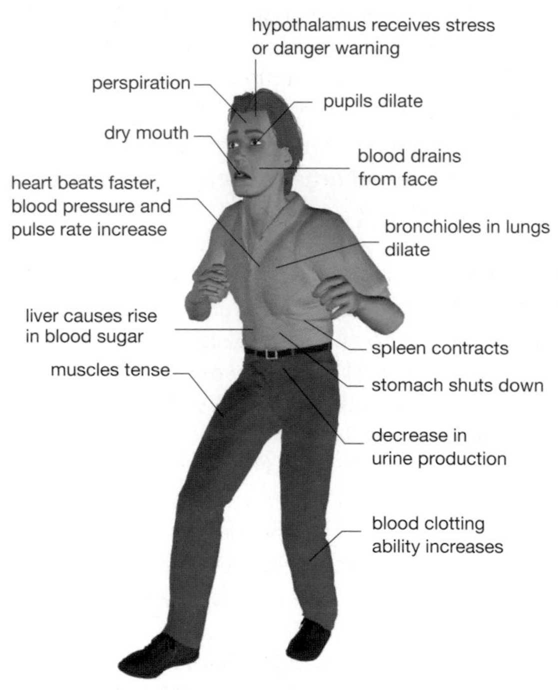

■ The physiological effects of stress on the body.

stress
Worry and pressure that can prove too much for some people. This can result in stress-related illnesses such as **heart disease**, **diabetes** and digestive disorders. The body's response to stress is to produce **adrenaline** and prepare for 'fight or flight'; this can cause agitation and **anxiety** or panic attacks, when people may feel palpitations, short of breath and very frightened.

stress incontinence
Leakage of **urine** or **faeces** owing to poor control of the sphincter **muscles** that hold the **bladder** or **anus** closed. Incontinence of urine is by far the more common condition. The condition can be improved by strengthening the pelvic floor, and ultimately through **surgery** if no other approach is effective.

stroke
A condition that results from an interrupted **blood** flow, causing a lack of **oxygen** to the **brain**. The consequent destruction of the **nerve cells** in the brain can be reversible or permanent, depending largely on how quickly **treatment** is started.

subcutaneous
Beneath the **skin**. The term is usually used to refer to the administering of **medication** in a subcutaneous injection, where it is only necessary to get the medication below the skin rather than into a **muscle** or a **vein**.

substance misuse
Using substances such as **alcohol**, **drugs** and **solvents** to obtain a physical effect rather than for their original purpose. Misusing or abusing substances poses serious **health** risks.

sudden infant death syndrome
Also known as **cot death**, the sudden **death** of a **baby** with no obvious cause. **Research** has shown that the number of these deaths can be reduced if babies are put to **sleep** on their backs. Since the 'back to sleep' campaign was launched in 1991, there has been a 75 per cent reduction in sudden deaths. There are around 350 sudden deaths a year. There are key steps that appear to reduce risks:

- putting babies on their backs to sleep
- not **smoking** during **pregnancy** (this applies to both **parents**)
- not allowing smoking in the same room as a baby
- not letting babies get too hot
- keeping babies' heads uncovered – their feet should be at the foot of the cot to stop them wriggling down under the covers
- not falling asleep with a baby on a sofa or in an armchair
- parents not sharing a bed with their baby if they smoke, have been drinking alcohol, are taking drugs or **medication** that causes drowsiness, are excessively tired, or if the baby was **premature** or small at **birth**
- putting the baby's cot in the parent's bedroom for the first six months.

sugars
See **carbohydrates**.

suicide
The actions of a person to end his or her own life. Suicide can happen as the result of a **mental disorder** such as **depression**, but can also be a considered decision of someone who wants to end life because of his or her personal circumstances or because of a **terminal illness**.

suppleness
The body's ability to bend, stretch and move without damage.

superbug
See **methicillin-resistant *Staphylococcus aureus***.

supervision
Support and guidance for **professional practice**. All professional practitioners in **health** or **social care** should have **access** to a supervisor on a regular basis. This gives the opportunity to discuss specific issues and to seek guidance on development of practice.

A B C D E F G H I J K L M N O P Q R S T U V W XYZ

support
The assistance that people need in order to manage day-to-day living and to achieve the **outcomes** and **goals** they have identified. *See* **active support**.

supported living
An approach that allows people to live in an **independent** small group, usually of about four or five people. The group shares a house and has **access** to a **support worker** who will visit regularly and is on call for emergencies. This has proved useful for people with **learning disabilities** and those who have had **mental health problems**.

support groups
Set up to offer help to people in particular situations, for example: people who care for a relative with dementia or people who have **asthma**. Sometimes they can be self-help groups set up by people who have had the experience themselves or they can also be set up and assisted by health or care professionals.

Supporting People
A **government initiative** that provides **funding** for **housing**-related support **services** aimed at removing **barriers** for **vulnerable** people who want to live **independently**. **Local authorities** and **housing associations** work jointly on making **provision**. More information can be found at www.spkweb.org.uk (Supporting People: Communities and Local Government)

support networks
Groups of people who link together, either face to face or virtually, to share experiences and offer help and advice. They usually have an interest in common, such as having the same condition or having been through similar **treatment**, or have a similar **addiction**. **Networks** can be organised by **professionals** or can be on a **self-help** basis.

support plan
The agreed actions that have been worked out between the individual or **family** using a **service** and the **key worker** responsible for arranging the delivery of services. The plan is followed by all those involved in providing services and can be **reviewed** or changed.

support worker
A **professional** who offers practical assistance to people, usually in their own homes, but also in **resource** centres.

surgery
The **process** of **diagnosing** and treating disorders by accessing the internal **organs** of the body by incisions in the **skin**. Increasingly, surgery is carried out by making very small incisions and using remote instruments; this is known as laparoscopic or **keyhole surgery**.

survey
A means of collecting **data** from a range of people or sources for **research** purposes.

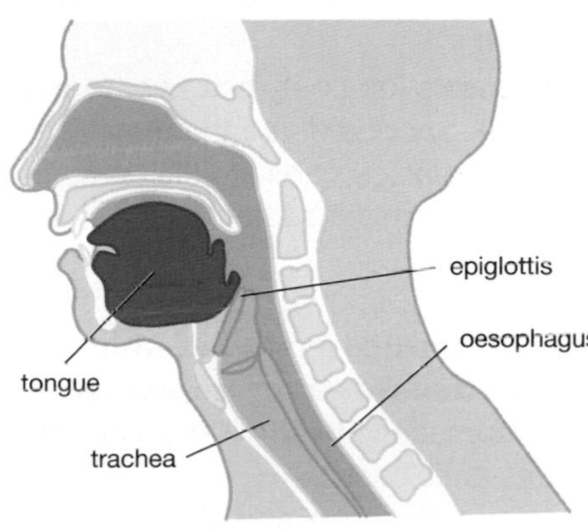

■ The swallowing process.

swallowing
The means of **food** getting from the mouth into the **stomach** through the **oesophagus**. After the food has been chewed and formed into a bolus the tongue presses against the roof of the mouth (and palate) and the muscular walls of the pharynx grip the bolus. The epiglottis covers the top of the trachea to ensure that food does not enter the **lungs**. It is pushed down the oesophagus by **peristalsis**. The swallow **reflex** is controlled by the autonomic **nervous system**.

sweat glands
Glands in the **dermis** of the **skin** that produce sweat. Sweat is secreted through a sweat duct to a pore opening on the skin surface. Sweat contains **urea**, **minerals**, salts and water. Sweat helps in regulating **temperature** by cooling the skin as it dries.

SWOT analysis
A useful exercise when planning new projects or ventures, this method of analysis aims to identify:

- Strengths
- Weaknesses
- Opportunities
- Threats.

sympathetic nervous system
Part of the autonomic **nervous system** which prepares the body for fight or flight. This happens without any voluntary action on the part of the individual; if a person is **stressed** or feels under **threat**, the sympathetic nervous system will pump additional **blood** to the **muscles**, raise **blood pressure**, increase **heart rate** and speed up breathing. Sympathetic nerves to the adrenal glands stimulate the release of adrenaline that further boosts the actions.

symptom
An indication of **disease** or illness that the patient complains of which assists with **diagnosis**.

synapse
A minute gap between the end of one neurone and another neurone or muscle/gland.

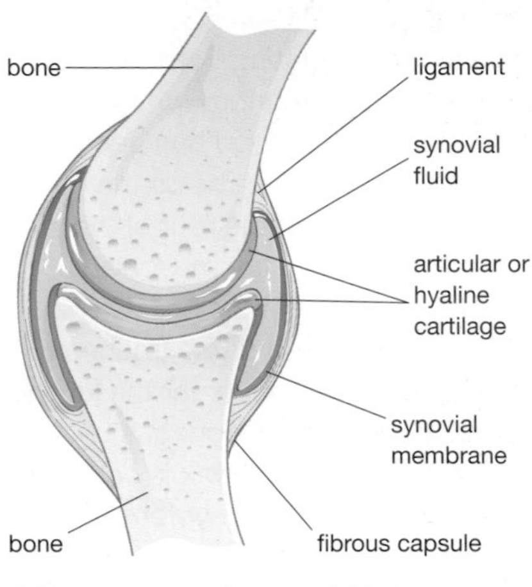

The structure of a synovial joint.

synovial joint
A freely moveable **joint** between two bones. The joint is encapsulated and the moving parts are protected by cartilage and synovial fluid, which lubricates the joint.

syphilis
A **sexually transmitted infection** caused by **bacteria**. The **disease** can cause serious permanent damage to **health** if left untreated, and requires antibiotics.
The **symptoms** are ulcers and blisters on the **penis** or **vagina**, sore throat and **fever**, and further ulceration. Ultimately the disease can affect the functioning of the **brain**.

syringe
A means of injecting **medication** through the **skin** into the body. The syringe is attached to a hollow **needle** so that the skin can be pierced.

system
The structures and **processes** that **support** the functioning of **society** or an **organisation** or a **community**. There is a theory that suggests systems also work in **families**, and that each family has its own system and structures that make it function.

systolic
The phase of circulation when the ventricles of the heart are contracting and actively pumping blood so the pressure of the blood against the heart is at its highest. Also refers to the upper figure in a blood pressure measurement.

T

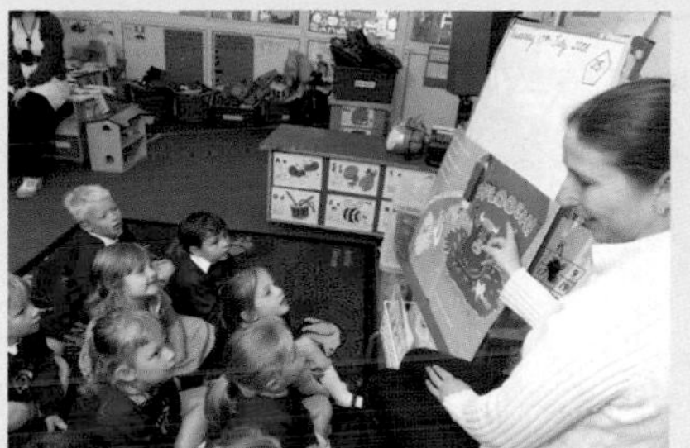

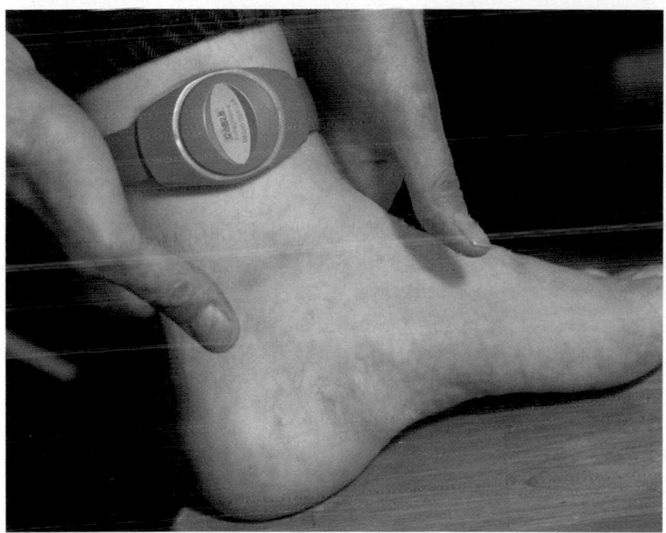

Tagging is an electronic means of keeping track of people, used by the police and prison authorities.

tagging
An electronic means of keeping track of people, used by the **police** and prison authorities. It is sometimes used for people on parole, or people who have had restrictions placed on their movements.

tantrum
An uncontrolled outburst of rage involving behaviour such as screaming, crying, physical aggression, lying on the floor and kicking Tantrums are commonly seen in young children between the ages of 1 and 3 years. At this stage they are testing out the limits and **boundaries** of the world they are discovering. Children need to have boundaries and dislike the feeling of being out of control that comes with having a tantrum. Most children move on from this after the age of about 3 years; however, some will carry on even into **adulthood**, although the behaviour may be different and not so public.

target
A **goal** to aim for. Targets may be set by others, such as **government** targets for reducing **social isolation**, or can be personal, such as those set in a personal development plan or during an **appraisal**. Targets showed always be SMART. *See* **objectives**.

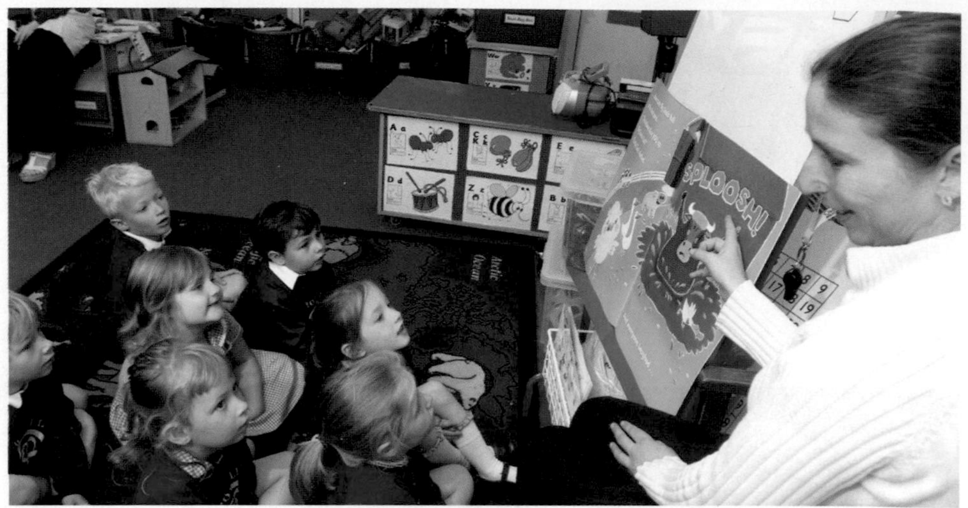

Teaching.

teaching

Sharing knowledge so that others can **understand** it. Teaching is the major part of delivering formal **education** for children, although **learning** continues and people can learn at any time of life. There is a **National Curriculum** that sets out the formal teaching that must be delivered for all children, but informal teaching is carried out by many people who come into contact with a child, including parents, friends and relatives.

team

A **group** of people who share joint aims and work towards achieving a common **goal**. Teams share resources and work together; they can be found in most **workplaces** but also in sports and in **leisure** activities.

teeth

The means of biting and chewing **food** in order to prepare it for **digestion**. They are made up of an outer coating of enamel and an inner core of dentine. The sensitive inner cavity of the tooth contains the **blood** vessels and **nerves**. Teeth appear between the age of about 6 months and 2 years. The first set are called 'milk teeth'. There are 20 of them and they will start to fall out around the age of 5 or 6 years to be replaced over time by 32 permanent teeth.

temper

The open expression of frustration, anger and rage. This can involve raising the voice, increased **respiration**, flushed face, sweating and **threatening** or **violent body language**. Some people have **personality traits** that mean that they readily express anger and frustration in response to quite minor incidents, while others very rarely display temper in public.

temperature
The measurement of heat in the body or the environment, showing how hot or cold a person, thing or place is. In the UK, temperature is measured in degrees Celsius, where water freezes at 0 degrees and boils at 100 degrees. In other countries, such as the US, temperature is measured in degrees Fahrenheit where water freezes at 32 degrees and boils at 212 degrees. *See* body temperature.

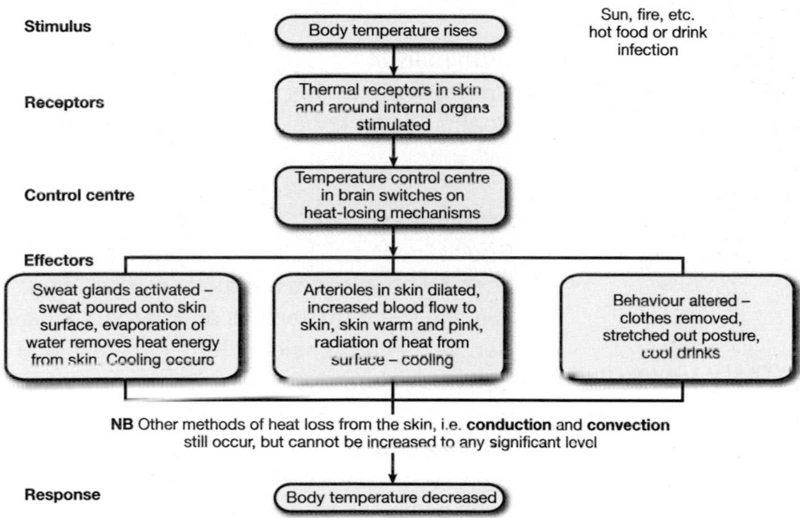

Control of rising body temperature.

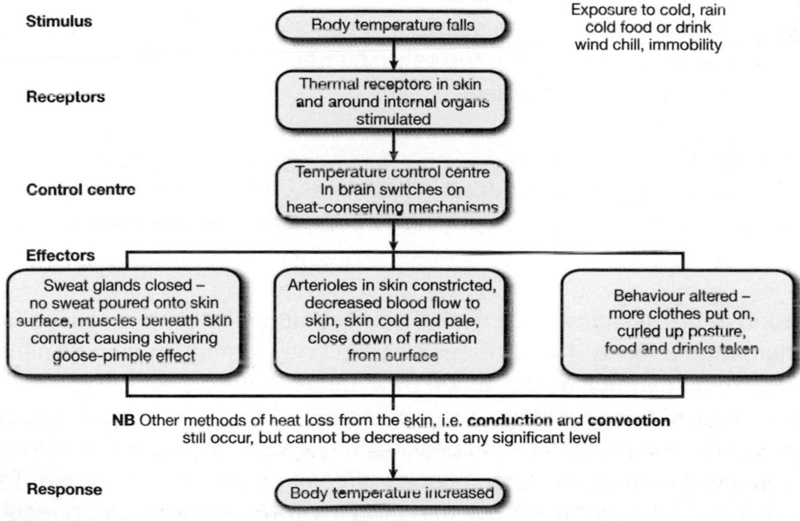

Control of falling body temperature.

A
B
C
D
E
F
G
H
I
J
K
L
M
N
O
P
Q
R
S
T
U
V
W
XYZ

tenant
A person who pays **rent** to live in a house that he or she does not own. The rent is paid to the owner, who can be a private **landlord**, a **housing association** or a **local authority**.

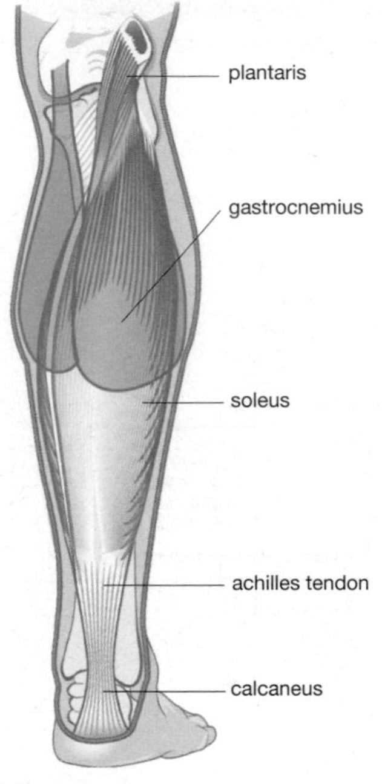

A tendon.

tendon
The tough cord of **tissue** that attaches **muscles** to **bones**.

terminally ill
Having an incurable **disease** that will result in **death**. The timescale, or prognosis for this, will vary.

terminology
Specialised vocabulary or expressions that are used by people in a particular work setting. There is a fine line between this and '**jargon**' where people use **professional** terms that exclude or confuse others.

tertiary care
Specialist **health care** provided in specialist units, such as spinal, **stroke rehabilitation** and **oncology** units.

testes
The male **gonads** contained in the **scrotum**, a sac that hangs between the legs. **Spermatozoa** are produced by the testes which need to be slightly below **body temperature** for normal development.

testosterone
The male **hormone** primarily produced in the testes. The hormone provides male characteristics such as facial and body hair, deep voice and muscular strength.

tetanus
An **infection** of the **muscles** in the neck, back and upper limbs. It is caused by anaerobic **bacteria** found in the soil entering the body through broken **skin** primarily in long deep wounds such as that made by a garden fork or a rose thorn. It is also known as 'lockjaw' because the muscles of the neck and jaw can tighten so far that they lock and make eating and speaking impossible. The main life-threatening effect is paralysis of the respiratory muscles affecting the ability to breathe. There is a preventive **vaccine** against **tetanus** and protection should be renewed regularly, particularly for people who work outdoors.

thalidomide
A drug given to **pregnant** women in the late 1950s to early 1960s to counteract morning sickness. The drug resulted in serious **birth** defects, particularly affecting the limbs, and many **babies** were born with missing or damaged limbs. The drug was withdrawn from the market, but is now used for the **treatment** of some **cancers** such as multiple myeloma. There are extensive safeguards around its use.

therapeutic
Designed to be of benefit. The term can refer to any **treatment** or **intervention**, such as a massage or **relaxation** session, **medication**, or **physiotherapy**. It can also apply to interventions such as a supportive **interview** with a **social worker** or **psychologist**.

therapeutic activities
Actions with a purpose that are designed and carried out by a qualified professional therapist in order to provide emotional or psychological benefit. Therapeutic activities can be provided in a one-to-one session or in a group.

third sector
Voluntary and **community organisations**. Many of these organisations are involved in delivering **health** and care **services** or in working to develop communities so that people can be **independent**.

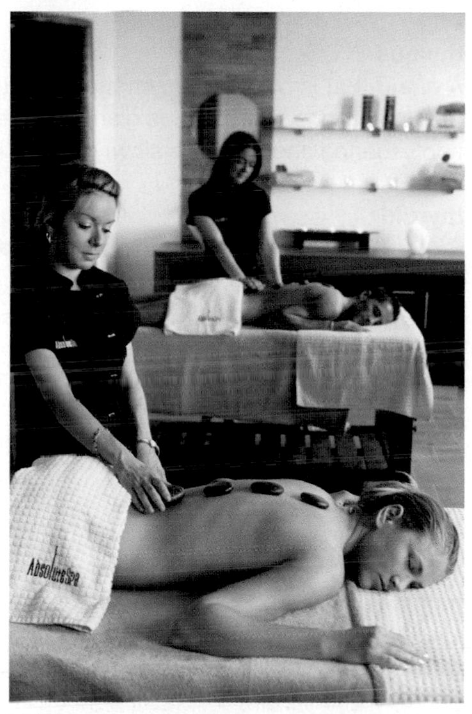

A therapeutic hot stone massage can aid relaxation.

thoracic cavity or thorax
The air-tight space containing the **lungs** and **heart**, protected by the **ribs** and bounded by the **diaphragm** and the neck.

thought processes
Ways of using the mind to gather **information**, consider something carefully and reach a conclusion, solve a problem or make a decision.

threat
A risk, possibility or likelihood of **harm**. Humans respond to a threat to their **safety** by the body preparing for 'fight or flight' with increased **blood** flow to the **muscles**, increased **heart rate** and **respiration**.

A B C D E F G H I J K L M N O P Q R S **T** U V W X Y Z

thrombosis
A **blood** clot. This can occur anywhere in the body when a small amount of blood becomes semi-solid and causes a blockage in an **artery**. This will stop or decrease the blood flow to **tissues** and can cause major problems depending on where it occurs; for example, a coronary thrombosis affects the heart. Blood in veins can also clot and the leg veins are particularly vulnerable in a patient confined to bed.

thymus
A **gland** that is part of the **lymphatic system**. It is situated in the **chest**, just behind the breastbone. The thymus gland reaches maximum size and activity during adolescence and declines slowly in function thereafter.

thyroid
A **gland** that produces the thyroid **hormone**, which affects growth and **metabolism**.

time management
The process and skill of being organised and making the best and most efficient use of available time, by planning work and not becoming distracted. Setting **targets** and **goals** and checking progress are helpful tools when planning and managing time.

tissues
A group of similar **cells** with a specific purpose, for example, **nervous tissue**, **muscle** tissue, epithelium, and so on.

toilet
The acceptable place to discharge body waste such as **faeces** and **urine**. Some people may have problems in reaching a toilet to perform these functions; this is referred to as **incontinence**. Some people require assistance to use the toilet, and this must be done sensitively.

tongue
The muscular **organ** attached inside the mouth. It is important for mechanical **digestion** as it rolls **food** into a bolus, mixing it with saliva ready for **swallowing**. The surface of the tongue contains taste buds and is also sensitive to **temperature** and texture of food. The tongue also has a role in speech.

total hearing loss
Profound **deafness** where no sounds can be heard. People who are **profoundly deaf communicate** through signing or lip reading.

A B C D E F G H I J K L M N O P Q R S T U V W XYZ

touch
One of the special senses. Where the sense of touch is lost through nerve damage, people are vulnerable to **injury** because they are unaware of pain.

toxic
Poisonous or **harmful** to living **organisms**. Substances may be toxic if **swallowed**, or fumes can be toxic if they are inhaled.

toxins
Toxic substances. Bacteria cause disease by secreting toxins.

toy library
A lending library for toys or **equipment**, intended for **families** who are not in a position to purchase the items they need. These libraries provide specialist equipment and toys for **disabled** children as well as a wide range of other toys.

trace elements
Elements that are essential for a balanced, healthy **diet** but are required only in minute amounts; for example, chromium, copper, selenium and zinc.

trachea
The windpipe in the form of a tube made from **cartilage** and lined with a mucous membrane that extends from the **larynx** to the **bronchi**.

training
Education and instruction to teach a new skill or increase knowledge.

training and development
Teaching and **mentoring** with the aim of improving someone's **skills** and **practice**. The need for training and development is identified and planned through **appraisal**. Much training is carried out in house, while some **organisations** may **support** staff to **access** outside training.

trait
A distinguishing feature of an individual, usually with a **genetic** base in **personality**.

tranquilliser
A drug that relieves **anxiety**, sometimes given to people suffering from **depression**. There are two types: benzodiazepines help **relaxation** and are normally used over a short period of time, and beta blockers are given to treat **symptoms** of anxiety such as palpitations and shaking.

A B C D E F G H I J K L M N O P Q R S T U V W XYZ

Transfer boards come in different sizes, shapes and colours.

transfer board
An **aid** used to assist someone to move from a bed to a chair or a wheelchair. *See* also **moving and handling**.

transition
A **change** or movement in a person's life, especially a child's. Usual and expected transitions are when a child goes to **school**, changes school and then leaves school. There can also be transitions from being a well child to a sick child, from an able child to a **disabled** child or from a child with two **parents** to a child with one parent. All transitions require planning, if possible, and **support**.

translate
Interpret spoken or written **communication** into a language that can be understood by the person for whom it is intended.

transmission model
A **model** of **communication** and development which suggests that **information** is passed from the 'transmitter' to the 'receiver' like a radio signal, and that it can be interfered with by external factors. There is a theory of development that believes children are like a blank sheet (*tabula rasa*) ready to 'receive' information.

transplant
The surgical transfer of an **organ** (such as **heart** or **lungs**) from one person (the donor) to another (the recipient). There is a national transplant list, so that people in need of a new organ may be matched (in terms of **blood** and **tissue** types) with a suitable donor. Nearly all recipients must take immuno-suppressive drugs after transplantation to avoid rejection.

trauma
An upsetting or distressing emotional experience, or a physical **injury** affecting a particular **organ** or part of the body.

treatment
An **intervention** designed to improve an illness or medical condition.

trigger
The immediate cause of an allergic **reaction**, for example pollen is a common trigger of hay fever, and peanuts are a common trigger for nut allergies.

tripod
A **walking aid** similar to a walking stick, but with three feet to provide more stability.

truancy
Not attending **school**. This can be as the result of **phobia** or because a **young person** has not been engaged by the teaching at a school, or has chosen to be involved in other activities during school time. It is **illegal** not to attend school in the UK between the ages of 5 and 16.

tuberculosis
A **bacterial disease** initially affecting the **lungs**, but capable of spreading throughout the body. It is infectious and there is an **immunisation** programme across the UK targeted particularly at vulnerable people.

tumour
A swelling, lump or growth in any part of the body. It always requires investigation to establish whether it is **benign** (non-invasive) or **malignant** (invasive).

twins
Two people who were born together as the result of a double **pregnancy**. This can happen after the **fertilisation** of a single egg which then splits into two before **implanting** in the **uterus**; this will produce identical twins who share the same **genetic** features. Alternatively, two eggs can both be fertilised and implanted during the same cycle; this results in non-identical or 'fraternal' twins who have different genetic features and may be different genders.

type of support
Could be at different levels and will take account of the strengths, vulnerabilities and breaking points of individuals, **families**, **carers**, groups and communities.

typhoid
Serious infection that causes inflammation of the intestine. It is caused by salmonella typhi which may be in food or water.

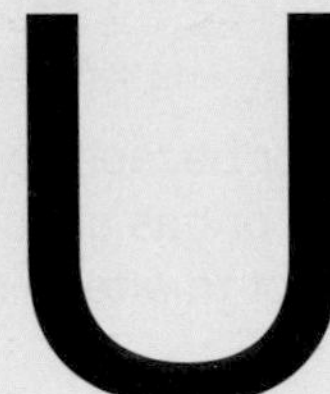

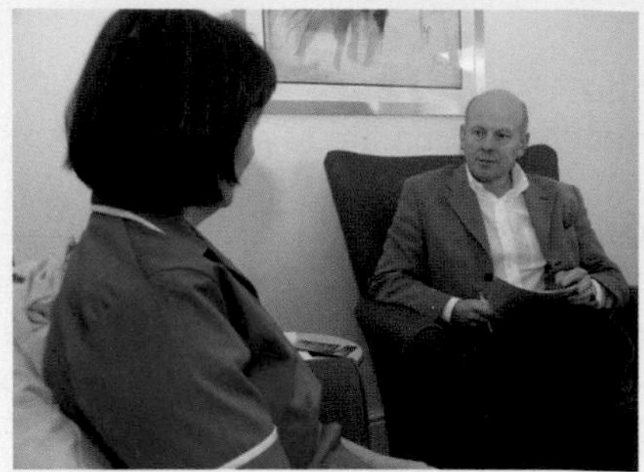

ultra filtration
Filtration carried out under a higher pressure than normal. This happens in the first part (the Bowman's capsule) of the kidney nephrons.

ultra-high temperature (UHT)
A method of preserving **food** (including milk) by exposing it to extremely high temperatures for short periods. The food is heated to 145 degrees Centigrade for about 2 seconds. This makes it possible to keep the food for longer periods before it deteriorates – for example, milk can be kept for up to a year.

ultrasound
An imaging technique that aids **diagnosis**. It uses high-frequency sound waves that bounce off parts of the body to produce images. It is used during **pregnancy** to check the developing **foetus**, and also to identify cysts and gall stones. It is particularly useful for obtaining images of fluid-filled organs.

umbilical cord
The cord that attaches the **foetus** to the **mother**. It is about 20 inches long and **blood** circulates through it, carrying **oxygen** and **nutrients** to the foetus and removing waste. Inside the cord are one **vein** that carries oxygen and nutrients from the mother to the foetus, and two **arteries** that return de-**oxygenated** blood and waste products to the mother. These umbilical blood vessels are protected by a sticky substance called Wharton's jelly, which is covered by a membrane called the amnion. The umbilical cord also passes **antibodies**, which are in the blood, from the mother to the foetus to enable it to fight **bacteria** and **viruses**.

umbrella body
An **organisation** that represents and supports a group of other, smaller organisations, for example a local council of voluntary service may represent many small voluntary organisations.

uncommunicative behaviour
An unresponsive way of behaving where someone fails to react or respond to **communication**. The person may be unwilling to join in communication for a variety of reasons, including illness or **disability**, anger, shyness and feelings of awkwardness.

unconditioned response
A sudden and unplanned response to an event, such as jumping at a loud noise.

unconscious
A state of having no awareness of surroundings or of sensory stimuli such as sounds or **touch**. In **psychodynamic theory**, the term is used to describe the **memory** of past events that have an impact on behaviour, but are not controlled by the individual nor is he or she aware of the existence of these memories.

under-represented groups
Population groups who have little **access** to positions of **power**, influence or authority. This includes: women, **disabled** people and black and minority **ethnic** groups. Employers and public **organisations** are attempting to encourage more representation from under-represented groups.

understanding
Recognising the implications of **information**. This can be applied to **learning**; it is only when the implications are recognised, as opposed to simply having memorised some information, that people can be said to have understood what they have learned. The concept is also important in **communication** between people, and means recognising and caring about the circumstances of another person.

unemployment
Not having a job.

unfamiliar and different environments
The areas in which people wish to be able to travel and move around independently and that are unfamiliar and different and maybe only occur occasionally, so they require strategies, techniques and skills over and above those required for people negotiating familiar environments.

United Nations Convention on the Rights of the Child
The first legally binding international instrument, agreed in 1989, that incorporates the full range of **children's rights**: civil, cultural, economic, political and social. This key instrument has been agreed by 192 of the 194 countries of the world. The only countries not signed up are Somalia and the United States.

Universal Declaration of Human Rights
Adopted by the United Nations in 1948, the declaration covers the full range of **human rights** and contains 30 specific rights that are the entitlement of all people.

universal precautions
The use of protective **barriers** such as **gloves**, gowns, aprons, masks, or protective eyewear which can reduce the risk of exposure of a **health care** worker's **skin** or **mucous membranes** to materials potentially infected with **HIV** or other **blood-borne viruses**. In addition, it is recommended that all health care workers take precautions to prevent **injuries** caused by **needles**, scalpels and other sharp instruments or devices. Universal precautions apply to blood, other body fluids containing visible blood, **semen**, and **vaginal** secretions, and also to **tissues** and to cerebrospinal, synovial, pleural, peritoneal, pericardial and amniotic fluids.

unpaid care
Care provided by **family** and friends rather than paid **carers**.

unstructured interview
A **research interview** that does not follow a rigid set of questions, but can be changed or adapted in order to respond to the interviewee.

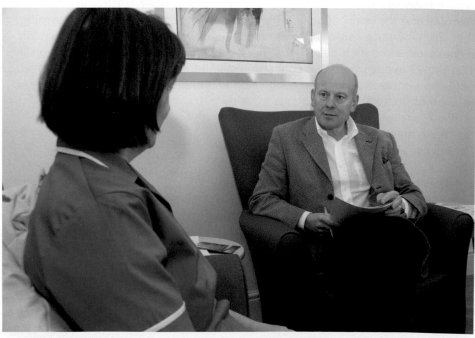

Unstructured interview in progress.

unwanted behaviour
Challenging behaviour can include verbal abuse (racist comments, threats, bullying others), physical abuse (such as assault of others, damaging property), behaviour which is destructive to the child/young person and behaviour which is illegal.

urbanisation
The **process** of people moving to live in cities and large, built-up **communities**.

urea
A toxic waste product produced by the **liver** from the breakdown of surplus amino acids. Urea is removed from the body in **urine** produced by the **kidneys**.

ureter
The tubes that carry **urine** from the **kidneys** to the **bladder**.

urethra
The tube leading from the **bladder** to the outside of the body. It is much longer in males than females and is inside the penis. In males it has the dual role for passing both urine and semen.

urge incontinence
The inability to contain **urine** in the **bladder** until reaching a **toilet**.

urine
The pale-yellow fluid containing waste products dissolved in water which is produced by the **kidneys** and stored in the **bladder** until it can be expelled from the body. It is the only means of eliminating potentially toxic urea from the body and if urine flow is reduced (or stopped) serious life-threatening illnesses will follow.

uterus
The female reproductive pear-shaped **organ** that is contained in the **pelvic cavity**. It is designed to accommodate a developing **foetus** for the length of a **pregnancy**, and contracts to push the foetus out when its development is complete.

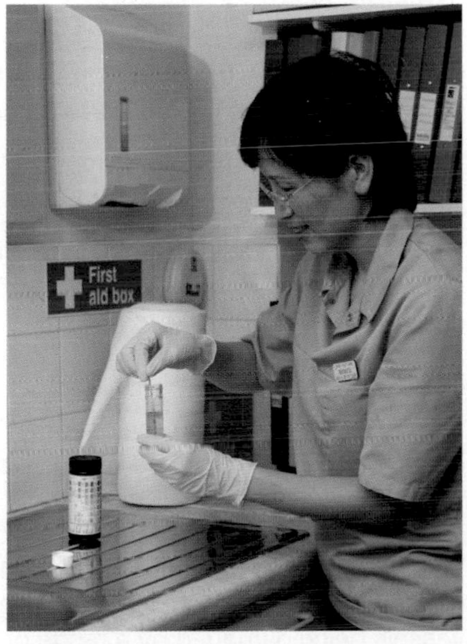

Urine sample.

V

vaccination
A means of protecting against **disease** by the introduction of a very small quantity of severely weakened or dead **pathogens** in order to stimulate the development of **antibodies** to a particular disease, thus creating **immunity**. Vaccinations may cause a short period of feeling unwell in many people but cannot cause disease.

vaccine
The substance containing the severely weakened or dead **pathogens** that is introduced into the body, usually by injection, but it can also be by mouth, in order to create **immunity** to a **disease**.

vagina
The muscular tube in the female body that leads to the **cervix** and the **uterus**. It provides the route for the male **penis** to enter the female body as part of sexual intercourse and the reproductive process, and also becomes the **birth** canal for the **foetus**.

valuing
Recognising and acknowledging uniqueness and importance, especially of individuals. The abilities, **culture** and differences of individuals all contribute to **society**.

values and principles
The **beliefs** behind professional **practice**. The way in which **professionals** work in each sector is underpinned by basic beliefs that influence working practices.

vascular dementia
The second most common form of **dementia** after **Alzheimer's disease**. It is caused by the decreasing **blood** supply to the **brain** resulting from small blood vessels being damaged by a range of different causes, such as high **blood**

pressure, **stroke**, **heart disease**, high **cholesterol** and **diabetes**. The **symptoms** include difficulty concentrating, **memory** loss and confusion. It affects people in different ways and there is no set pattern for the development of symptoms.

vascular disease
A general term meaning diseases associated with blood vessels such as narrowing, calcifying (hardening), inflammation etc.

vein
A **blood** vessel that carries de-**oxygenated** blood to the **heart**. Veins have valves to prevent blood from flowing in the wrong direction. The **pulmonary veins** are the only veins that do not carry de-oxygenated blood; they carry oxygenated blood from the **lungs** to the heart.

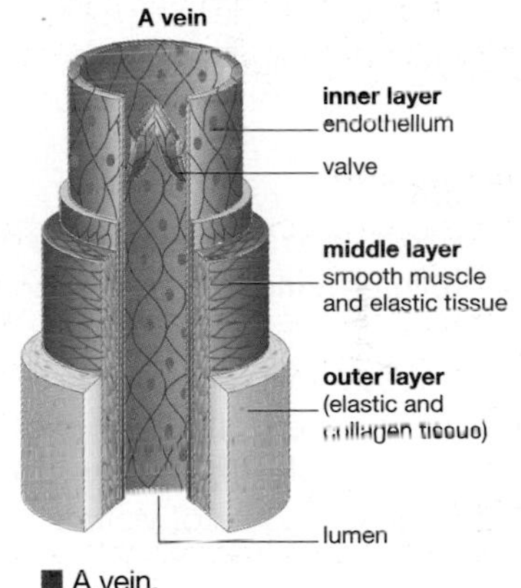

■ A vein.

venae cavae
Large **veins** that return de-**oxygenated blood** to the **heart**. There is a superior and an inferior vena cava; the superior vena cava returns blood to the heart from the head, neck and upper limbs, and the inferior vena cava returns blood from the lower part of the body.

venflon
See **cannula**.

venous
Relating to veins.

ventouse
A method of assisted delivery of a **baby** that involves attaching a vacuum cap to the baby's head in order to help its progress through the **birth** canal. This method is less likely to cause **injury** to the **mother** or the baby than the use of forceps.

ventricle
A fluid-filled cavity in an organ. The ventricles of the **heart** are the two lower chambers that pump **blood** into the pulmonary artery and the aorta. The left ventricular wall is much thicker than the right as it drives blood around the whole circulation whereas the right only sends blood to the nearby lungs. There are also ventricles in the **brain**.

verdict
The **outcome** of a court hearing. A **jury** listens to all the evidence and the members are then able to discuss what they have heard until they reach a conclusion about the guilt or innocence of the accused person.

A B C D E F G H I J K L M N O P Q R S T U V W XYZ

vertebrae
The **bones** of the spine that link together, separated by discs of cartilage, to form a strong but flexible column that enables movement and protects the **spinal cord**.

vertebrates
Living **organisms** with a backbone (spine).

vetting and barring
The **process** of maintaining a list of people who are not suitable to work with children or **vulnerable adults**. This **system** was introduced in 2006 and replaced the separate systems that were in place for working with adults, children or in the education sector.

victim
Someone who has been the target of, or affected by, criminal or **anti-social behaviour**. More information can be found at www.victimsupport.org.uk

Victim support
An independent charitable organisation which helps people cope with the effects of crime. It provides free and confidential support and information, and works to advance the rights of victims and witnesses.

violence
Physically **aggressive behaviour**.

viral infection
Illness caused by a **virus**.

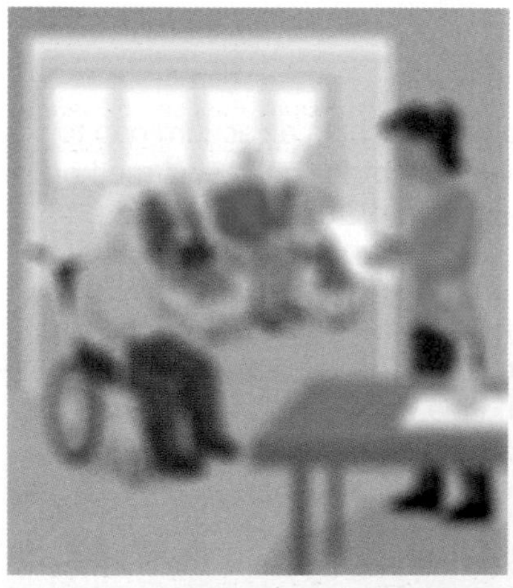

■ Imagine trying to find your way around a busy care home with poor vision like this.

virus
A minute **organism** that can only be seen through an electron **microscope**. It causes **disease** in humans by invading **cells** and multiplying. Unlike **bacteria**, viruses can only multiply inside human cells. Antibiotics are of no use in the **treatment** of **viral infections**, but the **immune system** will usually fight and overcome a viral infection.

visual impairment
The partial or complete loss of sight. More information can be found at www.rnib.org.uk (Royal National Institute for the Blind)

visual learners
People who learn through pictures, diagrams and watching demonstrations.

vitamins
Nutrients found in a range of **foods**; a balanced diet should provide sufficient amounts of each vitamin. Some of the main vitamins are shown in the table below.

Nutrient	Where found	Purpose
Vitamin A (fat-soluble)	Liver and fish oils, milk, butter, eggs and cheese; can be made by the body from carotene which is found in carrots, tomatoes and green vegetables	Protects from **infection** and contributes to growth. A lack of vitamin A can cause eye problems.
Vitamin B group (there are several) (water-soluble)	Cereals, liver, yeast and nuts	This is a large group of complex vitamins, all of which are essential for maintaining a good **skin**. It may be that a lack of vitamin B is responsible for some **diseases** of the **nervous system.**
Vitamin C (water-soluble)	Citrus fruits, strawberries, potatoes and some green vegetables	Vitamin C cannot be stored so it must be taken each day. A lack of vitamin C can cause **scurvy**, a serious disease which affects the gums and causes bleeding. People who have a lack of vitamin C are also more likely to be affected by **viral** infections and coughs and colds.
Vitamin D (fat soluble)	Eggs and fish oils, and made by the body when the skin is exposed to sunlight	Vitamin D enables calcium to be absorbed to strengthen and develop **bones** and **teeth.** A severe shortage of vitamin D will lead to **rickets**, a deforming disease seen in children where bones do not develop adequately.
Vitamin E (fat-soluble)	Wheatgerm, cereals, egg yolks, liver and milk	This helps prevent **cell** damage and degeneration.

vocational qualifications and training
An approach to **learning** and **qualifications** that is based on practical **skills**, supported by underpinning knowledge. Most vocational qualifications require a certain period of time to be spent in the **workplace**. Qualifications such as **NVQs** and BTEC or City & Guilds Diplomas and Certificates are vocational qualifications.

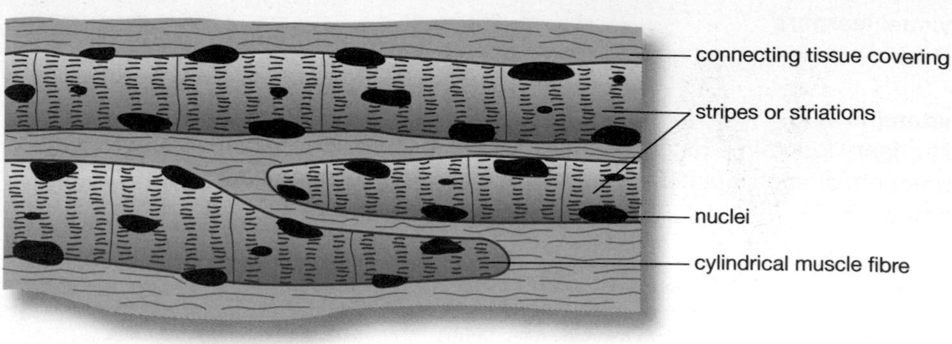

■ Appearance of striated muscle.

voluntary muscle
The most common muscle, also called 'striated', 'striped' or 'skeletal', as it is attached to bones; a muscle that is moved consciously, to make the body walk, run, jump, throw, catch or any other type of movement. Messages are sent from the **brain** via the **central nervous system** to make voluntary muscles contract. Composed of long cylindrical fibres with many nuclei and a striped appearance.

voluntary sector
Non-**statutory** and **not-for-profit organisations** that deliver **health** and **social care services** for adults and children, or campaign about related issues. Some parts of the voluntary sector are **charities**.

volunteer
Someone who offers to provide help or support for no charge.

vomiting
The **process** of the stomach's contents being ejected from the body through the mouth. This can be the result of an **infection** or **toxic** substance in the stomach, or it can result from an inner ear condition where the balance is affected, such as motion sickness.

vulnerable
A state in which being physically or emotionally hurt is more likely.

vulnerable adult
Someone over the age of 18 who is less able to protect himself or herself against harm or exploitation as a result of **mental health problems**, or physical or **learning disabilities**.

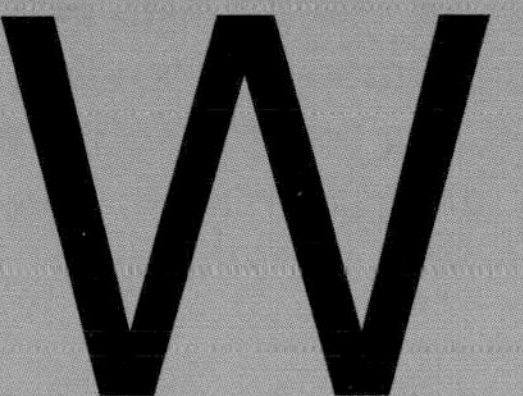

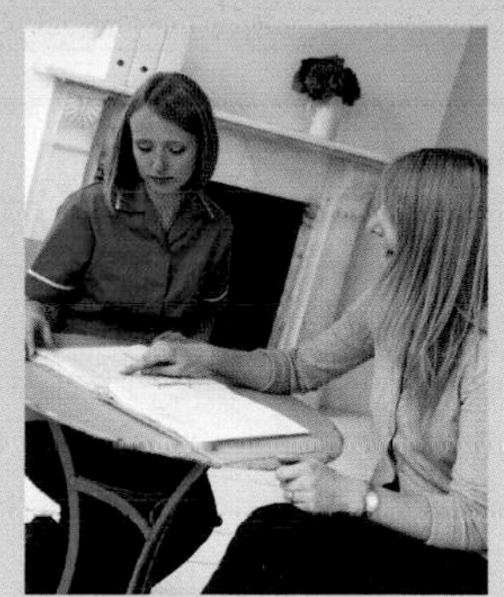

walk-in centres
Clinics that give people fast access to treatment and health advice, without an appointment.

walking aid
Any **equipment** that assists with walking. This can include full walking frames, or walking sticks and **tripods**.

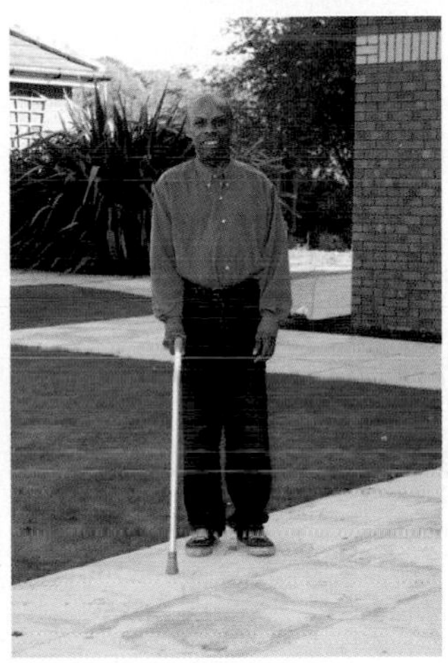

1 Move the stick forward, slightly to one side.

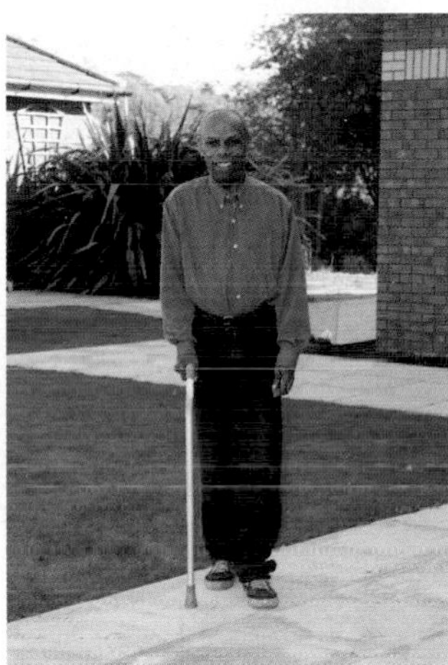

2 Take a step with the opposite foot, going no further forward than the level of the stick.

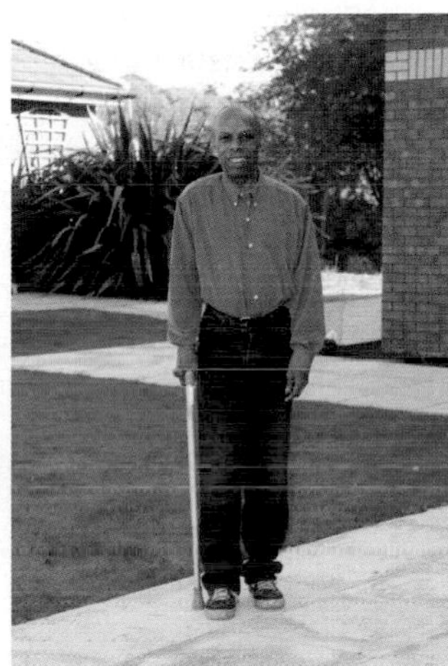

3 Take a step with the foot on the same side as the stick. This should go past the position of the stick. Then move the stick again so that it is in front of you, and repeat the sequence.

A B C D E F G H I J K L M N O P Q R S T U V W X Y Z

wandering
A behaviour usually seen in people who have **dementia**. People with dementia may walk around not really knowing where they are going, although often they may have in mind that they are going to a place they used to live or **work**. People who do this are at serious risk of **harm** as they do not have any **understanding** of their actual whereabouts, and are unlikely to be able to find their way back home, or even to be able to tell anyone where they live.

warehousing
The indiscriminate placing of people in residential or **hospital environments** in order to provide 'care' on a cost-effective and convenient basis. This practice was common until the 1990s, when attitudes began to change as a result of the demands of **disabled** people and people with a **learning disability**.

waste disposal
The **process** of safely getting rid of any **hazardous waste**, including human waste and contaminated waste resulting from **treatments**. There are procedures that must be followed to ensure that all waste is disposed of correctly so that it does not pose a risk to others. All **needles** and other sharps, for example, must be disposed of in a specially labelled container that can be sealed; clinical waste must be sorted into marked bags and soiled bed linen must also be sorted into specially marked bags that can be washed without the bedding having to be handled.

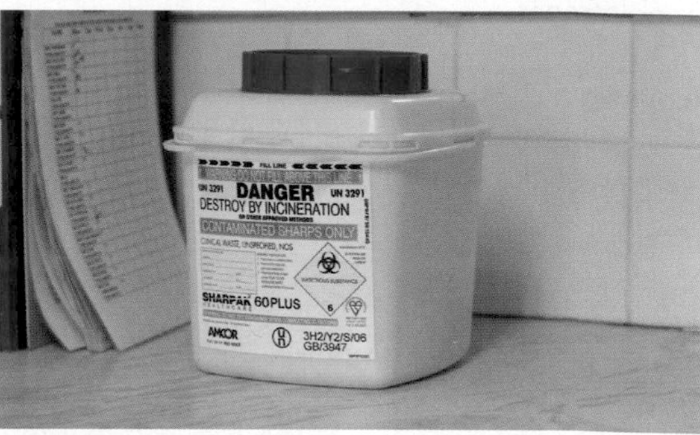

Yellow sharps box.

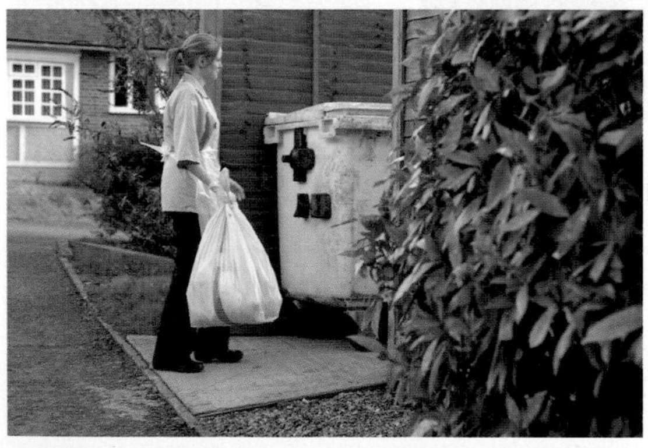
Yellow bag – used for clinical waste such as pads, nappies, wound dressings, used gloves.

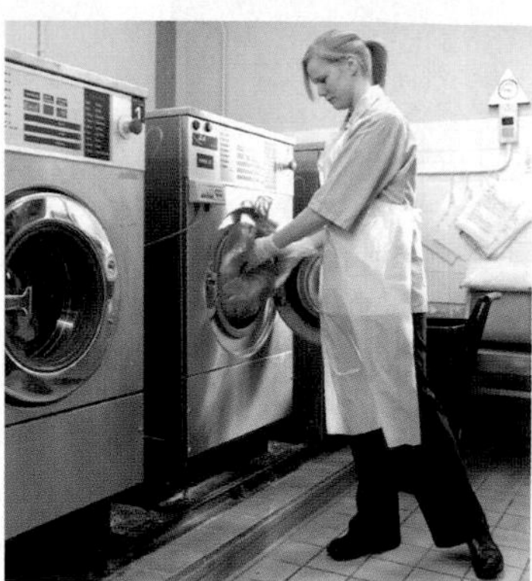
Red bag – dirty linen, soiled sheets and linen go in these bags.

weaning
The gradual **process** of introducing **babies** to solid **food** to replace milk feeds. When a baby is eating solid foods for all main meals, he or she is said to be 'weaned'.

welfare
Health, happiness, well-being.

welfare rights
The rights people have to financial **benefits** and **support** from the **state**. Most local areas have **organisations** that work to provide advice and **advocacy** to assist people to claim their rights and ensure that they are getting the financial and other support to which they are entitled.

Welfare State
The system set up in 1948 when, for the first time, the **government** ensured that everyone would have a minimum level of **income** and **access** to **health care** provided by the **state**. The principles of the Welfare State do not directly **discriminate** between 'deserving' and 'undeserving', and the **benefits** are available to all.

well-being
The quality of all aspects of an individual's life, including physical and **mental health**, emotional and intellectual fulfilment, and overall contentment.

wheezing
A whistling sound from the **chest** caused by a narrowing of the bronchioles, which makes it more difficult for air to pass through the breathing tubes. Narrowing is caused by **inflammation** causing swelling of the linings of the tubes, or by thickened mucous secretions. Both of these conditions are most commonly caused by **asthma** or **bronchial infections**.

whistleblowing
The **process** of reporting poor **practice, abuse** or corruption in the **workplace**. People who 'blow the whistle' are protected by **law** through the Public Interest Disclosure Act (1998).

white blood cells
Blood cells that form part of the **immune system** and do not contain **haemoglobin**. There are several different types but neutrophils (known as granulocytes or polymorphs) are the most numerous. They function by engulfing **bacteria** and destroying

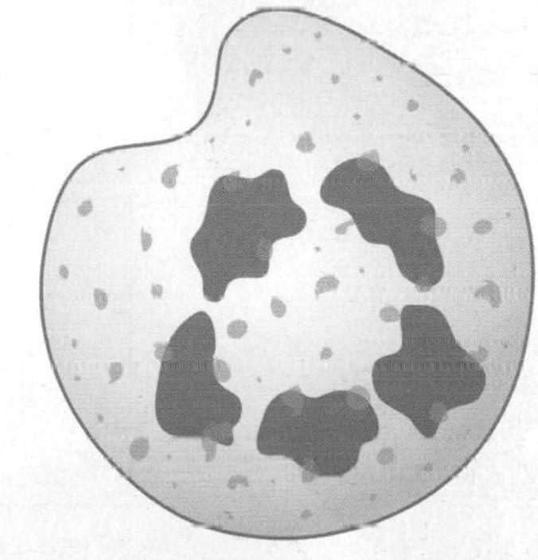

■ A white blood cell: neutrophil.

them (phagocytosis) and are made in bone marrow. Lymphocytes defend the body by producing **antibodies** to fight **infection**. They are produced in lymphoid tissue.

withdrawal
The **process** of stopping the use of an addictive substance. This can be drugs, alcohol or **nicotine**. Withdrawing will usually produce physical and emotional **symptoms**, which vary depending on the substance, but can be unpleasant and may be so hard to deal with that the withdrawal fails and people return to using the substance. **Babies** born to drug- or alcohol-addicted **mothers** will also suffer withdrawal after **birth**.

witness
A person who has **observed** an event or has knowledge about it. Witnesses may play an important part in the gathering of evidence for a criminal **prosecution**. Witnesses are also important when candidates are gathering evidence of **performance** for **vocational qualifications**.

womb
See **uterus**.

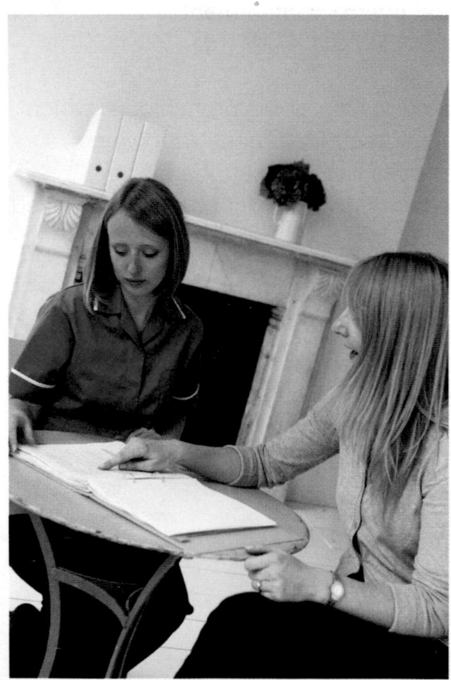
■ Work-based learning.

work
Paid **employment**.

work-based learning
Learning that takes place in the **workplace** and is assessed through **observing performance** and **questioning** to ensure that candidates have the necessary knowledge. **Qualifications** such as **NVQ** and SVQ are gained through work-based learning.

work experience
A period of time spent working while being **supervised** to find out what it is like to work in that setting, and whether a person is likely to be successful working in the sector.

workforce
All the people who work for a particular **organisation** or in a particular sector.

working practice
Any activity, procedure, use of material or equipment and working technique used in carrying out a job. It also covers any omissions in good working practice which may pose a threat to health and safety.

workplace
Anywhere that people carry out their **work**. This could be a residential setting or a **hospital**, but it could also be an individual's home.

workplace policies
Statements and plans from an employer about the position of the organisation on key issues. It is likely that workplaces will have policies about issues such as health and safety, equality of opportunity, the environment and anti-bullying.

World Health Organization (WHO)
The **public health** arm of the United Nations. It is responsible for taking a lead on **health** globally, for **monitoring** the spread of **disease**, and for key health issues around the world. The WHO provides public health programmes in many countries. More information can be found at www.who.int/en

wounds
Breaks in the **skin** caused by **accident**, **injury** or as the result of **surgery**.

XYZ

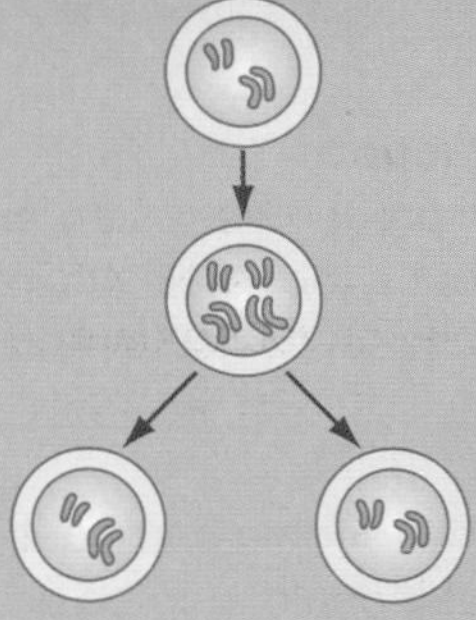

X chromosome
X and Y chromosomes are designated the sex chromosomes because females have two X chromosomes, while males have one X and one **Y chromosome**. When abnormal recessive genes are carried on X chromosomes the genetic condition is said to be sex-linked. Males suffer from the condition as they have no normal gene to counteract the abnormal gene. Females having two X chromosomes will nearly always have a dominant normal gene and carry the hidden condition but do not suffer from it. Additional chromosomes result in syndromes causing disorders such as XYY syndrome (affecting males with an extra Y chromosome); this results in extensive growth. XXY also affects males, and results in under-developed genitalia and some female characteristics. The diagram above shows a normal body cell at the top which has four chromosomes in two pairs. As cell division starts, a copy of each chromosome is made. The cell then divides in two (lower part of the diagram) to form two daughter cells. Each daughter cell has a nucleus containing four chromosomes identical to the ones in the original parent cell. *See* **chromosomes**.

xenophobia
Fear of people from another country; this term is also commonly used to describe people who dislike foreigners.

X-ray
Electromagnetic radiation of very high frequency. When used in low doses it creates images of the inside of the body, because the waves pass through **tissue** and **bone** in different ways and enable the bones and other body structures to be seen. The radiation is used in higher doses to treat **cancers**.

Y chromosome
One of the sex chromosomes that determines **gender**. Only found in males. *See* **chromosome** and **X chromosome**.

young carer
A person under the age of 18 who is caring for a **parent** or other **family** member or friend. Often quite young children provide care for ill or **disabled** parents. There is help available for young carers, but many are not known to **local authorities**. More information can be found at www.youngcarers.net

young offenders
Young person between the ages of 10–17 years who has been found guilty of a crime.

young person
There is no precise legal definition of the term, but it is usually taken to mean people who are aged 13 to 19. However, state **benefits** may define a young person as aged between 16 and 18.

youth court
Part of the **Magistrate's Court**, but more informal and run by specially trained **magistrates**. Almost all cases involving **young people** aged 10 to 18 are heard here. The court is not open to the public, but **victims** of crimes may attend and may have an input into any **sentence**.

youth justice system
The overall approach (and different parts of the system) designed to reduce youth **offending** and **anti-social behaviour**. All aspects, including prevention, pre-court, **court** and **sentencing** are part of the system.

Youth Offending Team (YOT)
All **local authorities** in England and Wales have a YOT. They are integrated and have workers from the **police**, **social services**, **education**, drugs and alcohol misuse, **health**, probation and **housing** teams. There is a YOT manager who is responsible for co-ordinating the work of the youth justice **services**.

youth service
Services for **young people** provided by **local authorities**, which vary depending on what is needed in a particular area. Some young people just want someone to talk to. Services are usually provided for young people from the age of 13 to 25.

youth work
Work with **young people** in either **local authority** or **voluntary organisations**.

zero tolerance
A policy which states that individuals have the right to be protected from abusive or violent behaviour.

zimmer frame
A metal walking frame.
See **walking aids.**

zygote
Formed by the fusing of one spermotozoon nucleus with one ovum nucleus at fertilisation. The zygote, if implanted in the female's uterus, will eventually form the embryo.

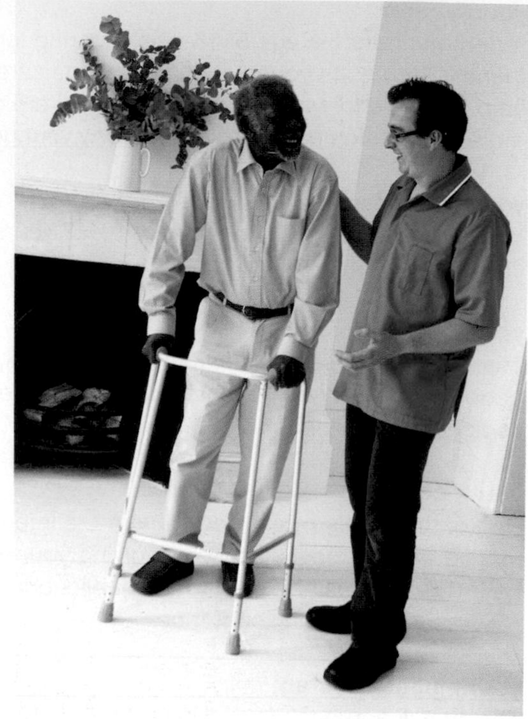

■ There are many types of walking frames.

Relevant legislation and organisational policy and procedures

Laws, in their simplest form, can be defined as society's behavioural rules on how people can live orderly, safe and peaceful lives. The process of making these formal rules is usually through primary legislation – the passing of laws by Act of Parliament. These Acts, or Statutes, come into force when a majority of Members of both Houses of Parliament vote them in.

The original idea for a law can come from one of several sources. These include the Government, advisory agencies (such as the Commissions for Equal Opportunities or Human Rights), pressure groups and charities supporting a particular cause or interest (like Age Concern) or individual Members of Parliament (MPs) who promote certain issues (such as the quality of care in nursing homes or whether young people should be prosecuted for carrying knives).

Ideas for new laws are first aired in an open-ended discussion document entitled a Green Paper. If it is decided to take them further, the discussion produces a set of proposals which is published in a White Paper, as a Bill. The Bill is discussed, voted on, amended and consolidated during three separate debates in Parliament, and then passed to the House of Lords for final approval. When everyone agrees that it says what's needed, it goes to the Queen for Royal Assent. At this stage it passes from a Bill to an Act, and becomes law.

Within Europe the European Union adopts legislation in the form of Directives and Regulations. These Directives and Regulations must then be adopted by European member states within their own domestic legislation.

In Scotland health (and social care) are the responsibility of the Scottish Parliament so legislation and policy differ from England, Northern Ireland and Wales. These variations are shown in blue below.

Legislation policy procedure	Website	Relevant content	EU directive implemented by the Act
Children Act (2004)	www.ecm.gov.uk	• Introduced Children's Comissioner, Local Safeguarding Children Boards and provided legal basis for Every Child Matters	
Children (Leaving Care) Act (2000)	www.ecm.gov.uk	• Requires local authorities to plan for children leaving care. • Must provide support for housing and preparation for independence. • Must have a personal adviser. • Can remain looked after if in full time education until 21 years.	

Children Act (1989) Children (Scotland) Act (1995)	www.desf.gov.uk www.scotland.gov.uk	• Major change in childcare practice. • Concept of 'significant harm' • Concept of 'parental responsibilities' rather than 'rights' • Wishes and interests of the child paramount.	
Data Protection Act (1998) Access to Medical Records 1988	www.dh.gov.uk	The protection of the individuals' personal data with regard to processing and safe storage: • storing confidential information • protection of paper based information • protection of information stored on computer • accurate and appropriate record keeping.	95/46/EC
Freedom of Information Act (2000) Freedom of Information (Scotland) Act 2002	www.dh.gov.uk	Introduced to promote a culture of openness within public bodies. Allows anyone the right of access to a wide range of information held by a public authority. Access to information is subject to certain limited exemptions, such as information about an individual. It is under this Act that individuals can access their health records. In Scotland this Act established the office of Scottish Information Commissioner who is responsible for ensuring public authorities maximise access to information.	95/46/EC
Health and Safety at Work Act (1974)	www.hse.gov.uk	• Ensuring the environment is safe and free from hazards. • Assessing risks before carrying out tasks. • Checking equipment for faults before use. • Use of appropriate personal protective clothing. • Handling hazardous/contaminated waste correctly. • Disposal of sharp implements appropriately. • Shared responsibilities – employers/employees.	89/391/EEC
Manual Handling Regulations (1992)	www.hse.gov.uk	• Preparing the environment before moving or handling anything. • Checking equipment is safe before use. • Safe moving and handling of patients. • Safe moving of equipment/loads.	90/269/EEC

Legislation policy procedure	Website	Relevant content	EU directive implemented by the Act
Control of Substances Hazardous to Health (2002) (COSHH)	www.hse.gov.uk	• Storing cleansing materials correctly. • Labelling of hazardous substances correctly. • Appropriate handling of bodily fluids such as blood and urine. • Appropriate handling of flammable liquids/gases. • Appropriate handling of toxic/corrosive substances/liquids.	67/548/EEC
Reporting of Injuries, Diseases and Dangerous Occurrences Regulations (1995) RIDDOR	www.hse.gov.uk	• Reporting accidents and injuries objectively and accurately. • Reporting diseases to the appropriate bodies. • Reporting dangerous occurrences to the appropriate bodies. • Completion of relevant paperwork.	89/391/EEC
Lifting Operations and Lifting Equipment Regulations (1998)	www.hse.gov.uk	The Lifting Operations and Lifting Equipment Regulations aim to reduce risks to people's health and safety from lifting equipment provided for use at work by ensuring it is: • strong and stable enough for the particular use and marked to indicate safe working loads • positioned and installed to minimise any risks • used safely, that is the work is planned, organised and performed by competent people • subject to ongoing thorough examination and, where appropriate, inspection by competent people.	89/655/EEC amended 95/63/EC
Environmental Protection Act (1990, section 34) and the Environmental Protection (Duty of Care) Regulations (1991)	www.dh.gov.uk	Section 34 of the Environmental Protection Act (1990) imposes a duty of care on persons concerned with control of waste. It places a duty on anyone who in any way has a responsibility for control of waste to ensure that it is managed properly and recovered or disposed of safely.	2006/12/EC